China
Interrupted

China Interrupted

Japanese Internment and
the Reshaping of a Canadian
Missionary Community

Sonya Grypma

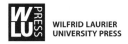

WILFRID LAURIER
UNIVERSITY PRESS

This book has been published with the help of a grant from the Canadian Federation for the Humanities and Social Sciences, through the Aid to Scholarly Publications Program, using funds provided by the Social Sciences and Humanities Research Council of Canada. Wilfrid Laurier University Press acknowledges the financial support of the Government of Canada through the Canada Book Fund for its publishing activities.

Library and Archives Canada Cataloguing in Publication

Grypma, Sonya, 1965–
      China interrupted : Japanese internment and the reshaping of a Canadian missionary community / Sonya Grypma.

Includes bibliographical references and index.
Issued also in electronic formats.
ISBN 978-1-55458-627-1

      1. Women missionaries—Canada—Biography. 2. Women missionaries—China—Biography. 3. Missions, Canadian—China—History—20th century. 4. United Church of Canada. 5. Nurses—Canada—Biography. 6. Nurses—China—Biography. 7. Gale, Betty. 8. World War, 1939–1945—Prisoners and prisons, Japanese. 9. Concentration camps—China—History—20th century. 10. World War, 1939–1945—China—Sources. I. Title.

BV3415.G79 2012   266'.0237105100922   C2012-903284-0

Electronic monograph.
Issued also in print format.
ISBN 978-1-55458-643-1 (PDF).—ISBN 978-1-55458-847-3 (EPUB)

      1. Women missionaries—Canada—Biography. 2. Women missionaries—China—Biography. 3. Missions, Canadian—China—History—20th century. 4. United Church of Canada. 5. Nurses—Canada—Biography. 6. Nurses—China—Biography. 7. Gale, Betty. 8. World War, 1939–1945—Prisoners and prisons, Japanese. 9. Concentration camps—China—History—20th century. 10. World War, 1939–1945—China—Sources. I. Title.

BV3415.G79 2012   266'.0237105100922   C2012-903285-9

Cover design by Sandra Friesen. Cover image: *Mishkids Travelling across the Da Min Hu Lake, Jinan,* photo by E.B. Struthers (courtesy Mary Struthers McKim). Text design by Sandra Friesen.

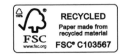

For Iona, Sylvia, and Mike

Contents

Illustrations

All illustrations courtesy of Margaret Gale Wightman unless otherwise noted.

Foreword

My friendship with Dr. Sonya Grypma first began with her telephone call, nine years ago. As a nurse historian, she was researching the work of the Canadian missionary nurses in China, which included my mother, Betty Gale. I could not have predicted, at the time, how interlaced our lives would become. As we spoke further, I began to realize what an opportunity this would be for my family. For many years, my brother Kendall, my sister Patricia, and I, together with our families, had discussed how to make our mother's story known to a wider audience. Through Sonya's research, this could now be possible. Canada has been quiet for too long on the nurses' contributions to the development of western health care in China. She has reopened this chapter in our history.

Sonya's first book, *Healing Henan*, was published in 2008. Meanwhile, we continued to discuss her research into the life and experiences of my mother, both as a missionary nurse and as a civilian internee during the Second World War. Born to missionary parents in China in 1911, she later received her professional training in Toronto and returned to China in 1939 as a missionary nurse. China was already at war. Although the Canadian nurses were separated geographically, they were part of a large and cohesive missionary community. *China Interrupted* describes their lives in China during this time, how they were able to deal with their war experiences, and how these experiences influenced their life decisions. Sonya has meticulously reviewed all the available records and has met or corresponded with many members of the missionaries' families, including my own.

When she asked me to write the foreword for *China Interrupted*, I was reminded how lives can suddenly be altered by world events over which one has no control. My parents met in China in 1939. My father, Godfrey Gale, was an English missionary doctor who was practising in Qilu. They were married in 1940 and I was born in July 1941. Pearl Harbor was bombed five months later. We were immediately placed under house arrest by the Japanese and spent the duration of the war in civilian internment camps in eastern China. Newly married and with the added responsibility of caring for a young child, my parents endured years of confinement, deprivation, and uncertainty.

During their captivity, my mother kept a diary. She was a caregiver by nature and wrote from her unique perspective as a woman, a wife, a mother, and a nurse, committed to ensuring the well-being of my father, myself, and the other internees. Now that we more fully understand the importance of the early years in a child's development, we realize the extent to which children interpret the world through the eyes of the adults closest to them. My mother instinctively understood this and was able to hide from me any sense of loss. While she and my father coped with the challenges of daily survival and attended to the diverse medical needs of the internees, I spent my time playing with my friend Eli, the daughter of two English doctors who had been with us since the beginning of our internment. Eli and I were the same age and these camps were the only homes we had ever known. Although I had never spent a day at the beach or had an ice cream cone, these simple childhood pleasures had been described to me by my parents as things yet to come.

As an adult, I have few memories of internment. My most vivid recollection is the day of our release. I was four years old. The war was over and the Japanese guards had gone. The camp was in turmoil as the internees were packing their belongings and saying their tearful goodbyes. I can remember the wild excitement and wondering what was happening. When we left the building, Eli and I ran ahead of our parents towards the gate, which had been left wide open. As we hesitated at the threshold and looked back, my mother reassured us that "it was okay" and that we could now go through to the outside.

My mother condemned all acts of violence, including those committed by the Allies. Her war experiences never changed her world view. Her love of China remained with her throughout her life. She followed the changing developments there with intense interest, but always with conflicting emotions. She never returned.

At the same time that Sonya was starting her research into my mother's China experiences, I was sorting through forgotten files and I discovered old photographs and letters from years ago, some of which I had never seen before. In my attempts to provide her with as much family information as possible, I became reacquainted with the details of my own history. It was time to go back.

In 2003, I returned to China. Sonya and her husband agreed to join me. As they were living out West and I was in Ontario, we finally met for the first time. I was impressed with her powers of quiet observation and her attention to detail, how suited she seemed for her vocation.

In 2006, Sonya and her husband and I returned to China, accompanied by my sister, Patricia. We had been included in an invitation from the staff of the Weihui hospital in Henan, to help them celebrate the 110th anniversary of the establishment of their first hospital by Canadian missionaries in 1896, and the opening of a museum in the original building, which was located on the same grounds. As we and the other invited Canadians arrived, we were greeted by hundreds of people, including a sea of nurses, all in white uniforms. It was a well-organized and extremely elaborate event, as they expressed their appreciation towards these men and women who had come to China to offer their assistance, so many years ago. The ceremony closed with fireworks.

As Sonya and I spoke more about her plans to write *China Interrupted*, I became aware of the similarities between her life and that of my mother. Both were Canadians, Christians, nurses, mothers, and wives of doctors. How providential it was that our paths had crossed!

Kendall, Patricia, and I and our families want to thank Sonya for telling this story. I know how humbled and honoured our mother would have felt. I wish that she and Sonya could have met, so that she could thank Sonya personally. I'm sure that they would have become good friends. However, through this intimate portrayal of her life, I believe that they actually have. I will always think of them that way.

—Margaret (Gale) Wightman

Foreword

In *China Interrupted* nursing scholar Sonya Grypma skilfully analyzes the intertwined social history of a Canadian missionary community and the personal story of missionary nurse Betty Gale, one of its members. Born and raised in China as a daughter of Canadian missionaries, and determined to continue her family's legacy of missionary work, Gale returned to China as a registered nurse in 1939, as did two of her nursing friends from this same community. Two years prior the Japanese had invaded China. Gale and her fellow nurses arrived in a war-torn country. Despite their professional commitment, religious calling, and personal determination, they never got the chance to take up their missionary pursuit among the Chinese population. Instead, they, with the new families they had formed, became imprisoned in a series of Japanese internment camps in China from 1941 to 1945.

By probing the history of one Canadian missionary community in China, while foregrounding the life history of Gale, Grypma points out how this community's dramatic, complex, and contradictory life in China during the Japanese occupation not only represents a broader story of Canadian "mishkid" nurse internment but also a broader social Canadian missionary history. Therefore, this very fine historical account and clear analysis goes much beyond a personal story. It is a social history about an entire missionary community, about the end of an epoch in Canadian missionary history, and the end of an era in the history of Canadian nursing and health care. In foregrounding Betty Gale's multi-faceted China life, and in reconstructing the shared identity of an entire, albeit small, community of Canadian missionaries and their mishkids, Grypma depicts, in vivid detail, the broader social meaning of the internment of Western missionaries and nurses. The internment of many members of the missionary community by Japan in 1941 symbolically and in reality represents the coming to an end of Canadian missionary work in China.

This work complements existing historical scholarship on the imprisonment of Western military nurses under the Japanese in Asia, and of internment experiences more generally. It also significantly adds to Canadian missionary history. To date, little has been written on civilian internment experiences in China. In writing this social history, based on a captivating collection of primary documents and personal stories, Grypma has created an intriguing and significant book that will help shape our collective memory of this important period in international nursing and missionary history.

—Geertje Boschma

Geertje Boschma, PhD, RN, is Associate Professor at the School of Nursing, University of British Columbia. Her current scholarship focuses on the history of nursing and mental health care in western Canada.

Acknowledgements

A project like this, spanning nine years and two continents, would not be possible without the goodwill and support of many individuals and organizations. First and foremost my gratitude goes to Margaret Gale Wightman, daughter of Betty and Godfrey Gale and collaborator extraordinaire. Margaret generously provided me with hundreds of pages of (meticulously organized) family documents, photographs, films, books, tape recordings, and her mother's original diary. She also introduced me to her surviving aunts and uncles, paving the way for me to conduct interviews with relatives in Ontario and the UK. We travelled together twice to China, where Margaret invited me to come alongside her to revisit her birthplace (Jinan) and the site of her last two years of internment (Pudong, in Shanghai). I cannot overstate the value of Margaret's contribution to this project; it simply would not have happened without her.

There are a number of other China-born missionary kids (or "mishkids") who were unfailing in their support and enthusiasm. I am especially grateful to the late Ruth Thomson Laws, Murray Thomson, Muriel Thomson Valentien, Mary Struthers McKim, Norah Busby, the late Arthur Menzies, and Mavis Knight Weatherhead. Particularly memorable is an evening spent as a dinner guest of Murray Thomson in Ottawa in 2005. Murray also invited Mary McKim, whom he had not seen for many years. Along with a lovely dinner I was treated to candid reminiscences of hilarious and frightening childhood events, recounted with great relish. In Alberta, Mavis Weatherhead gained the honorific "granny" from my children just hours after she came to our home for a visit with Chinese dignitaries. My observation of the depth of China-bred relationships extended into China, where I travelled with Margaret, Mary, Norah, and Mavis and other missionary relatives in 2006 at the invitation of the president of the former mission hospital in Weihui, Henan. Bearing witness to that historic return "home" was a privilege unmatched by anything in my career so far.

A number of former internees provided insights into life in internment camps in China. Most notable are Greg Leck and Desmond Power who, in addition to painstakingly compiling a database of over 13,500 internees held in China and Hong Kong, responded enthusiastically to my enquiries. Other former internees who pointed me in helpful directions include Ron Bridge, Alexander (Zandy) Strangman, and Donald Menzie.

I am grateful for the support we received in China from individuals who put considerable effort into bringing the story of Canadian missionaries back to Henan and Jinan. I am especially indebted to Song Xianzhong (President of Anyang People's Hospital), Zhang Xinzhong (President of First Affiliated Hospital of Xinxiang Medical University), Ren Jijuan (in Xinxiang), Li Xiandong (Beijing), Lucy Lu (Weifang), and Sophia Sun (Beijing) for their efforts and goodwill. I am also grateful for those who have assisted with English–Mandarin interpretation and translation along the way: Huihui Li and Jing Zhu (University of Lethbridge) and Na Wu (Trinity Western University). Research assistants Lyndsay Payne and Lydia Wytenbroek provided invaluable help with organizing material. Filmmaker Mike Visser, who also accompanied me on one of the more complex trips to China to help produce a documentary, was an invaluable accomplice. He is a gifted filmmaker, and a fine brother to boot.

One of the pleasures of being a historian of nursing is being part of an extraordinarily supportive community of scholars, nationally and internationally. When this project developed into a sshrc-funded, two-year postdoctoral fellowship at the University of British Columbia School of Nursing, I had the distinct privilege of working closely with Geertje Boschma. Geertje asked difficult questions, pointed me to significant publications, and provided consistent encouragement. I am grateful for our innumerable lunchtime conversations outside the Regent College bookstore. Similarly, I have valued the many opportunities to discuss my ideas formally and informally with Canadian historians of nursing, especially with members of a related sshrc (Social Sciences and Humanities Research Council of Canada) project on nationalism and colonialism in nursing: Meryn Stuart, Cynthia Toman, Jayne Elliott, Kathryn McPherson, Laurie Meijer-Drees, Myra Rutherdale, Marion McKay, and Johanne Daigle. The Canadian Association for the History of Nursing and the British Columbia History of Nursing Society have also been supportive, and I am especially indebted to Glennis Zilm, Shirley Stinson, Verna Huffman Splane, Janet Beaton, Florence Melchoir, Susan Armstrong-Reid, and Sioban Nelson for their keen interest and timely advice at different stages of this project.

The international community of historical scholars in health and nursing has been equally supportive. Members of the American Association for the History of Nursing, the University of Pennsylvania Barbara Bates Center for the Study of the History of Nursing, and the University of Virginia Center for Nursing Historical Inquiry provided opportunities to speak, study, and collaboratively wrestle with concepts. I am particularly indebted to Barbra Mann Wall and Barbara Brodie who opened their homes to me while also organizing incredible opportunities for me to engage with their students and local scholars. It was Barbara Brodie, Arlene Keeling, and graduate faculty and students at the University of Virginia who suggested that the real story here was about missionary kids. They were right; I am grateful.

Colleagues and students at universities in Canada have provided invaluable opportunities over the years for me to test early ideas in the lunchroom, classroom, and boardroom. I am grateful to the University of Alberta (especially Janet Ross Kerr), the University of Lethbridge (especially Judith Kulig, Jean Harrowing, and Chris Hosgood) and Trinity Western University (especially Sheryl Reimer-Kirkham, Allyson Jule, Rick Sawatzky, Robynne Healey, and Landa Terblanche) for providing practical support and advice related to the development of missionary and nursing history into a program of research. I am grateful also for funding from the Social Sciences and Humanities Research Council of Canada, the University of Lethbridge, and the University of Virginia Center for Historical Inquiry (Barbara Brodie Fellowship).

Finally I wish to acknowledge my children Mike and Janessa, parents Henk and Cobi Visser, Ann de Hoop, siblings Mike Visser and Sylvia Slagter, sister-in-law Martha Grypma, and especially my incomparable husband Martin Grypma for mustering an extra measure of enthusiasm for my preoccupation with China missionaries. It is admittedly an odd pursuit for a child of Dutch immigrants with no connection to China or the United Church, and yet my family has been actively supportive of this work. My children have grown up on tales of China; my husband, brother, and daughter have accompanied me there at different times; and my parents have stepped in with practical support along the way. My family continues to listen—to my excitement at new discoveries, my descriptions of research trips, and even to my public lectures. They affirm for me in a million tiny ways that this research is important. Who could ask for more?

Abbreviations

CCC	Columbia Country Club
GMA	Glenbow Museum and Archives
ICN	International Council of Nurses
ICRC	International Committee of the Red Cross
LAC	Library and Archives Canada
LMS	London Missionary Society
MWPC	Margaret Wightman Private Collection
NAC	Nurses Association of China
NCM	North China Mission
PUMC	Peking Union Medical College
RVH	Royal Victoria Hospital (Montreal)
TGH	Toronto General Hospital
UBC	University of British Columbia
UCCA	United Church of Canada Archives
UWO	University of Western Ontario (London)
VGH	Vancouver General Hospital
WCM	West China Mission
WGH/HSCA	Winnipeg General Hospital/Health Sciences Centre Archives
WMS	Woman's Missionary Society

China Interrupted

Yesterday, December 7, 1941—a date which will live in infamy—the United States of America was suddenly and deliberately attacked by naval and air forces of the Empire of Japan.

—US President Franklin D. Roosevelt, radio address, 8 December 1941

Margaret weighs 15 lbs to-day! Is that more important—that I write it down first, before saying that Japan declared War in the United States, and Britain, last night? It helps to keep me from panicking, in any case— thinking of those pounds. "War is declared to-day!" "Yes, I know, but Margie weighs 15 lbs."

—Canadian nurse Betty Gale, "Journal," 8 December 1941

At 9:15 a.m. on Monday, 8 December 1941, Canadian missionary nurse Betty Gale walked through the Shandong Christian University "Qilu" campus gates into four years of internment under the Japanese in China. She was returning home from the Qilu University Medical School and Hospital where she had been supervising registration exams for her nursing students. Her house, like the houses of all missionaries on staff at Qilu, was located a few blocks from the hospital, within the walls of the large, beautifully treed campus. Betty Gale was heading home to feed her infant daughter Margaret (Margie) before returning to work. Her British husband, Dr. Godfrey Gale, was at the medical school, presenting a lecture to his medical students on spinal cords, membranes, and nerves. As Betty Gale drew close to the campus, a "lorry unloading dozens of [Japanese] soldiers—all armed to the teeth"[1]—appeared between her and the campus gates. Betty paused, "a moment of wild panic" overcoming her as she realized, "Margie is inside the gates":

Frantically I rush across the road and "join the [Japanese] Army" [entering through the campus gates]—and the gates clang shut behind us. In the general excitement and confusion, no one notices me—and when the army turns left by command, I disobey the order and march right, and keep on going—running like mad—to get home to our baby … I snatch her to me and hold her fast while my heart thumps and my mind races.[2]

The much-anticipated war had finally come to the Gale family at Qilu—and with it, nine months of house arrest followed by three years of imprisonment in civilian internment camps created for enemy aliens, that is, citizens of Allied nations at war with Japan.

This is the story of the richly interwoven lives of Canadian North China missionaries and their "mishkid" (missionary kid) offspring whose lives and mission were irreversibly altered by their internment as "enemy aliens" of Japan from 1941 to 1945. Rooted in the context of missionary nursing as a viable career option for China-born missionary daughters desiring to return to the land of their childhood, *China Interrupted* foregrounds the perspectives of Canadian mishkid Betty Thomson Gale,[3] a second-generation missionary nurse whose internment represented an irreversible interruption in the remarkable phenomenon of missionary nursing in China and marked a final epoch in the sixty-year history of China missions. It offers important insights into the ways in which Canadian missionary nursing extended from, and depended on, the small, tight-knit Canadian missionary community that had planted itself in the "Middle Kingdom" decades before. During Betty Gale's China childhood, the United Church of Canada North China Mission in Henan province had developed from a primarily evangelistic enterprise led by a tiny cadre of itinerant ministers and physicians to a well-organized humanitarian and educational network that included modern hospitals, training schools for nurses, and Qilu University.

When Betty Gale and five other North China mishkids returned to Henan as missionary nurses in the 1920s and '30s, modern nursing was becoming firmly established in China at the same time that the future of missionary work was growing increasingly uncertain. The missionary enterprise in China was under very critical scrutiny in both Canada and China as members of both countries questioned its ties with imperialism. While missionary nurses were still held in extraordinarily high regard in Canada, interest in joining the overseas missionary movement was waning. Fewer barriers to professional careers for women meant that missionary work was no longer the most attractive avenue open to educated religious women. Furthermore, China had entered one of its most traumatic periods—one that culminated in an eight-year war against Japan. China was thus becoming an increasingly dangerous place to live.

Viewed mainly, but not exclusively, through the lens of Betty Gale and her family, this story of a small Canadian missionary community in China during the Japanese occupation reveals how the internment of mishkid nurses (and other missionaries in the field) not only profoundly altered their understanding of their calling but also ultimately marked the effective end of the Canadian Christian missionary endeavour in China. All fifteen Canadian missionaries living in Japanese-occupied regions were arrested when Japan declared war on the United States and Britain on 8 December 1941. Of the ten who were subsequently interned, three were Canadian mishkid nurses, including Betty Gale.

The mishkid nurses' grounding in missionary values (in particular, acceptance of peril and tribulation as part of the job, and a trust that God would see them through difficult times) played a significant role in three aspects of the story told here: first, the decision made by the Gales (and others) to remain in China against consular advice; second, their ability to survive the privations and emotional challenges of internment; third, the way they understood and actively shaped a narrative of these experiences—namely, that good things ultimately came out of the hardships they experienced.[4]

The central thesis of this foray into the largely unexplored territory of Canadian internment under the Japanese is that the story of mishkid nurses is integral to a fuller understanding of the history of Canadian missionary nursing in China. Most of the nurses hired at the North China Mission after 1922 were mishkids. Five of these six mishkid nurses married in China and resigned from the United Church of Canada North China Mission to join their husbands' missions. When the North China Mission was evacuated between 1939 and 1945, the historical record from China became silent. Although the five married mishkid nurses remained in Japanese-occupied China—three were interned for the duration of the war—they were no longer part of the North China Mission; their war experiences were not included in the United Church of Canada mission record. This story sheds light, then, on an elusive component of China missions and missionary nursing largely inaccessible through public records. Based mainly on a wealth of sources from private family collections—including Betty Gale's diary of internment—and supplemented with archival documents, this book is about the end of an era in a Canadian missionary community, and how that community dealt with—and was reshaped by—war and separation.

As a social history, *China Interrupted* emphasizes social structures and the interactions of missionaries as a social group in Japanese-occupied China. It uses a chronological structure to frame the narrative of wartime missionary work (emphasizing the years that the mishkid nurses were employed as missionary nurses), while exploring analytic themes of gender, religion, culture, and the transnational development of modern nursing. Highlighting the experiences and perspectives of Betty Gale and those closest to her, it argues that disregarding consular advice in 1941 provided second generation missionaries with an unprecedented opportunity to test an emerging premise of medical missions—that Christian nurses and physicians were uniquely suited to alleviate suffering in unstable regions, no matter what the conditions. Eventually cut off from the Chinese populace they had come to serve, their internment unhinged existing notions of what it meant to be missionaries. To remain relevant, they would have to refocus their gaze onto a diverse and desperate new micro-society of imprisoned Western expatriates representing over thirty nationalities. To survive, they would have to adapt to their increasing privation by reapportioning their limited resources, both material and social, and reconstructing the narrative of their lives along the way.

Upon their release, the interned Canadian missionaries departed China, some with vague plans to return when their health was restored. Postwar attempts by the United Church of Canada to rehabilitate the North China Mission were quickly abandoned in the face of a new civil war in 1947, rendering the last few months of Canada's sixty-year mission in China a mere epilogue to the epoch of internment. Internment marked the end of the mishkid nurses' China careers and, as it turned out, of missionary nursing in China as a viable branch of Canadian nursing.

Finding the Story: The Invisibility of Canadian Missionary Nurses

Although numerous memoirs and books have been written by and about civilian internees in China and prisoners of war in the Pacific region as a whole,[5] none has focused on civilian nurses or nursing, Canadian or otherwise. Here the term "internees" is used to refer to civilian enemy aliens incarcerated in Japanese internment camps, whereas "prisoners of war" refers to military personnel, generally incarcerated in POW camps specifically intended for military prisoners. While both involved imprisonment, neglect, starvation, and privation, the POW camps, which were administered by the Japanese military, were characterized by additional layers of abuse and atrocities not generally experienced in civilian internment camps in China (which were administered by civilian authorities—for example, Japanese Consular Police).[6] There are a number of explanations for the paucity of scholarship on interned civilian nurses. These include the general invisibility of history in nursing curricula,[7] the lack of research on missionary nursing in China, and the silence that has surrounded China missions after the expulsion of all foreigners from China after 1949.[8] Furthermore, comprehensive and analytic studies on civilian internees are rare. Perhaps most importantly, there were very few nurses interned. Compared with the eighty-three American and sixty-four Australian military nurses in the Philippines and Indonesia, the numbers in China were small: two military nurses, thirteen non-missionary nurses, and five missionary nurses. That is, out of 13,544 civilian internees in China, only seventeen were Canadian nurses (see Appendices A and B). Yet out of these, three were North China mishkids. As Hamish Ion has argued, although the numbers of Canadian POWs and internees are relatively small, the significance of the Canadian experience in Japanese camps lies not in its scale, but in what can be garnered from it about broader issues—in this case, the larger narrative of Canadian missions, missionary nursing, and the reshaping of a Canadian missionary community.[9]

The Silencing of Missionary Nursing

For a period of almost sixty years following the expulsion of foreigners from China after the Communist victory in 1949, a veil of silence shrouded the history of Canadian missionary nurses in China. Theirs was a rich history encompassing six decades of nursing service and education in nine provinces of China—most notably the United Church North China Mission in Henan and Shandong, and the United Church West China Mission in Sichuan. From the arrival of the first Canadian missionary nurse in 1888 until the abrupt closure of the war-ravaged North China Mission in Henan in 1947, approximately one hundred Canadian missionary nurses contributed to the establishment of a Nightingale-style, hospital-based system of nursing practice and education that continues to this day.[10]

During the early years of China missions, Canadian missionaries enjoyed strong public support in Canada. Their reputation as self-sacrificing servants of God grew out of stories of danger, disease, and death. The narrative of triumph over tragedy associated with events like the Boxer Uprising of 1900, the murder of Dr. James Menzies in 1920, and the Nationalist army march to Nanjing in 1927 resonated among the Canadian churchgoing public who actively promoted and financed missionary endeavours. However, the Great Depression of the 1930s and the increasing debate over the morality and viability of missions tempered the public appetite for missions, and the outbreak of war in Europe preoccupied the attention of most Canadians between 1939 and 1945. By the time the North China Mission sites closed during the Communist-Nationalist civil war in 1947, missionaries had already fallen out of favour among the Canadian public.[11] A sense of exhaustion and failure coupled with public critique of the global missionary movement gave second-generation Canadian missionary women little desire to publicize their China experiences beyond their immediate circles.

The Hidden Record

Given the social context that served to silence missionary nursing, it is not surprising that little attention has been paid to the handful of Canadian missionary nurses who were interned under the Japanese in China. But there are a number of other factors that have also contributed to their invisibility. First, missionary nurses who married in China are difficult to trace in mission records. Because married women were not allowed to work as nurses in Canada, and because the United Church of Canada Woman's Missionary Society (wms) only supported unmarried women, missionary nurses who married in China were expected to give up their vocation and resign from the wms. Married nurses took on their husbands' surnames and mission organizations, which were expected to take over financial responsibility for the women. Thus one would not easily recognize Mrs. Godfrey Gale of the London Missionary Society as Canadian mishkid Betty Thomson, Mrs. John Stanley of the American Board of Commissioners for Foreign Missions as Mary Boyd, or Mrs. John Lewis of the American Baptist Society as Georgina Menzies.

For a similar reason, the identity of these three Canadian missionary nurses is obscured in official internment camp lists. Of the 13,544 civilian internees in China meticulously listed by the Japanese, only Hilda Elizabeth McIllroy is listed as a "Canadian missionary nurse."[12] Betty Gale is listed as a British missionary nurse, Mary Stanley as a Canadian housewife and Georgina Lewis as a Canadian wife.[13] Canadian missionary nurse Susie Kelsey—who was repatriated before the camp lists were compiled in 1943—is not listed at all. Thus, of the five Canadian missionary nurses confirmed through this study as civilian internees, four are not listed as such in the most comprehensive camp lists available. And of Hilda McIllroy, little is known except her name and sponsoring mission—listed as the Church Missionary Society, which is an English organization.[14]

My own discovery of these nurse-internees began during my previous study of Canadian missionary nursing at the North China Mission,[15] when a participant alerted me to the existence of Betty Gale's diary, kept during her internment. I suspected that other North China missionaries were interned, but this was not confirmed until I found Mary Boyd Stanley's name on the list of internees engraved on a memorial wall at Weixian Camp in

Shandong province. At about that time, a former British civilian internee emailed me to confirm Georgina Menzies Lewis's internment at Ash Camp, and a letter published in the *Canadian Nurse* journal in 1943 alerted me to the internment of Susie Kelsey.

While it is possible that additional Canadian missionary nurses were interned in China, it is unlikely. The majority of Canadian missionary nurses in China were employed by the United Church of Canada, and there is no record of internment of nurses from either the West China Mission in Sichuan or the South China Mission in Guangdong. Only the North China Mission was in Japanese-occupied China; internment of Canadian missionaries in China was, it appears, a North China Mission phenomenon.

The Visibility of POWs

An additional reason for the invisibility of interned Canadian nurses is that they did not belong to any single *publicly identifiable* group during the internment years. Unlike American military nurses in the Philippines[16] or Australian military nurses in Indonesia,[17] whose collective identity catapulted them into public consciousness during and after the war, the five interned Canadian missionary nurses were officially identified with five separate mission organizations from the United States, Britain, and Canada. They lived in different cities in China and were arrested and interned separately. Once interned, moreover, they had virtually no contact with each other.

This is in sharp contrast to the shared history of imprisoned American and Australian military nurses, who experienced internment as distinct groups identifiable by their citizenship, occupation, and gender. The eighty-three American nurses, for example, went to war in the Philippines as a group, and subsequently experienced Japanese attack, were imprisoned, and were liberated as a group. When they were taken captive after the fall of Corregidor in 1942, media reports brought their imprisonment to public attention. Their plight caught the imagination of military propagandists in the United States, who portrayed the nurses' captivity as evidence of their patriotism and promoted their story as motivation for others to take up the call to arms. For example, a Second World War poster featuring the POW nurses from Corregidor portrays a group of six nurses immaculately clad in blue caps, white uniforms, and blue capes behind a barbed-wire fence guarded by a sallow-faced Japanese soldier brandishing a bayonet. The caption reads: "Work! To get them free. Work! To keep 'em fighting!"[18]

The nurses of Corregidor also caught the attention of Hollywood. In 1943, Universal Studios released a full-length feature film based directly on their story, albeit a romanticized version with a fictitious ending. What is especially striking about the film *So Proudly We Hail* is that the nurses were still imprisoned during its creation, and would be for two more years after its release. When all eighty-three nurses were liberated in February 1945, news crews captured the event on camera. Hailed as heroines, these nurses later expressed astonishment at the celebrity status awaiting them back in the US; they were embarrassed by the inaccuracies of the film that had been made about their capture and fictionalized release.[19] Four decades later Elizabeth Norman's *We Band of Angels*, a scholarly account of the nurses' ordeal, revived public interest in the story, as did a patriotic documentary produced by the United States Department of Defence called *They All Came Home*.[20] The story of imprisoned American nurses, then, has been firmly established in public consciousness.

Australian military nurses who were prisoners of war in Indonesia have also received tremendous public attention. Not only were published memoirs of nurses widely circulated after the war, but the Australian nurses also continue to hold a place of honour in the Australian Nursing Services War Memorial in Canberra.[21] Tragically, in contrast to the American story of survival, only a third of the Australian nurses survived. Of the sixty-four nurses who were aboard a military ship that was bombed by the Japanese, eleven drowned. Twenty-two others who made it to shore were lined up at the water's edge by Japanese soldiers, shot, and left for dead. Vivienne Bullwinkle survived and escaped. She was the only living witness of the beach massacre, and she was later caught and imprisoned with thirty-three other surviving military nurses from her unit. By the end of the war, eleven more had died from the stark camp conditions. In total, only twenty-two of the original sixty-four Australian military nurses survived.

Canadian military nurses Kathleen Georgina Christie and Anna May Waters were also POWs. Arriving in Hong Kong with Canadian troops only six weeks before the unexpected 8 December attacks, the women were captured with 1,900 other Canadians after the Japanese won the battle for Hong Kong on 25 December 1941. While their story is not the subject of this book, it is important to note that it, too, has received little attention. Originally imprisoned at the Bowen Road Hospital, Christie and Waters were relocated to a civilian internment camp, called Stanley Camp, in August 1942 before being repatriated in September 1943.[22]

The main difference between the military nurse (POW) experience and the civilian (internee) experience was the intensity of trauma that preceded imprisonment as well as the collective lack of psychological preparedness for the reality of warfare and imprisonment. In general the military nurses were not apprised of their top secret destinations until shortly before deployment from their home countries. Most arrived at their destinations only weeks before war broke out, and all suffered direct and horrifying attacks by the Japanese military before their surrender. In contrast, civilian nurses in China had made their homes there for years, even decades, before their arrests. The mishkid nurses' transition to civilian imprisonment was not accompanied by the violence and violation experienced by the military nurses. While both the military and the missionary nurses spent most of their imprisonment in civilian internment camps with similar levels of neglect, the missionary nurses entered with a sense of relief, having anticipated much worse in the months leading up to their arrest, whereas the military nurses entered with a level of psychological and physical trauma that threatened to unhinge them—and sometimes did.

Unlike the punitive nature of Japanese POW camps, the purpose of internment camps was to neutralize the possibility of enemy aliens spying or otherwise hindering local war efforts. It was in the POW camps that prisoners were required to engage in forced labour, the act of which was utilized as a propaganda tool to demonstrate Asia's liberation from Western imperialist rule.[23] Japanese prison camps, civilian and military, fell under the 1929 Geneva Convention on the treatment of POWs. Under the convention, the Japanese were ostensibly responsible for the provision of food, water, shelter, and the distribution of mail and Red Cross parcels. They were also required to allow a neutral observer—a Swiss consul in this case—into the camps to ensure that these obligations were being met. Prisoners were left to organize their own cooking, cleaning, laundry, entertainment, education, and health care. In short, prisoners in civilian internment camps were neglected rather than abused. As the war progressed, however, the conditions worsened for POWs and civilians alike. As Hamish Ion has noted, the Japanese ignored or abandoned the Geneva Convention in many cases, claiming that they were not bound by it because it had never been officially ratified.[24]

Finally, Canadian missionary nurses were no strangers to China; it was their adopted home. While their internment in 1941 was an act of Japanese aggression, it was not a sudden one. They and their families had become accustomed to the looming Japanese threat from as early as 1928, when Japanese soldiers bayonetted a hospital full of patients near Qilu, three years before the Japanese invasion of Manchuria.[25] Furthermore, Japanese aggression was seen not so much as a new threat against enemy aliens as an extension of the ongoing threat against the Chinese. By choosing to stay in China against consular advice in 1941, missionaries like Betty Gale, Mary Stanley, and Georgina Lewis knowingly put themselves at risk. While their job as they perceived it was to provide medical assistance where it was needed most, they had not anticipated that their care would be to the population *within* their walls rather than the one *outside* them—that is, to the prisoners within the barbed wire fences rather than the Chinese who lived outside the mission compound walls. They would have to develop a revised version of their missionary calling.

Nursing and the United Church of Canada North China Mission

When mishkids and friends Betty Thomson, Mary Boyd, and Dorothy Boyd returned to China together as missionary nurses with the United Church of Canada Woman's Missionary Society in 1938, they were continuing a tradition that had started fifty years earlier. The first American missionary nurse went to China in 1884; the first Canadian nurse in 1888.[26] Canada occupied a special place within the phalanx of China missions.[27] As a colony of both France and Britain, Canada had a unique history as both a missions-receiving and missions-sending nation, in two languages, cultures, and religions (English Protestants; French and English Roman Catholics).[28] In 1919 more than one quarter of British missionaries were, in fact, Canadian. In proportion to their size and resources, the churches of Canada sponsored more missionaries at home and abroad than any other nation in Christendom.[29]

The Canadian presence in China as a whole was most recognizable through six main missions: the Presbyterian Church in Canada mission in Taiwan (est. 1871), the Presbyterian mission in North Henan (est. 1888), the Methodist Church of Canada mission in Sichuan (est. 1891), the Presbyterian mission in Guangdong (est. 1902), the Catholic Scarboro Foreign Mission Society in Zhejiang (est. 1902), and the Anglican Church of Canada mission south of the Yellow River in Henan (est. 1910).[30] The Presbyterian mission in Taiwan was the first overseas field of the Canadian Presbyterian Church, but the eccentricity of its founder, George Leslie McKay, its remoteness from Mainland China, and its continuance with the Presbyterian Church after "Union" kept Taiwan on the fringe of Canadian missions.[31] The union of all Canadian Methodists, Congregationalists and most Presbyterians into one United Church of Canada in 1925 set the United Church apart as the largest Canadian mission in China, with the North China Mission in Henan, the West China Mission in Sichuan, and the South China Mission in Guangdong. The United Church was the largest employer of Canadian missionary nurses.[32] An estimated one hundred or more Canadian nurses worked in at least nine provinces of China during this period.[33] By the time the three mishkid nurses signed up to work at their parents' United Church of Canada North China Mission in Henan province, Canadians had already established four hospitals and the first nursing school there and had been training nurses for sixteen years.

Missionary nurses were thus an integral part of the Canadian missionary community in North China. Furthermore, missionary nurses played a key role in the establishment and incipient growth of modern nursing in China. When the first American and Canadian "trained" nurses arrived in China there was no equivalent in Chinese culture to the conceptualization of nursing popularized by Florence Nightingale—that is, as a noble profession suitable for unmarried, God-fearing ladies.[34] In late-nineteenth-century China, it was inconceivable that Chinese ladies "of good family" would care for the sick, other than their own relatives.[35] Nor was there an equivalent of "the Christian ethic in which caring could be lifted onto a plane of moral obligation" to become a "respected profession in which the most unpleasant work could be ennobled."[36] The missionary ideal of nursing as an honourable profession was "so novel" that "the Chinese had no word in their language to express the concepts 'nobly' and 'properly' for the nursing pioneers."[37] By the 1910s there was a small but growing cadre of Chinese women and men poised to enter missionary-sponsored nurses training.[38] In 1914 the modern Chinese nurse was named into being when American missionary nurses in the newly-established Nurses Association of China (NAC) adopted the term *hu shih* (literally, "caring scholar") to describe the new professional role being taken up by their Chinese proteges. In 1922, eight years after its inception, the NAC joined the International Council of Nurses, bringing China into the growing imagined community of women from around the world with a shared identity of woman-as-nurse.[39] That same year, the United Church of Canada North China Mission opened its first modern hospital and training school for nurses, at Weihui, Henan— and Toronto General Hospital graduate Jean Menzies became the first of six mishkid nurses to return to North China.

North China mishkid nurses found a natural fit between the goals of their profession and that of their missionary community; sharing the gospel of soap and water, light and fresh air was no less valued than sharing the gospel of Christ. By the 1930s the North China Mission no longer viewed evangelism as the primary aim of missionary physicians and nurses. Rather, compassionate care of patients was seen as a meaningful expression of Christianity in action—a worthwhile endeavour in and of itself.[40] North China missionaries, having defined themselves as credible contributors to the burgeoning development of hospital-based health care by Christian missionaries around China, were committed to the development of nursing service through the education of Chinese nurses. But they needed nurses well-versed in modern nursing practices to do the teaching, and these were hard to find. Mishkids who had completed their nurses training in Canada were the best hope for the future of health care at the new Canadian hospitals in North China.

Telling the Story: Advantages of Social History

Using a social history approach to explore the story of Canadian mishkid nurses in North China during Japanese occupation allows us to analyze the social structures and relationships of the Canadian missionary community across two distinct time periods: pre-internment and intra-internment. Tracing the richly interwoven lives of Betty Gale and other mishkids from their China childhoods through internment allows us to consider how the experiences of Japanese internment altered their lives, relationships, and sense of communal mission. Having access to archival *and* private papers is key to making this possible: whereas the mission record becomes silent after internment in 1941, private letters and diaries bridge that silence and keep the narrative moving past house arrest and into various prison camps over the next four years. In this way, social history allows us to consider internment as a continuation of the history of Canadian missions in North China rather than as a separate phenomenon.

A second advantage to using a social history approach to the study of mishkid nurses is that it allows identity to be placed at the centre of analysis. It allows us to explore how gender, religion, culture, professional, and other social constructions influenced relationships and decision making. Through it we can examine the "seamless interconnection" between the mishkids' private and public lives; how personal and family experiences shaped public choices.[41] In China, missionary nursing was not confined within the walls of mission hospitals, nor was it carried out only within boundaries of paid employment. As Patricia D'Antonio has noted, women's culture and experiences can never be completely understood just in their relationship with paid labour; understanding women's places within the social fabric of their communities, neighbourhoods, and families is key to understanding their consciousness, role, and agency.[42] Social history invites reflection on how individual mishkids' self-identity was influenced by the well-established social identity of North China missionaries as devout and highly educated risk-takers. And it helps to explain why second generation missionary nursing was not an independent career so much as an extension of the family business: becoming a trained nurse was one of the few ways that mishkids could reunite with their missionary parents and return to their childhood home.

Perhaps nowhere is the link between China missions and the development of Canadian identity more evident than in the lives of China mishkids. Bilingual and bicultural, mishkids had a particular view of the world and a unique understanding of their place in it. The strong representation of mishkids in missionary nursing between 1922 and 1941 demonstrates how nursing was understood not merely as congruent with missionary ideals but as an embodiment of them. The collective identity of missionary nurses at the North China Mission after the 1920s was shaped in large part by the childhood experiences of six girls who came of age there, including Betty Gale.

Sources

This study is based on a wide range of material from public (archive) and private (family) collections. Private sources were primarily obtained from China mishkids and their families—particularly members of the Thomson/Gale family—whose cache of original documents became central to this study. These sources included Betty Gale's China journal, diary and diarized notebook (described further below), hundreds of pages of family letters to and from China, photo albums and loose photographs, memorabilia (immunization certificates, nursing certificates, graduation and wedding programs), newspaper clippings, annual hospital reports, drawings, internment camp newsletters, and one eight-millimetre film (Gale wedding in Tianjin, in 1940). The United Church of Canada Archives provided missionary biographical files, official mission communiqués, and photographs from the North China Mission. Library and Archives Canada provided International Committee of the Red Cross reports on conditions at China's internment camps.

Other sources included a variety of China memoirs, both in the form of written and oral histories. Oral histories included taped interviews of six internees (including Betty Gale and Kenneth and Frances McAll) recorded by Margaret Gale Wightman in 1991, plus my own interviews with three of Betty Gale's surviving siblings. Written memoirs included published autobiographical sources such as Marion F. Menzies Hummel's *Memoirs of a Mishkid*, Peggy Abkjazi's *A Curious Cage*, and Frances and Kenneth McAll's *Moon Looks Down*. Self-published biographical sources were typically comprised of transcribed and dated missionary letters and diaries, supplemented with memories recorded by their children—including Murray Thomson's *A Daring Confidence* (Andrew Thomson) and *Mother, God Bless Her* (Margaret Thomson), and Preston Robb's *Flowers Amongst the Debris* (Clara Preston).

Additional insights were gleaned from innumerable informal conversations with China mishkids, including those who accompanied me to China on research visits to Anyang, Weihui, Jinan, and Shanghai—most notably Betty Gale's daughter Margaret, whose generosity and support were primary. While the study draws on formalized records and recordings, these informal conversations and related insights have inevitably influenced my interpretation of the material, whether consciously or not.

Because much of this social history focuses on memory work, including diaries, memoirs, and oral interviews (Betty Gale's and others'), it is important to note that I approached this study with sensitivity to the ways in which the process of narrating lives may itself serve to write a particular identity into being. Because reminiscences reflect the subjectivity of the narrator, these sources are sometimes dismissed as unreliable because they are seen as coloured by egocentrism, hyperbole, and selective memory.[43] M. Louise Fitzpatrick, for example, suggests that recollections are best suited to fill gaps left by existing documentation rather than as principal sources. Alice Wexler is less skeptical than Fitzpatrick, suggesting that recollections are valuable as long as the researcher is clear about the distinction between the memory of a life and the life actually lived.[44] I agree with Wexler, who argues that the real value of recollections lies in how they represent a person's construction of self and give insight into the ongoing tension among people's gendered, racial, economic, and cultural selves—that is, their multiple identities. Geertje Boschma and others also agree, adding that oral history also serves to create history of ordinary people's lives, countering the hegemonic record documented by those in power.[45]

In the study of missionary women like the mishkid nurses of North China, memory sources are of particular importance. Although much has been done over the past twenty years to restore "to their rightful place" Victorian women missionaries "who have been ignored, misunderstood or forgotten,"[46] the historical record on second-generation missionary women remains scant.[47] Not only are nurses subsumed into the historical records of their husbands, as noted earlier, but also missionary nurses are often "rendered invisible" within the rubric of missionary medicine.[48] While the omission of nurses in medical histories has been attributed to gender biases which privilege the voice of (male) physicians over (female) nurses,[49] one cannot get away from the fact that there are, as Christoffer Grundmann has noted, simply a lack of "documents and biographies" related to missionary nursing.[50] Memoirs and oral recollections, then, serve as more than gap-fillers to the mission record; in many cases they *are* the record. By supplementing narrative accounts with official mission and governmental documents rather than vice versa, this study provides a descriptive context of China-as-observed by foreigners who lived there, as well as individual and collective interpretations of China-as-lived by them.

In relying on recollections as a predominant source of information from within the camps themselves, it is important to acknowledge, as oral historian Sally Chandler has noted, that "subjectivity—both our subject's and our own—shapes the content and interpretation of our work."[51] Just as historians must be sensitive to the ways in which subjects bring their particular values and beliefs to their writing, so researchers must be sensitive to how our own location and perspective might influence our work. To Boschma, interpretation of sources, be they written records or evidence generated by oral interviews, always reflects the subjective position of the researcher.[52] Pamela Sugiman's study of interned Japanese Canadians in Canada illustrates this well. As a third-generation Japanese Canadian of working-class parents who were both interned in British Columbia after the attacks on Pearl Harbor, Sugiman was conscious of the importance of self-reflexivity in the research process. Situating herself as a co-constructor of the narratives that emerged through her oral interviews, Sugiman acknowledged the need to consider her own motivations and needs alongside those of her subjects.[53]

With that in mind, I am not sure that I would have been invited into the lives of China mishkids and their families if I did not share some of the characteristics of the mishkid nurses who are at the centre of this study—that is, as a Canadian, Protestant nurse who has worked in foreign mission settings. Our relationships developed slowly over the course of nine years as I met surviving relatives of the Canadian missionary nurses, who then introduced me to others in their circle. Eventually these relationships led to two research trips to China involving twelve relatives of Canadian missionaries, four of whom were mishkids returning for the first time in six decades—including Betty Gale's daughter Margaret, then in her sixties. We shared stories during our travels across China, while gazing over the Great Wall, Shanghai Bund, Yellow River, Qilu university campus, Weixian internment camp memorial, and the former Weihui mission hospital. In addition to this, some missionary family members communicated with me by email, letter, or telephone; others sent me published and unpublished memoirs, letters, and photographs. Each of these contributed to my developing understanding of mishkids and the story of Japanese internment and the reshaping of a Canadian missionary community.

Sugiman describes oral interviews as conversational narratives benefiting both the interviewer and the interviewee. So, too, were the letters, diaries, recorded interviews, and written recollections conversational narratives benefiting both them and their audience—in the case of mishkid nurses like Betty Gale, mostly their families. Ultimately the historian must respect what the narrator says and writes. Sugiman notes that there is always self-selection by narrators in terms of the memories they wish to share. Thus, while many of the missionary descriptions of events and their responses to them were written as they occurred, their renderings were nonetheless self-selected. Private anxieties and frustrations were tempered by a desire to reflect qualities considered admirable and consistent with their religious upbringing. Sugiman asserts that narratives "contain a message that the narrator wishes to communicate to a wider audience—a message that is moral rather than empirical."[54] Mindful of the need to situate the narrator in her cultural and historical context, part of my aim in the following pages is to decipher and explicate mishkids' moral message(s) and the underlying social values that stimulated their creation.

A few sources deserve special mention. The chapters dealing with the last years of internment (particularly Chapter 7) draw almost exclusively on material authored by Betty Gale. The main source was Betty Gale's unpublished journal, handwritten some time later in her life as a gift to her daughter Margaret. Comprised of a transcribed collation of entries from her diary, notebook, and letters home, the journal is a diarized account of Betty Gale's life in China from the day of Margaret's birth (in July 1941) until their release from Pudong Camp (August 1945). Divided into four sections based on internment sites (Qilu, CCC, Yangzhou, Pudong), this 231-page work incorporates introductory comments by Godfrey Gale, and numerous photos and illustrations of camp life, many drawn by fellow internee Ken McAll. The dated entries include a snapshot description of daily events and Betty Gale's responses to them. Best viewed as a memoir rather than a diary, the unpublished "Journal of Betty Gale" (hereafter "journal") is similar to other unpublished memoirs written by missionaries at the time. For example, Godfrey Gale wrote a thirty-seven page (undated and unpublished) manuscript he entitled "Pacific War," based on his China diary and prefaced with the comment "let me [now] take up my diary, very much as I wrote it at the time and on the spot, except for an occasional expansion or word of explanation or additional note, and let me start with our last day of freedom, Sunday December 7th [1941]."[55] Betty Gale's journal was both an impetus and a key source for this study.

Years after my study was under way, the Gale family discovered tucked away in storage two invaluable sources, which they mailed to me. One was Betty Gale's original leather-bound Five Year Diary, started the day she commenced her journey back to China, and filled with short descriptions of daily events (from 15 February 1939 to 31 December 1943). The other was a fragile, yellowed, and mouldy notebook, with pages missing but with longer, detailed descriptions of events during Betty Gale's last years of internment (from 1 January 1944 to 2 October 1945). The surviving notebook consists of eighty handwritten pages. When her children found the notebook they also discovered seventeen additional pages of handwritten notes tucked into it—an undated, rough draft of Betty Gale's post-liberation reflections (possibly notes for a speech, apparently written nine and a half years after liberation, thus in 1955). Betty Gale kept the diary and notebook with her through her entire internment. Taken together, Betty Gale's primary sources (letters, diary, notebook, journal, notes) corroborate each other. Because the journal, diary, and notebook contain dated entries, it is possible to get a sense of what Betty Gale edited out or added to the journal (memoir) she painstakingly prepared as a gift to her daughter Margaret. The journal, then, is not only a record for posterity, but also an illustration of the moral message(s) and underlying social values she wished to pass along to her children. In this sense Betty Gale's journal is an expression of the values of the missionary community she so closely identified with.

There are some noteworthy differences between the sources. Whereas the diary contains brief descriptions of Betty Gale's daily social activities and the people she visited, the notebook and journal contain fuller descriptions of her responses to the people and events. When transcribing events from her notebook to her journal, she took care to change the full names of some internees to initials only, especially when describing difficult people or interactions. She glossed over details that could be construed as disparaging or damaging to someone's reputation (e.g., when a minister was "accused of being a hypocrite and other juicy names" after acting in a controversial camp play; or details of conflicts between internees). She excluded at least one intimate expression of her love for her husband (identified as "Private!" in the margin of her notebook). In both her notebook *and* journal Betty Gale expressed ways in which she found her internment experiences valuable; framing her internment in positive terms was not something she only did in retrospect. For example, on 22 January 1945 she wrote in her notebook: "This internment has been marvellous for me in some ways, and I'm very sure that God intended Margaret and me to stay here with Godf[rey]"—a message consistent with her post-liberation reflections. Finally, Betty Gale excluded from her journal some reflections on her interior spiritual life. For example, in her notebook on 21 August 1944, she extrapolated personal meaning from a sermon on how Peter, a disciple of Jesus Christ, had to "be changed in all his ideas of things—what Christianity really is" because of his trials in life (trials which culminated in his martyrdom).

Betty Gale's journal, then, was not quite as candid as her notebook. Nor was it always accurately transcribed. For example, according to her notebook a memorial for Eric Liddell was held before 16 April 1945; according to her journal it was held after 17 April. Both sources note that the memorial was on Good Friday, which was 30 March 1945; the original source is correct. Such inaccuracies notwithstanding, the journal of Betty Gale is an invaluable historical source, particularly as a reflection of her social values and identity. What she excluded in the journal (but included in her diary and notebook) provides insight into how she differentiated her private, interior life from her less private role as mother. What she included in her journal (and memoir draft) provides insight into the social values of her missionary community; the moral message(s) she passed along reflected both her personal values and those of her social group. For our purposes, Betty Gale's journal is a reliable source of her own perception of events and her responses to them. Except where there is a discrepancy noted between sources, the journal is used interchangeably with sources penned at the time.

Overview of Chapters

A central theme of this book is the intersection between mishkid nurses' social identity and the increasingly fragmented and isolated nature of second-generation Canadian missionary nursing in China both before and during the Japanese occupation. Narrated mostly from the perspective of Betty Gale, it is arranged chronologically with 1941 as the pivotal year, the point of no return for those who decided to stay in China against consular advice. The book is thus divided roughly into two parts: before internment and during internment. The first part examines the social context that shaped China mishkid identity. China mishkids embodied a combination of cavalier ease in China with a desire to create a China mission narrative that was as thrilling and dangerous as their parents', but one they could call their own. The second part is the evolution of that very narrative, exemplified mostly by the life of mishkid nurse Betty Gale during Japanese internment between 1941 and 1945.

This book is organized into seven chapters, each including both description and integrative analysis. Chapter 1 examines the childhood experiences of Betty Gale and her contemporaries at the United Church North China Mission between 1911 and 1934, exploring how a mishkid elite emerged from Henan province. Chapter 2 examines how mishkids' decisions to return to China as missionary nurses reflected the expectations and realities of the subculture of second-generation missionaries coming of age during the early war years in China between 1935 and 1938. Chapter 3 explores mishkid nurses' early experiences, between 1939 and 1940, as part of the "new" generation of China missionaries, suspended in exile in a protected world of parties, romance, and marriage, while the mission hospitals they had come to China to work in were attacked and evacuated. Chapter 4 critiques Betty Gale and other missionary nurses' pivotal decision to remain in China against consular advice in the months leading up to Japan's attack on Pearl Harbor in 1941. Chapter 5 considers how Betty Gale and other "enemy aliens" adapted to life under house arrest on the Qilu campus, as the Japanese experimented with their new role as prison camp administrators for a population of civilian prisoners. Chapter 6 examines Betty Gale's search for meaning between 1942 and 1943 as she and her family were moved from North China to Shanghai—not for freedom, as they assumed, but for internment, first at a Civilian Assembly Centre with 350 other enemy aliens, then as medical-staff prisoners in charge of a remote civilian camp in Yangzhou. Finally, Chapter 7 explores how two years of increasing privation and danger in a condemned tobacco warehouse in Pudong with 1,200 other internees confined Betty Gale's personal sense of mission to ever-diminishing social circles as she slowly withdrew into herself during the months of incessant air raids over Pudong that preceded liberation in 1945. The conclusion highlights salient themes and new insights, asserting that the life that Betty Gale and other missionaries composed through their letter writing, diary entries, and post-internment memoirs and reflections was informed by a collective missionary belief in a grand redemptive narrative. Being able to make sense of internment was strengthened by close identification with, and as, China missionaries.

Developing a Mishkid Elite (1910–1934)

We must both have China blood right in us, I think.

—Canadian missionary nurse Mary Boyd Stanley,
letter, January 1941

Theirs was an unconventional childhood. To Canadian missionary children born in early-twentieth-century China, rickshaws, chopsticks, and "*amahs*" (nursemaids) were as familiar as Brontë novels, piano lessons, and Christmas plays. While their parents immersed themselves in the Christian service they came to China to fulfill, North China mishkids immersed themselves in "everything dusty and heavenly"—not realizing that riding donkeys on the beach at Beidaihe, absorbing the work songs of "coolies" (unskilled labourers—hereafter "labourers"), poling up the Wei River on barges, and purchasing Chinese delicacies from the street vendors outside the mission gates were unusual activities for Canadian children.[1]

Between 1923 and 1939 six daughters of Canadian North China missionaries returned to China to join their parents as missionary nurses. Each of these six mishkid nurses was born in Henan province to long-serving Canadian missionaries. Jean Menzies (b. 1898) and her sister Georgina Menzies (1906) were born to James R. and Davina Menzies. Florence Mackenzie (1911) was born to Hugh and Agnes Mackenzie. Betty Thomson (1911) was born to Andrew and Margaret Thomson. Dorothy Boyd (1913) and her sister Mary Boyd (1916) were born to H.A. and Jessie Boyd.[2] These six mishkid nurses were bound by similar world views, difficult circumstances, and a genuine need for each other. They shared formative years at the North China Mission which bred in them a unique bicultural, bilingual understanding of the world. They also shared formative nursing years at the Toronto General Hospital Training School for Nurses, where each had studied before returning to China. Their lives were inextricably linked. It was during their childhood that nursing shifted from the margins to the centre of missionary interest at the North China Mission. Their decisions to return to China were part of this shift.

The North China Mission did not always value nursing. In the earlier years of the mission, some of the most influential Canadian missionaries viewed medicine (and by extension, nursing) as little more than a means to an evangelical end. That is, because the primary purpose of missionaries was understood as bringing Chinese people to a belief in the Christian gospel message, pioneer missionaries only reluctantly accepted the treatment of patients as part of the Canadian mission to China. In this context, medical care was viewed primarily as a way to win the trust of potential converts; healing bodies was a means to saving souls. It took the vision and persuasive powers of missionary physicians to catalyze nursing and move it onto a modern and organized pathway. Although a missionary nurse was among the first group of Canadian missionaries (then Presbyterian) commissioned to work in Henan in 1888, it was not until 1911—the year of Betty Gale and Florence Mackenzie's birth—that the North China Mission began strategically to include missionary nurses in their overall plans.

Three socio-political factors converged in 1911 to provide a favourable climate for the development of nursing at the North China Mission: a widespread acceptance of Western ideas in China after Sun Yat-sen came to power, publicity by the Christian Medical Association of China for better nursing services, and the vision and persuasive power of North China missionary Dr. Fred Auld. In 1911, China was in the midst of a national crisis. Ever since foreign powers had defeated a violent movement against non-Chinese commercial, religious, and political influence in China (the 1900 "Boxer Uprising"), the Chinese government under the Manchu Qing dynasty had been considered hopelessly feeble and out of step with the rest of the world. The Empress Dowager and her nephew, the Kuang-hsu Emperor, had died in 1908, leaving two-year-old Aisin-Gioro Puyi to ascend the Qing throne. A series of anti-dynastic movements in 1911 culminated in the overthrow of Qing dynasty, and Dr. Sun Yat-sen was elected first president of the new Republic of China. That same year a pneumonic plague was raging in northern China. Medical missionaries from all over North China offered their services to the new government and, according to historian Yuet-wah Cheung, helped to get the plague under control.[3] Western medicine, Cheung asserts, was officially recognized in China after its worth was proved during the pneumonic plague of 1911.

The successful treatment of the pneumonic plague opened up new opportunities for medical missions in general, and for nursing in particular, since medical missionaries across China were starting to recognize a need for nurses to staff the new Western-style hospitals they were developing.[4] The Christian Medical Association of China, in an article on "The Work of Medical Missions in 1911" that identified nursing as the "weakest side of

Medical Mission work," reported that only one in two hospitals in China had even one nurse.[5] Foreign nurses were needed to teach Chinese nurses and to oversee the nursing work at men's and women's hospitals. In Henan, Dr. Fred Auld considered the recommendations of the Christian Medical Association of China and, after making a careful study of what was going on in the large hospitals of other missions, concluded that Henan needed to move beyond what was largely an outpatient practice, to organized inpatient services. He recommended the appointment of Mrs. Jeannette Ratcliffe, a widowed graduate nurse who was already living in Henan, as superintendent of the new North China Mission hospital at Weihui once it was built.[6]

Although Jeannette Ratcliffe's position would not officially start until the hospital was ready (in 1922), she was, in the meantime, meticulous in her preparation for her new role. While she waited for the construction of the hospital to be completed, she undertook postgraduate education in Toronto, as well as hands on experience as the Acting Matron at the University Hospital in Jinan. She also studied the Chinese language. She was joined by a second nurse, Janet Brydon. Their plans were interrupted by the First World War when most of the male missionaries at the North China Mission went to France to help with the war effort between 1918 and 1919. When the men returned, the North China Mission was finally poised to move forward with nursing development. Meanwhile, the vision for medical and nursing services had grown. Plans included opening new hospitals at three of the mission sites, one of which would also serve as the first training school for Chinese nurses in Henan, at Weihui. Together with the (Chinese) Church of Christ in China, the Canadians initiated plans to recruit Christian nursing students from local Chinese congregations. Once again, however, the plans to advance hospital-based care in Henan were interrupted—this time by the murder of Dr. James R. Menzies, in 1920.

Pioneer Canadian missionary James Menzies was shot by "bandits" while coming to the aid of Janet Brydon and her housemate Sadie Lethbridge, who had called out for help from their balconies when their house was being stormed. The tragedy devastated the small North China missionary community. Although the community had experienced its share of violence and *illness*-related death in its thirty-year history, this was the first violent death. Sadie Lethbridge who, it was said, never fully recovered from the shock, died a few months later of dysentery. Janet Brydon remained at Henan, working at the mission hospital at Huaiqing while assisting with plans to open the new hospital and nursing school at nearby Weihui. Three years later she and Jeannette Ratcliffe were joined by three new nursing recruits, including the first North China mishkid nurse, Jean Menzies— daughter of the slain James Menzies.

The Phenomenon of Mishkid Nurses

The phenomenon of mishkid nurses can be best traced back to the year of James Menzies' death.[7] Menzies' wife, Davina R. Robb Menzies, was living temporarily in Toronto with her three daughters when the telegram bearing the tragic news arrived on 26 March 1920. Twenty-two-year-old Jean Menzies, the oldest daughter, had just started nurse's training at the Toronto General Hospital nursing school. Fourteen-year-old Georgina Menzies was in secondary school. Although we do not know why Jean Menzies made the remarkable decision to return to Huaiqing to work at the newly named Menzies Memorial Hospital where her father had laboured for thirty years, we do know that her decision was received with unmitigated delight by the missionary community in China and Canada. Through Jean Menzies and fellow mishkid Dr. Bob McClure—who agreed to return to take James Menzies' place—Jean's beloved father's work would live on.

When Jean Menzies arrived at the North China Mission in 1923 with her mother and sisters, the five girls who would later follow in her footsteps would have been well aware of the excitement caused by her arrival. At the time, Jean's sister Georgina was seventeen, Florence Mackenzie and Betty Thomson were twelve, and Mary and Dorothy Boyd were ten and seven years old respectively. Having borne witness to the outpouring of grief at the "martyrdom" of James Menzies, these young girls were doubtlessly caught up in the enthusiastic reception of the first "one of our own" as a missionary. To North China missionaries who felt devastated by the traumatic loss of James Menzies, the return of his daughter was reassuring: who better to take up the legacy of missionary work than the children of the missionaries themselves? If Jean Menzies was willing to return to the very hospital where her father had worked, to be supervised by the very woman her father had tried to rescue, and to work alongside the physician who took her father's place, then any missionary child could continue the legacy.

Jean Menzies' return—even more than the return of the esteemed Bob McClure—reinforced the notion that the value of missionary work was proportionate to the level of self-sacrifice involved. Committing to work at the scene of her father's tragedy meant that Jean Menzies was willing to place herself in jeopardy, just as he had. James Menzies had sacrificed his life; Jean was prepared to do the same. To the five young girls watching from the sidelines in 1923, two messages were clear: first, missionary work by its very nature involved risk and self-sacrifice, and second, the North China Mission community would always embrace its own. The arrival of Jean Menzies and Bob McClure ushered in a new and vital generation of missionaries—those who had the inherent respect of the older generation of conservative, evangelically minded missionaries, *and* of newer missionaries who had both the desire and passion to see medical services developed in Henan. Furthermore, Jean Menzies and Bob McClure were bred-in-the-bone Chinese: they spoke the language and understood Chinese culture intrinsically, in a way that neither the older nor the newer generation of Canadian missionaries ever would.

Perhaps not surprisingly, Jean Menzies did not last long at Huaiqing. Historical sources are silent on her decision to transfer to the mission hospital at nearby Weihui, but it seems reasonable to presume that the emotional toll of working in a place still filled with her father's presence was too much to bear. Nor is there evidence on how the missionary community responded to her decision to leave Huaiqing. When Jean Menzies later decided to marry Dr. Handley Stockley of the English Baptist Mission, she unwittingly set two other standards for younger mishkids to follow: marry a China missionary and establish roots in China, regardless of any political instability there. The couple had planned to be married in 1926, but Handley Stockley was "shut up for eight months in the siege of [Xian]" by Nationalist army forces[8]—part of Chiang Kai-shek's "Northern Expedition."

Chiang Kai-shek, a close ally of Sun Yat-sen, took his friend's place as leader of the Nationalist Party (the Kuomintang) when Sun Yat-sen died in 1925. Communist and Nationalist factions in the fragile new government became increasingly polarized.[9] The year 1926 was marked by increasing national upheaval, student demonstrations, turbulence, and warfare between "warlords" who vied for control of various regions around China. In an effort to unify China under the Nationalist banner, Chiang Kai-shek led a two-year military campaign called the "Northern Expedition," starting in 1926. The related military conflict prompted foreign consulates to order their missionaries to evacuate from interior regions. All ninety-six North China missionaries evacuated Henan. Over two hundred missionaries evacuated the West China mission at Sichuan. Interestingly, however, five Canadians refused to leave Sichuan, defying consular orders even after receiving a telegram asking "Whatinthehellisdelayingyoufivemen?"[10] That they were later honoured as "gold star missionaries" exemplified the fine line between disobedience and heroism in crisis situations. Refusing to evacuate could be considered foolhardy, or a sign of one's depth of commitment to the cause. In the middle of the turmoil, Jean Menzies and Handley Stockley were married, in January 1927.

In what became known as the "Great 1927 Exodus," over eight thousand Protestant missionaries (including Betty Thomson and her family) evacuated China; three thousand never returned. The United Church of Canada's North China Mission in Henan lost twenty of their ninety-six missionaries.[11] The Canadians who stayed in China bided their time in Tianjin while the crisis played out. It was in Tianjin that fifteen-year-old Florence Mackenzie first met Eric Liddell of the London Missionary Society. Liddell was also a mishkid, born in Tianjin in 1902. He had gained notoriety in Scotland as an Olympic gold medalist before returning to China; his refusal to run on the "Sabbath" during the 1924 Olympics would later become the subject of the film *Chariots of Fire*. Florence Mackenzie and Eric Liddell became engaged in 1930, shortly before Florence's departure for Toronto, for nurse's training. Although Florence's parents approved of the match, her father, Hugh Mackenzie, presciently believed that all women should have some kind of training before marriage—just in case something happened to their husbands.[12] Florence Mackenzie was in the third year of her nursing program when her best friend and fellow mishkid Betty Thomson started in the first year of the same program. Florence returned to China to marry the thirty-one year old Eric Liddell after her graduation, in 1933—the third mishkid nurse to return to China. Georgina Menzies had returned two years earlier, in 1931.

Nursing and the Sino-Japanese War

Jean Menzies's younger sister Georgina was the second mishkid to return to China as a missionary nurse. She returned to the North China Mission in Henan province after graduating from the Toronto General Hospital nursing school in 1931, and she nursed at the Canadian mission hospitals at Anyang and Weihui for eight years. Georgina Menzies's 1936/37 report from the Anyang Women's Hospital report offers a glimpse into the harsh reality of daily life on a mission hospital ward during this period.[13] In it, Menzies described seven patients who were hospitalized for long-term treatment of severe burns, gunshot wounds, opium addiction, smallpox, and Kala Azar (a systemic disease mostly of the spleen, liver, and bone marrow, caused by tiny protozoa and transmitted by sandflies). An eight-year-old child and a sixty-year-old woman had been shot by bandits. The child had been taken captive after bandits raided his village; he was kept in an empty pit, where one foot and hand became frozen. Chinese soldiers eventually rescued him, but he was shot in the elbow during the fight. The woman had also been shot in the arm, but it had taken two weeks before she was taken to hospital, and "now her upper arm [was] just pouring pus."[14] One of the "burn cases" was a ten-year-old beggar lad who had lain down by an open Chinese stove during a cold night. His "rags caught on fire, and his arm and side were badly burned before the blaze was extinguished." The opium addict was a twenty-year-old woman whose husband admitted her because of "a new ruling of *shooting* all drug addicts [which] comes into force with the new year."[15]

Georgina Menzies was working at Anyang on 7 July 1937 when a full scale war broke out between China and Japan. As Japanese armies advanced from northern regions of China towards Henan, refugees started pouring into Henan from the north. In October 1937 Anyang was heavily bombed. Missionary women were evacuated to Weihui. As physicians and nurses took care of the wounded at Weihui, three thousand refugees jammed into the compound seeking a safe haven. At Huaiqing, Japanese planes dropped bombs on Chinese soldiers and civilians alike, and, within one twenty-four-hour period, one hundred and two seriously wounded were operated on by a staff of two doctors and two missionary nurses.

Within weeks, Japanese troops entered Henan and Japanese bombers started flying overhead. Missionaries at Anyang, Weihui, and Huaiqing were warned to evacuate because of the fighting between Japanese and Chinese troops, but this time most chose to stay. Because the Japanese had promised not to target British property, the North China missionaries began to fly British flags. They also painted large Union Jacks on the roofs of all the buildings and on the outside of the Weihui mission compound wall. Missionary physicians and nurses filled their days caring for the wounded and for refugees. According to North China Mission historian Margaret Brown, Chiang Kai-shek praised their decision, proclaiming that "thousands of people had escaped pain, suffering and death as a result of the missionary effort, and girls and women have been saved from a fate worse than death."[16] The idea that defying consular orders could be valorous was becoming well ingrained.

By this time, the nursing situation in the North China Mission was becoming dire. The three mission hospitals continued to offer outpatient services to ill and injured ambulatory patients, and they continued to admit those who required more intensive care and surgery to the in-patient wards, but there were not enough nurses to adequately care for all of the patients. As in the West, modern hospitals in China depended on nursing students to staff the wards in exchange for nurses training and room and board, while graduated nurses worked in administrative and teaching roles. Under normal conditions, eight Canadian nurses and two Chinese graduates would be teaching and supervising thirty Chinese nursing students across three hospital sites. However, by the end of October 1937, most of the Chinese staff had abandoned the mission—at least at Weihui. In a letter published in the *Canadian Nurse* journal in 1938, Jeannette Ratcliffe lamented: "Planes carrying bombs droned and roared overhead, and victims were carried into the operating theatre. The infection of fear spread, and on one never-to-be-forgotten day twenty of our staff left [to join fellow Chinese at military and Red Cross hospitals]. Within two weeks our staff was reduced to one Canadian doctor, two Canadian nurses and seven Chinese graduates and pupils."[17]

By early January 1938 most of the Chinese staff had returned, and a graduation ceremony was held for three nurses. The mission took in ten more students: "not that we wanted to have more young women to care for right now," wrote Jeannette Ratcliffe, "but because these graduates of Middle and Normal schools are refugees, and are homeless like so many thousands more."[18] By 1938 there were only five Canadian nurses left in the North China Mission; three had resigned to get married.[19] One of these was mishkid nurse Georgina Menzies who, in 1938, was engaged to Baptist Missionary Society physician Dr. John Lewis.[20] The volume of work was becoming overwhelming.

Not surprisingly, the North China Mission was having difficulty finding replacement missionary nurses for the three who resigned. Not only were parents loathe to allow their daughters to go to war-torn China, but Canadians were starting to question the value of the missionary enterprise. Alvyn Austin notes, that, between 1927 and 1935, articles in *The Christian Century* testified to the growing anthropological and sociological critique of missions as culture destroyers. In 1930 an article asked, "Can a Missionary Be a Christian?"[21] In response to the mounting criticism (and a related "alarming" drop-off in charity gifts to missions),[22] a group of American Baptist laymen initiated a commission to review the work of missions in Eastern Asia, including China. The "Appraisal Commission" consisted of members of seven leading denominations in the United States and the Associated Boards of Foreign Missions of the United States and Canada. After nine months of touring Eastern Asia they began releasing their report to the public in instalments. Their final report, published in 1932 as *Re-Thinking Missions: A Laymen's Inquiry after One Hundred Years*, concluded that missions, if they were to remain relevant, would have to change to systems that were less evangelistic (not having preaching as their main focus) and more practical (being service-oriented), integrated (working in cooperation with multiple denominations, organizations, and religions), and indigenous (having the goal of transitioning program responsibility to nationals).[23]

The United Church Board of Overseas Missions[24] was appalled by the inquiry. Some responded to what they considered a decade of financial and spiritual depression by renewed conservatism and back-to-basics evangelism.[25] In 1937 retired pioneer North China missionary physician Dr. James Fraser Smith (also an early supporter of missionary nursing) published an autobiography to rally public support for evangelistic Christian missions. Entitled *Life's Waking Part*, it provided a fifty-year overview of the missionary work in Henan. Its Foreword makes clear that the book was intended as a pointed response to *Re-Thinking Missions*, as well as to a recent mission critique by Professor of Law (and later President of the University of Toronto) Sydney Smith that missions were a fanciful dream. The Foreword says: "There is ground for the fear often expressed that experts at the home-base who have been *re-thinking missions* have given an unfortunate impression regarding the value of World-wide Evangelization, inclining some even to Sydney Smith's view that 'missions are the dream of a dreamer who dreams he has been dreaming'" (italics added).[26] While the North China missionaries believed in the ongoing value of their mission, the combined economic concerns of the Great Depression, fears over growing unrest in Europe and Asia, and church members' doubts about the nature of evangelistic missions meant that fewer Canadians saw China missions as worthy of their attention and support. All of this made it difficult to recruit nurses.

Dr. Bob McClure, who was briefly in Canada in 1937 after having been seconded to the International Committee of the Red Cross in China, took it upon himself to make an urgent plea for more nurses. He appealed to Toronto General Hospital nursing school superintendent Jean Gunn, as well as to the United Church community in Toronto. Looking for four nurses to work in Henan, Bob McClure recognized that "Betty and some of her pals in nursing were possible candidates."[27] Desiring to get Betty Thomson and other potential candidates released from their positions at the Toronto General Hospital, Dr. McClure visited Jean Gunn. But she was "not keen on the girls going to China."[28] He later recalled,

We were in her office and I felt quite intimidated by her austere manner. When I told her what I wanted she told me frankly why she did not like the idea of "her nurses" going out to a strange country on such a glamorous but risky job of work. She climaxed her talk by saying, "It's all very well for you, Dr. McClure, to offer this kind of glamorous work for my girls but suppose anything should happen to them? Suppose they were wounded or get sick on the job. What insurance coverage do you have in all this romantic sort of a job? Who would look after them if they were permanently injured?" For a moment I did not know what to say. Then I looked up on the wall above her desk. There was a picture of Florence Nightingale hanging on the wall. I had an inspiration. Looking Miss Jean I. Gunn straight in the eye and pointing up to that picture above her desk I said, "Miss Gunn, these girls will have the same provision for their work as that lady had and they will do much the same kind of work."[29]

Jean Gunn gave her permission.

Bob McClure also pled his case at the kitchen table of the Thomson family home, where Betty Thomson had lived since evacuating China in 1926 (as part of the Great 1927 Exodus). According to her sister Ruth Thomson Laws, the idea that Chinese children were starving and suffering ultimately nudged her sister Betty to the offices of the United Church

Woman's Missionary Society to sign up, along with her childhood friends Mary and Dorothy Boyd.[30] With parents still in China, an understanding of Chinese culture, and education in a practical profession, the three unmarried women were ideal missionary candidates. They made a pact to return to China together. The three sailed together for China on the *Empress of Asia* on 4 March 1939.[31] There would now be six North China mishkid nurses in China.

To understand what it was about their North China childhoods that shaped these six missionary nurses into independent-minded women who were willing to return to and stay in China at a time when few others would consider it, we turn now to an exploration of the nature of their upbringing. The following section examines three aspects of a mishkid childhood that left indelible—if not unintended—marks on the lives of Canadian mishkid nurses: intimate and forbidden relationships with Chinese people and culture (becoming Chinese), a boarding school upbringing with painful separations from one's parents (becoming Canadian), and living among China missionaries in Toronto (becoming a nurse).

Becoming Chinese: Developing Language and Relationships

> So through a process of osmosis, we grew up feeling comfortable in both Western and Chinese ways.
> —Marion Menzies Hummel

Living in enclaves created by and for foreigners, North China mishkids grew up in a world that was at once sheltered and dangerous, structured and unpredictable. As "British subjects" (as Canadians were formally termed before the Canadian Citizenship Act of 1947), mishkids enjoyed the privileges granted their parents and other missionaries, including the privilege to move freely around China. In practical terms, however, mishkids grew up within the boundaries (later walled and gated) of mission compounds, self-contained foreign enclaves that were eventually comprised of rows of Western-style homes with flourishing gardens, tennis courts, chapels, and hospitals. Formally separated from the Chinese—and, as will be seen, from their parents—mishkids nonetheless found ways to skirt around the social barriers, listening in on private adult conversations on the one hand, and engaging in forbidden conversations with Chinese staff and children on the other.

Mishkids were curious bystanders to the world of missionary work, watching as their parents preached in tent meetings set up at Chinese festivals, hosted British-style tea parties in their homes, led singsongs, and agitated with other missionaries over the political situation in China. Mavis Knight Weatherhead, daughter of Weihui Hospital administrator Norman Knight, recalls listening in on animated discussions in her parents' living room:

> We kids had a front row seat when the meetings were held in our living room. Our bedroom that was directly above had a hole in the corner of the floor that was formerly used for a heating pipe. We used to lift the cover to peek though the opening and to hear what was going on. The end of the meeting was signalled by a sudden silence followed by the words, "Let us pray." Then we would eagerly wait through the first few minutes of mumbled prayers until we heard a familiar rumble that began to build in volume. It only lasted a few seconds until it ended with a sharp snort. Someone had dutifully poked our dear friend Miss McLennan in the ribs to wake her up.[32]

Similarly, Betty Thomson recalled attending tent meetings with her parents when she was not in school: "I can remember often going with mother and Dad out into the country places for days at a time. Dad would conduct the meetings while Mother played the small, portable organ and led the singing. My sister Peggy and I would sit up on a flight of stairs and listen, sometimes staring back at people who had poked a hole in the paper windows to stare at us!"[33]

As young bilingual children, mishkids gravitated to the hidden spaces that separated Chinese and Canadian life. They conversed fluently in Chinese on the back porch with their amahs and cooks—and in the yard with Chinese playmates—and then sat at formally set dining room tables eating Western-style meals prepared and served by Chinese servants. Language was the key to moving between these worlds. The language of these encounters was a very practical (if not vulgar) form of Chinese—which included some words that young Bob McClure's father, upon hearing, forbade him to speak.

While missionary parents took advantage of their children's fluency—for example, in Marion Menzie's case, "translating Chinese into English and English into Chinese for my grandmothers and [my amah] Shen Dasao"[34]—they also worried about their children's eventual transition to Canadian life when they were grown. Dr. William McClure "used to draw a chalk line across the door," Bob McClure recalls, "and he'd give me a real good spanking if we spoke a word of Chinese inside that chalk line because he said 'you're speaking Chinese all day, you're playing with Chinese and he said if you're going to learn English, you'll have to learn English before we go to Canada.'"[35]

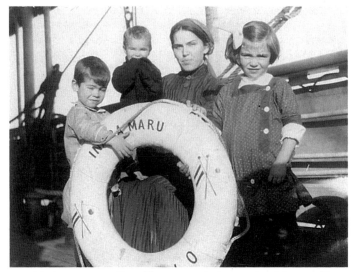

Fig. 1.1   Mackay, Betty, and Jean Thomson with their mother, Margaret Thomson, aboard a Japanese steamship, c. 1917

Their parents' suppression of the Chinese language bothered mishkids like Bob McClure. It seemed strange to him that their daily family Bible reading and prayer, joined in by the Chinese amah, cook, and gardener, was always in Chinese, and yet he was forbidden to speak Chinese within the walls of his home. Chinese was his first language, and there were some Chinese words for which there were no English equivalents.[36] As he described it at age seventy-six: "Chinese is my natural language and, today if I get angry, I get angry in Chinese. I don't get angry in English."[37]

Despite parental efforts to contain it, mishkids found creative ways to learn and use Chinese, using the forbidden words with particular relish at opportune times. Mavis Knight, the only child of Norman and Violet Knight, used her knowledge of prohibited Chinese words to her advantage during the Japanese occupation. Walking along the tops of the compound walls, Mavis would call out "naughty words" in Chinese. Desiring in her child's mind to push the boundaries of family rules while also distinguishing between "our" Chinese soldiers and the "enemy" Japanese, Mavis could tell by the reactions whether the soldiers below were Chinese or Japanese: the Japanese would not respond.[38]

In addition to learning spoken Chinese, mishkids cultivated a taste for Chinese food, and they developed an intrinsic understanding of certain aspects of Chinese philosophy and values, including the importance of saving face. As Marnie Lochead Copland commented:

An American mission board secretary once remarked to us that of all the missionaries he deals with [around the world], the old China hands are the most clannish and the most devoted to their adopted country. From whatever part of the Western world we come, and in whatever part of China we have lived, we are united in our love of that country and in our loyalty to each other. This secretary said that we have come to think like Chinese. Our real meanings lie not in our spoken words but in the implications behind the words.[39]

Although missionary parents placed restrictions on their children's development and use of language, they were not opposed to all cultural influences. Missionary parents who perceived China as their adopted home desired that their children also view China as home. For example, in 1911, when Bob McClure was eleven years old, he accompanied his father back to China while his mother remained with her parents in Canada. William McClure did not want his son to be separated too long during these formative years from his natural environment. As Bob McClure's biographer later noted, "it is highly significant that in the minds of both Dr William McClure and his son, Bob's 'natural environment' was unquestionably accepted as being North Henan, China."[40]

Becoming Canadian: Boarding School at Weihui

For mishkids with no first-hand experience with Canada, the notion of being Canadian was a strange one. It was through encounters with Canada—either directly through furlough or indirectly through a Canadian curriculum—that mishkids began to conceive what the term "Canadian" actually meant, and how it applied to them. Marnie Lochead Copland pinpoints the moment "I became Canadian" as the day she made maple syrup in the Ontario woods with her relatives at age seven. Marnie recalled, "I had known my parents only in China, and was surprised to find that they had had a life of their own in Canada before I was born."[41] With furloughs only every seven years, missionary parents believed that the best way to develop "Canadian" children was to educate them using Canadian standards and curricula. Formal education, in China as in Canada, was the means through which children would learn not who they *were*, necessarily, but who they *should* be. Thus began years of learning English grammar, Canadian geography, and British history.

One of the overriding values of missionary parents was the education of their children. Missionary children would eventually return to Canada where they would be expected to meet the standards and requirements of

Canadian secondary schools and universities. By 1908 Weihui had become the centre for missionary children's education. In that year, ten-year-old Jean Menzies left her parents' home at Huaiqing to live with the McClure family at Weihui. Huaiqing was approximately one hundred and fifty kilometres farther inland from Weihui. Rather than teach her themselves, Jean's parents thought she would receive a better education as a member of the little group that was growing around a woman named Maria Sloan.[42] Jean Menzies joined the McClure household and grew up with Bob McClure, two years her junior. In 1910, Mrs. Jeannette Ratcliffe was invited to become the matron of the Weihui residential school for missionary children. Mrs. Ratcliffe held the position until she was appointed the first Nursing Superintendent of the Weihui Hospital and Training School for Nurses—a role that she did not officially take up until 1922. Thus the mishkids who returned to China as nurses already knew Mrs. Ratcliffe well.

The North China Mission compound at Weihui had a hospital, a middle school, a Chinese church, and approximately ten missionary houses, as well as the boarding school. Over the course of its service, the missionary children's school "never had more than twenty children—often less."[43] The school was housed in a two-story grey brick building, with a boy's dormitory in one wing and a girls' dormitory in the other. In-between there were bedrooms for a matron and a teacher on the second floor. Downstairs was a living room on one side of the central hall and two classrooms on the other side. It was not an extravagant place:

> There was no electricity or flush toilets. We carried candles up to our bedrooms each night. A holding tank of rainwater set near the ceiling over two washrooms provided us with cold running water to fill our hand basins. A communal bath system, where each of us bathed after the other, was in a cubicle to one side of the bathroom. Chinese servants brought up buckets of hot water for our baths … our meals were called by bell and we sat at one long table. Our diet was Western style, though at times we enjoyed Chinese food.[44]

Missionary children whose parents lived relatively close by could visit them every few weeks. For those further afield, visits home might occur only at Christmas and Easter, and on summer vacations.

Mishkids described their visits home as highly anticipated events. Betty Thomson recalled that, when she took the train from Weihui to Daokou, her father would be waiting for her and her siblings at the station on a bicycle: "We kids would ride in rickshas through the narrow streets of the city, always packed with people. Some of them would yell at us 'Foreign Devils' or some such term, but good naturedly and without apparent malice. My older brother Mac was their favourite target: Bao bay, Bao bay (his Chinese name) and he would happily acknowledge their greeting with those of his own."[45] Betty Thomson remembered what a "thrill" it was to arrive at the compound gate and walk up the tree-lined pathway to their home where her mother was "always waiting for us on the doorstep" with the youngest child, Muriel, "and what a welcome we received. We would dash into the house to see what new wonders she had created while we were away at school."[46]

Such nostalgic reminiscences provide important insight into how missionary children constructed the long separations from their parents. For China mishkids, separation from their parents started at a young age: Betty Thomson's brother MacKay, for example, left for Weihui in 1914 at the age of five. While some mishkids embraced the boarding school experience at Weihui, others were consumed by isolation and loneliness. If the familiarity of such separations accounts for the later decision by Florence MacKenzie Liddell to return to Canada without her husband Eric, the painfulness of childhood separations may equally account for the decision by Betty Thomson Gale, Mary Boyd Stanley, and Georgina Menzies Lewis to stay in China with their husbands.

From the perspective of a twenty-first-century emphasis on family unity as a goal and as a sign among Christians of a strong spiritual life, the degree to which China missionary families spent time physically isolated from each other is striking, even ironic. Parents spent years away from their children; couples from each other. Sometimes the separations were spurred by national crises or unrest in China, when local conditions were deemed too dangerous for Canadian women and children, who were evacuated. At other times they were triggered by personal or family illness. Missionary wives were often responsible for the convalescence of ill family members, including parents who were living in Canada. Most commonly, separations were prompted by the higher education needs of children. Prior to the development of the Canadian Academy at Kobe, Japan, missionary children would have to return to Canada to take the courses required for matriculation. During these periods of separation, Canadian missionary women typically resided with or nearby their parents—usually in or near Toronto. There, as in China, missionary families often supported, and socialized with, each other in tangible ways—including providing room and board for each other's children if necessary.

Marion Menzies Hummel experienced separation from her parents as a form of neglect. Born to Rev. James Mellon and Annie Menzies in 1913, Marion was a contemporary of Betty Thomson, Dorothy Boyd, and Mary

Boyd. She recalled a father who was both distant and severe. James M. Menzies (no relation to the murdered James R. Menzies) became better known for his archaeological passions than evangelistic ones. Stationed at the North China Mission site at Anyang, James Menzies discovered oracle bones—tortoise shells and other bone fragments inscribed with predictions by royal diviners from the Shang Dynasty (1300 BCE). He became increasingly preoccupied with what grew into a priceless collection.[47] From the perspective of his daughter Marion, Menzies was "strict and often angry, for he had migraine headaches, but I remember only once that he hit me and that is when Frances and I quarrelled so loudly that he took the flyswatter to our legs. When we were young our father did not write to us on a regular basis, leaving this to mother, but when he did write they were letters to remember."[48]

Because of the physical separation of missionary children from their parents, letter writing was an integral part of the missionary experience. Letters flowed regularly between missionary children and their parents regardless of whether they were separated by the Yellow River or the Pacific Ocean. As Marion Menzies Hummel described it, "I feel that, looking over our years in boarding school, in many ways we children were brought up by our mothers' letters. They were loving, instructive, urging us to do our best, to depend on God and to fortify ourselves with His promises in scripture, and to keep on striving."[49] The letters were also used to instill values and ethnic, religious, and national identity—not all of which the mishkids accepted. When Marion Menzies was at boarding school at age thirteen in 1926 her mother wrote:

> Just thank God you aren't a poor little Chinese girl. Do you remember Dung-Lai the girl in my school with the brown hair, who often came to the door for something. Well, she was married last week. Just fancy that! And to a man about 40 and of course whom she had never seen. Her mother got $150 for her. How would you like that, dear? She cried and cried and didn't want to go. I cried too … I know it is hard dearie to be separated from your mother so much but Maudie and Bertha had their mother taken from them when they were just 6 and 8 years old and you see had no mother to write to when they were unhappy. Count your blessings dear.[50]

Letters like this one attempted to construct a racial—if not national—identity that emphasized the notion of difference, of the superiority of Canadian over Chinese cultural norms, including a rationalization for missionary parent-child separation. Mishkids generally resisted—and resented—such claims of superiority, however. In fact, some denied experiencing any kind of racial inequality during their childhood in China, including discrimination aimed toward them. Bob McClure, for example, contended that his first encounter with what he called "racial prejudice" was when he attended Harbord Collegiate in Toronto in 1915. Here he discovered that he was considered a "WASP" (White Anglo-Saxon Protestant) and that WASPs did not associate with Jews or Catholics. To Bob, discrimination based on race or religion was a North American phenomenon: "I had never heard [nor was] aware of any racial stuff until I got to Canada [at age fifteen]."[51]

While Marion's mother's letter exemplifies a familiar theme in post-colonial studies—the imperialist or colonialist gaze—mishkid children did not take up the Chinese-as-other view in the same way that their parents had. Whether the resistance to the discrimination sometimes displayed by their parents was a form of adolescent defiance, or simply contrary to their sense of rootedness in the China that extended beyond the walls of the mission compound, mishkids did not define themselves in terms of how they differed from the Chinese. In this way, the China mishkid phenomenon complicates Edward Said's Orientalist gaze and Franz Fanon's colonizer/colonized sense of "us" and "them": for mishkids, "we" were the China-born; "we" moved fluidly between otherwise segregated Chinese and Canadian groups; "we" were puzzled by the rules of separation laid down by mission-

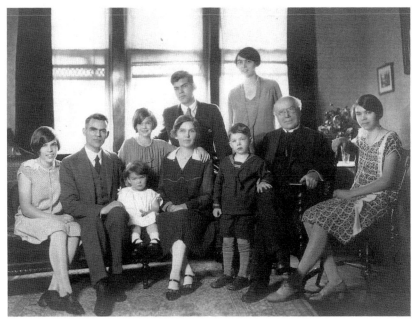

Fig. 1.2   Thomson family with R.P. MacKay

ary parents; and "we" resisted subaltern notions of superiority based on race, religion or nationality.[52]

If mishkids felt isolated during the regular school year, summer vacation was an entirely different affair. It is difficult to overstate the significance of summer vacations at Beidaihe, a seaside resort in Qinhuangdao municipality in Hebei province: without exception, North China mishkids considered Beidaihe the highlight of their childhood. Easily accessible by train from Tianjin, Beidaihe includes a beach that stretches ten kilometres and is covered with fine yellow sand stretching some one hundred metres to the sea. Of all the experiences recollected by mishkids, this was the one that most resembled a colonized, segregated space—that is, a place of privilege not easily accessible by the regular Chinese populace.

Beidaihe was a gathering place for expatriates from across northern China, including missionaries, business people, and diplomats. Mothers would come with their children for the entire summer, with fathers joining for weeks at a time. The days were filled with tennis, beach activities, social gatherings, and picnics. A number of North China missionaries built sum-

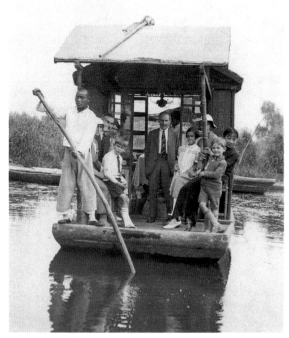

Fig. 1.3   Canadian missionaries crossing the Da Min Hu Lake, Jinan, in the 1930s
(Photo courtesy of Mary Struthers McKim)

mer homes at Beidaihe. Muriel Thomson Valentien recalled spending hours at the beach exploring and playing with her brother Murray. Supervised by "only a teenage brother or sister," Muriel and Murray would swim out to a raft "far beyond our depth" despite "meter-high breakers [that] came crashing in."[53] There were no lifeguards and only one "danger sign at one end of the beach: *Undertow, beware!*"[54]

What is striking about both the long separations and the Beidaihe vacations is how remarkably unperturbed missionary parents were by the notion of leaving their children in the hands of caregivers—be they Chinese amahs, surrogate missionary families, boarding school teachers, or teenage siblings. To be fair, water safety was not a major North American priority until after the Second World War (with the creation of YMCA and Red Cross swimming lessons as swimming became a more common leisure activity), nor were missionaries the only parents in the broader White Anglo-Saxon Protestant culture who left childrearing in the hands of boarding schools and governesses. The point is, as working men and women, missionary parents had a divine purpose into which the daily routines of parenthood did not easily fit. Perhaps more importantly, missionary parents held an essential belief that their children's fate was ultimately in the hands of an omnipotent, omniscient, and omnipresent God. As Muriel Thomson Valentien understood it: "Our parents trusted—in life, and in something higher than themselves; a spiritual reality guiding and sustaining them—and us. And this trust with which we were imbued, carried into our later lives."[55] Allowing one's children to swim unsupervised, to travel alone by train, or to be cared for by relative strangers may have been risky, but no more so than other aspects of missionary life. To North China missionaries and their children, missionary work was a dangerous calling.

Becoming a Nurse: The TGH Connection

In the summer of 1926 the Thomson family was evacuated to Canada as part of the Great 1927 Exodus. Margaret Thomson's father, Dr. R.P. Mackay, purchased a home for them at 33 Rose Park Drive, approximately five kilometres from the Toronto General Hospital and the University of Toronto. Betty, then fifteen years old, enrolled in her first Canadian school. In 1929, the year of R.P. Mackay's death, Andrew Thomson returned to China, leaving Margaret in Toronto with their seven children. Andrew Thomson worked alone at Daokou for two years before reuniting with his family in Toronto. A year later, in 1932, Margaret and Andrew Thomson embarked for China once again, this time with only the youngest three children; the older four remained in Toronto where Betty Thomson started nurse's training at the Toronto General Hospital School for Nurses, where she joined her best friend Florence Mackenzie.

In United Church missionary history, if North Henan was the "colony," the city of Toronto was the "metropole." Evacuation and education needs had brought a number of United Church missionary families to Toronto during those years; the missionary community in Toronto was almost as vibrant as in China. Toronto was the United Church of Canada headquarters and the city where most missionary families lived during furlough. It was also home to a number of respected educational institutions that served as training grounds for ministers, physicians, social workers, deaconesses, and teachers. These included the University of Toronto, Victoria University, the Presbyterian Missionary and Deaconess Training School, and the Toronto General Hospital (TGH). Because so many missionaries had trained at the TGH, there was a high regard for this hospital; missionaries entrusted their family members to the care of the TGH.[56] Perhaps this explains why all six mishkid nurses studied at the TGH School for Nurses: Jean Menzies graduated in 1922, Georgina Menzies in 1929, Florence MacKenzie in 1934, Betty Thomson in 1935, Dorothy Boyd in 1936, and Mary Boyd in 1937.[57] Missionary parents naturally urged their children to study and live at places that they approved of and where there existed a network of missionary families to provide support to the students when one or both parents were in China. This was the case with Muriel Menzies, whose father insisted she attend his alma mater, the University of Toronto. As she recalled:

> It had been arranged that I should live with one of our mission friends, the Boyds, who were on furlough and living in a mission house ... I was lovingly accepted by the Boyd family. Mary [Boyd] was in second year [taking public health at the University of Toronto] so we saw little of each other during classes. There were a number of other mishkids at Vic [Victoria College] from Japan, India and Africa—those who attended C.A. [Christian Academy] in Kobe—who formed a group called "The Chushinguru," a Japanese expression meaning "loyal companions."[58]

In this sense, Toronto was an extension of the mission field—and vice versa. While it is not surprising, then, that missionary parents would choose to send their children to Toronto for their education, social support was only one aspect of what their children required for academic success. The other was access to sympathetic administrative personnel who would be willing to be flexible about entrance requirements. For example, when Florence Mackenzie returned to Canada in 1930 to start nurse's training in Toronto, it at first appeared that her age and education might keep her from being admitted. According to Eric Liddell's biographer David McCasland, Florence was "still three months shy of her nineteenth birthday, the minimum age for applying. In addition, her academic work at Tianjin Grammar School did not meet Canadian standards for matriculation, and she had not taken Latin."[59] However, a "sympathetic letter" from the registrar noted that Florence had received the equivalent of a four-year high school program in Ontario and urged Helen Locke, the School for Nurses' Assistant Superintendent, to recommend Florence Mackenzie for admission, which she did.

Jean Gunn would have approved: seven years earlier Gunn had admitted Amy Hislop (later the wife of Dr. Bob McClure) into the TGH School for Nurses because Amy had told her that her desire was to go overseas and work in a mission hospital. Gunn, it seems, had a soft spot for missionaries: she reportedly "thawed" at the mention of missionary work.[60] If nursing work was the most legitimate way for a missionary daughter to return to China on her own, the Toronto General Hospital was the most expedient place to train.

There are few records from Betty Thomson's years in Toronto (1926–1938). It is of interest that through these years the ebb and flow of family separation and reunion continued. As always, family letters were a key source of communication and of maintaining relationships. When Betty Thomson was awarded a scholarship from a nomination by her peers in her second year as a nursing student, her three siblings immediately dispatched a letter to China to inform their parents. The scholarship, it seems, was awarded on the basis of one's character. On 15 June 1934 Margaret Thomson responded with a confidential letter to her daughter Betty. Writing on the premise that "you might not like to let the others [siblings] see how proud we are!" Margaret Thomson exuberantly poured out her admiration for her daughter.[61] Upon reading it, Betty Thomson could have had no doubt of her parent's high opinion of her:

> My own dear girlie ... Do you know my darling that ever since you went into hospital I have hugged to my heart the thought that you would get this very scholarship. I knew no-one could deserve it more, and I felt that if you did not receive it, it would be because the girls [Betty's classmates] had not such good judgment as they should have!! Dad almost wept he was so pleased! ... Well my dearie you have once more proved what we have always known, that you have great ability ... And of all scholarships, the one given by your classmates is, we think, the one to be *most coveted* ... Once more I realize that space does not separate us, we are very near in spirit ... Can you not feel Grandfather's [R.P. Mackay's] approving smile resting on you?[62]

It is not hard to imagine why this letter is among the few preserved from Betty Thomson's youth. Along with a few others on particularly significant milestones, it carried a parental blessing, the significance of which cannot be overstated. When Betty graduated from the TGH on 22 May 1935, both parents penned a separate letter from China on the very day of her graduation. Margaret Thomson wrote: "This is the date of your graduation so we are thinking of you this morning and hoping it will be a truly happy day for you."[63] And Andrew Thomson wrote: "It does not matter much to me whether you have been first or not, you have stood a far higher test than only the examinations, you have been helpful, cheerful, unselfish."[64] Like his wife, Andrew Thomson called into being Betty's ancestors and family members, suggesting that deceased relatives would provide support from the afterworld—a belief that, not incidentally, intersected well with Chinese culture: "I have no doubt that unseen presences will be there also—grandfather [Mackay], and my mother and others." Just as importantly, Andrew Thomson emphasized his daughter's heritage, pointing out what he saw as significant, inherited traits: "You resemble [my] mother [Elizabeth Durie] in appearance and in character; it is lovely that you carry her name also. She was a nurse to the neighbourhood [in Owen Sound]; nothing was too laborious, no task too gruesome even to preparing bodies for burial in the homes of the poor. In you her granddaughter, she is alive today."[65]

Both Andrew and Margaret Thomson recognized this period as a crossroads in their daughter's life. Both offered their opinions on what she should do next. In Andrew's opinion, his daughter had three alternatives: take up private nursing, stay at TGH for further training, or take a postgraduate course in "some allied subject such as Public Health."[66] For her part, Margaret thought her daughter should take postgraduate training at the University of Toronto but, based on the advice of United Church missionary nurse Clara Preston, she recommended that Betty wait a few months so that she could first recover from what had been a difficult program of study. Margaret Thomson also desired that her twenty-four-year-old daughter find a suitable husband; apparently Betty had had some disappointing experiences of late. "I am sorry that the course has not given you the true friendship of worthwhile men," Margaret wrote, "[but] you are *much* happier without the friendship of men who cannot leave drink alone."[67] To Margaret and Andrew Thomson, alcohol and Christianity were mutually exclusive. Andrew Thomson penned pamphlets such as *Alcohol or Christ?* and *Crusade for a Resurgent Church: Must Alcohol Win?* and he reportedly "achieved fame" within the United Church for his work "in the cause of temperance."[68] That their daughter demonstrated "highly principled" behaviour (by abstaining from alcohol) was a sign of their success as parents.

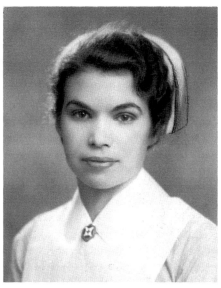

Fig. 1.4   Betty Thomson, TGH Graduation in 1935

In June 1935, a year after being awarded a scholarship for her virtuous character, Betty Thomson was again selected by her peers to receive "the highest award her fellow students could award her," the Gertrude O'Hara Prize for Efficiency in Bedside Nursing.[69] To her father, "the best of it is that you have never compromised your principles, you have consistently stood for what was highest and noblest. At the same time, you would not have received this award unless you had been an all-round friend, and had put your personality and accomplishments fully at the service of your teachers and fellow students."[70] Betty's mother was no less complimentary, writing to her on her birthday on 22 June 1935:

> It was a happy day which brought you into this world! All through these twenty-four years you have given nothing but pride and pleasure to your parents … We are *very* proud and happy because of this scholarship and because of the excellent work you have done in the Hospital, but we have *always* been proud of you … Any honours which you gain are deserved, because you are so genuinely good; not the sort of girl who is lovely to outsiders and selfish and cross with her own family. As Margaret [Betty's sister, in China] says, "She is *just Betty*, and you know what that means."[71]

Whatever the next stage in her life, Betty Thomson would be heading into it with enviable security in the knowledge of her family's deep love and support.

Summary

To be a North China mishkid in the early twentieth century meant being instilled with a sense of belonging to a broader missionary community that extended well past one's immediate family. The ease with which missionary children moved from home to home is striking. Travelling between their parents' mission station, missionary childrens' boarding schools at Weihui and Kobe (Japan), the summer resort at Beidaihe, and the large urban centre of Toronto, these children seemed surprisingly adaptive to disparate settings. The Thomson children, for example, felt an inordinate sense of security, learning early on that awaiting on the other side of their journey—be it by train, rickshaw, or donkey—were missionary adults (and children) whose values and beliefs they inherently understood and trusted. Equally remarkable is the seeming ease with which parents separated from their children, handing them over to surrogates and caregivers despite the considerable dangers this might expose their children to, be it train bandits, cholera, or the undertow at an ocean beach. Reliant on letters to communicate their values, parents must have been aware of the significance of their words; mishkids seemed to have developed a sense of self and security proportionate to their parents' ability and willingness to regularly commit pen to paper. A parent's love could be measured, in part, by the frequency, length, and tone of the letters they scribed.

The supportive nature of the Thomsons' letters contrasts with the admonishing tone taken by the parents of Betty Thomson's contemporary Marion Menzies. One feels a bit sorry for Marion, who remembers her father as distant and harsh; her upbringing as lonely. Her assertion that "we were raised by letters" rings true, and her recollection of a forlorn childhood is heart-rending, but hardly surprising. More surprising is the number of North China missionary kids—including seven of the eight I interviewed—who recalled having a close relationship with their parents, not to mention a pleasing childhood. The dissenter, well into his nineties when we spoke, criticized what he perceived as sanctified neglect by missionary parents of their children. He sardonically concluded that his parents' overriding concern with their missionary purpose in China distracted them from their central calling—that of loving their children and providing for their emotional needs. His feeling of abandonment lingered for eight decades. By all accounts this was not so for Betty Thomson: she felt loved.

Also noteworthy is the relative ease with which missionary children moved between Western and Chinese cultures. Although they spoke English, ate Western-style cooking, were educated using a Canadian curriculum, and perceived themselves to be as Canadian as their parents, mishkids also absorbed some of the values and customs of their Chinese amahs, house servants, and neighbours. A belief in wandering ancestral spirits, for example, was accepted without question. Betty Thomson seemed quite comfortable with the notion that her deceased maternal grandfather would be watching her from the hereafter, or that her deceased paternal grandmother could influence her decisions related to her nursing career. Although the notion of deceased relatives watching from another spiritual realm was not entirely outside of Christian traditions, the Presbyterian tradition from which Betty's parents came would not have supported the notion that deceased relatives could actually intervene in one's present life.

Perhaps most significantly, the mishkid's China childhood provided opportunity to develop strong ties with other missionary children. In this way the missionary network was often more important than extended family back in Canada; the relationships between missionary children had more opportunity to develop than between missionary kids and their cousins in Canada, for example. Betty Thomson and best friend Florence Mackenzie, for example, were both born in Henan in 1911. After a childhood of summers together at Beidaihe, Florence and Betty met up again in Toronto where Betty's family was temporarily living when Florence commenced nursing studies there in 1930. How much of Betty Thomson's decision to enter nurse's training two years later had to do with Florence's presence there is unknown, but for one year their studies at the TGH overlapped before Florence returned to China. When Betty sailed to China as a missionary nurse in 1939, she was greeted at the Tianjin harbour by the now-married Florence Mackenzie Liddell, and when Betty moved to Beidaihe that summer to continue private Chinese lessons, she moved in with Florence, who was vacationing there. The two would later consult each other for advice when faced with the difficult decision of whether to evacuate China. Over the course of their lifetime they had become kindred spirits, a relationship borne of similar temperaments, to be sure, but also of similar, extraordinary childhoods. The six mishkid nurses who, apparently, thrived during their childhood in China, were among a privileged few who considered themselves bred-in-the-bone, non-ethnic Chinese. They had, as Mary Boyd later put it, "China blood right in us."[72]

Chapter 2

"A Call to Live Dangerously" (1935–1938)

The call to the Christian adventure is always a call to live dangerously. Not foolishly dangerously, of course, but wisely dangerous, if that phrase can pass as not mutually contradictory!

—Rev. Andrew Thomson, *A Daring Confidence*

In our childhood "out there" we were surrounded by revolutions, conflicts between warlords, unrest also through periods of drought, floods, famine. We knew nothing of all this, although our adult world was fully involved in alleviating the suffering wherever possible. We had the perfect security of home, and—I speak now for myself—it was a basis helping me feel at home wherever my later life has taken me.

—Muriel Thomson Valentien, *A Daring Confidence*

The mishkid nurses' decisions to return to China during wartime countered Canadian societal expectations of women to avoid danger; women were to be protected from war, not to enter into it. As the political landscape of China became increasingly dangerous after Japan's 1937 invasion, the response of western governmental and mission agencies was to urge women and children to quit China. Why, then, did Betty Thomson and Mary and Dorothy Boyd head to China in 1938? In this chapter I argue that the mishkid decisions to return to China reflected the expectations of the missionary subculture as instilled into, and adapted by, this second generation of China missionaries. Danger was perceived as an unavoidable aspect of missionary work; if Canadian mishkids wished to carry on the family profession, they had to learn to take and accept risks—just as their parents had done.

Betty Gale's sister Muriel Thomson Valentien depicts their childhood in China as strangely idyllic—"strangely" because, in fact, they grew up against a backdrop of violence and suffering during one of the most traumatic periods in modern history. While their compound walls, boarding school existence, and resort summers undoubtedly buffered mishkids like the Thomsons from the intensity of the suffering encountered by the common people in China, they did not grow up in the westernized, cosmopolitan treaty ports: their childhood home was in a remote, rural village far removed from the luxuries of Beijing, Tianjin, or Shanghai. The Thomson children accompanied their parents on evangelistic excursions, listened to their father passionately speaking of the need for peace to be brought to China, and observed him being "reduced to tears" when confronted by what was best and worst in the world—be it intense beauty or injustice.[1]

Ruth Thomson, the sixth child, recalled an early memory of "seeing a small, badly burned Chinese boy brought to [Andrew Thomson] for healing."[2] Ruth was not supposed to watch, but before she was sent from the room, she caught sight of "what looked like a large feathered bird, with a small boy's face and head. The child had been burned from head to toe and his mother had covered the awful sight with mud and feathers. Infection and suppuration had followed and as a last resort she brought him to a foreigner. The stench from the festering sores was terrible."[3] Because there was no hospital at Daokou, Rev. Andrew Thomson prepared a bath of warm water and little by little, soaked off the mud and feathers. Each day a little more of the burn was exposed and treated with a healing salve. "I remember thinking, then," recalled Ruth, "that Dad could be a doctor, too."[4] In this sense, the Thomson children were not shielded from painful circumstances—they learned to take them in stride. Those within the missionary community perceived China missions as a risky business. As Bob McClure understood it, "there are risks, but missionaries have to take these risks. It is a part of the modern job."[5]

North China mishkid Marnie Lochead Copland's recollections of her childhood bring into sharp focus the ways that missionary kids were acculturated to a dangerous life. Recalling the tumultuous warlord period of the 1920s and '30s in China, Copland wrote:

> News on the street had it that two rival warlords were vying [with] each other for that section of the Peking-Hankow [Beijing-Hankou] railroad. Father [Arthur Lochead] decided that walking home would be preferable to spending the night at an inn. Before they had gone very far, bullets began to ping and raise spurts of dust around them ... Father and [my sister] Ruth found themselves in the middle of a [warlord] battle. An open grave happened to be conveniently near the road, so Father jumped in and pulled Ruth down after him ... After an hour or so ... Father said, "Dear, if it should happen that a bullet hits you, and if it should happen that I'm not able to help you, just take off your hair ribbon and tie it tightly above the hole. Do you understand?

Good! Now let's have some of this good lunch ... After a few moments Ruth said, "I can chew it, Daddy, but I can't swallow it."[6]

While compound walls and seaside bungalows represent the privileged status given Canadians and other foreigners in early-twentieth-century China, the *need* for such protection was not illusory: North China missionaries had experienced violence in many forms since their arrival in 1888.[7] While it is not clear from the record whether Betty Thomson considered her childhood at Daokou as particularly dangerous, her younger brother Murray Thomson described their family as being "only thinly protected from roving groups of bandits and warlords by an easily-scaled wall."[8]

On one occasion in 1924—when Betty Thomson and her sister Margaret were attending boarding school at Weihui—a warlord came up the railway towards Daokou from the south, while another warlord approached from the north. According to Betty's younger brother Murray, "both had the weapons necessary to ransack and destroy much of the city."[9] Their arrival terrified the city dwellers, some of whom sought refuge in the mission compound. Andrew Thomson, the Catholic priest, and city officials negotiated a three-day ceasefire, after which the southern warlord withdrew towards Weihui, "blowing up the tracks behind him."[10] Although this incident seared itself in Murray's memory, not once in their entire lives did his parents refer to it again in his presence. One can reasonably presume that the Thomson parents were scared—given that they had a five-year-old and a two-year-old at home, not to mention their children living in Weihui. Yet, according to Murray Thomson, his parents treated the five-day standoff as "just another day at the office."[11] Speculating that his parents would have felt a tremendous sense of relief at the thwarted violence, and wondering what his conservative parents would have done to celebrate this moral victory given their abstinence from cigarettes and alcohol, Murray wryly noted that his younger sister Muriel was born nine months after this incident.

So what *was* missionary life like for the mishkid parents? What was the cultural and religious ethos of the missionary community into which the mishkids were born? To get a sense of the social milieu and the values and beliefs instilled into North China mishkids, we shall turn our attention to Betty Thomson Gale's extended family as an exemplar of the Canadian approach to China missions as a family affair.

Betty Gale's maternal grandfather, Rev. R.P. MacKay, had an intense interest in China missions. In 1887 it was he and Rev. Charles Gordon (the clergyman and novelist known as "Ralph Connor") who persuaded a young seminarian named Jonathan Goforth to relinquish his plans to go to China with Hudson Taylor's China Inland Mission and instead to become the Presbyterian Church in Canada's first missionary to mainland China.[12] The fiery evangelist Rev. Jonathan Goforth would become one of the world's most recognized missionaries for his forty-seven-year tenure in China. Goforth survived a sword attack during the Boxer Uprising of 1900, buried five of his eleven children in China, and refused to join the newly established United Church of Canada with the rest of his North China missionary colleagues in 1925. R.P. MacKay would be remembered not only as Goforth's mentor, but also as a founder of the United Church of Canada—the very institution Goforth famously rejected. When MacKay's daughter Margaret married the Rev. Andrew Thomson in August 1906 with plans to go to China six weeks later, the Assistant Secretary of the Presbyterian Foreign Mission Committee noted, "Mrs. Thomson is the only daughter of the Rev. R.P. MacKay, D.D.," adding pointedly, "and has therefore the missionary spirit in an unusual degree."[13] Having grown up listening to her father talk about the struggles and triumphs of China missions, Margaret Thomson must have felt quite prepared for the road ahead.

Andrew Thomson: Defiant Innovator

On arriving in China in 1906, Andrew and Margaret Thomson first settled at the North China Mission compound at Weihui. However, within two years they had gravitated to the mission fringes, choosing to live as the only foreigners at Daokou, a small village about fifty kilometres east of Weihui. A stubborn, independent, and resourceful man, Andrew Thomson had little patience for mission politics. In his estimation, the purpose of missions was to respond directly to the urgent needs of the people he lived among, not to spend energies on building and supporting bureaucratic structures for missionaries, such as committees and presbyteries. His personal mission became to address meaningfully both spiritual and physical needs of the villagers around him whether this was the priority of the North China Mission or not. His "daring confidence" got him into trouble on more than one occasion.[14]

During his thirty-six-year tenure in China, Andrew Thomson immersed himself in diverse projects that included prison visits, planting gardens at garbage sites, building a road, and even opening a small hospital—despite the fact that he had no medical training or immediate access to nursing staff. Thomson's focus was to respond to the immediate needs of the Chinese people he lived among. When there was an extreme famine in Henan in 1936, for example, he made a radical decision to advance some of his own money to Mr. Hsieh, the Magistrate of Hwahsien, to help buy grain during the height of the crisis. His plan was to charge two percent per month—a rate set by the Chinese government—using the interest for "construction schemes" like road building by persons who had no land. His idea was that the scheme would "carry through about 1000 families until the wheat harvest."[15] Acknowledging that there was "some risk in what I am doing," including danger from communist forces in the neighbouring province of Shaanxi and the possibility of a crop failure, Andrew Thomson also reasoned, "if the crops fail another year it will result in social anarchy."[16] In his mind, he had nothing to lose.

When Andrew Thomson wrote the North China Mission treasurer Hugh MacKenzie in Tianjin to issue him with the necessary money, he was disappointed to hear that MacKenzie would not support his plan. Furthermore, Bert Armstrong, the North China Mission Foreign Mission Secretary in Toronto, agreed with MacKenzie: "I would think that it is not wise for any missionary to allow his generous impulse to make a loan of this kind, in view of the precedent it may thereby establish."[17] In a spirit of defiance Andrew Thomson decided to disregard this advice, finding instead an alternate way to secure the funds. In a 1936 report he wrote: "To the M$10,000 [approximately $3,000 CAD] borrowed from the Bank of Commerce in Toronto I added several hundred dollars, and in cooperation with Magistrate Hsieh and the Famine Relief Committee I bought four railway carloads of grain from southern Honan [Henan] and distributed it to the distressed people."[18] Three months later, after a bountiful harvest, Thomson repaid the loan to the Bank of Commerce, including interest. The number of people who received the grain was 11,576.[19] Thomson felt vindicated, and even more confident in his ability to make sound decisions with or without the approval of those in authority over him. He had been "quite aware" that "many people will think me foolish" for taking this risk. However, he mused, "I wonder if such critics make a close study of the New Testament. I do, for I have to teach it, and I cannot teach it unless I practice it."[20]

Andrew Thomson's defiance of the authority of his own mission was one of the most striking aspects of his missionary career. His independent-mindedness served him well in Daokou, as much of his time was spent as the only foreigner there. Thomson believed that his authority came from God alone, and that, when faced with various crises, the Bible would provide answers through Christ's imperatives to feed the hungry, heal the sick, and care for widows and orphans. For this reason, and with little fanfare, he also made the singular decision to start his own hospital in Daokou in 1933. Dysentery, typhus fever, and tuberculosis were endemic. And the closest hospital was the North China Mission hospital at Weihui, fifty kilometres away—too far to walk and too expensive for the poorest people to travel by train. His decision was hardly spontaneous: In 1918, he and his wife Margaret had decided to put aside three thousand dollars (Canadian) of their own money to help build and staff a hospital at Daokou.[21] Years later, their plans were interrupted, first by the Great 1927 Exodus, when they evacuated back to Canada, and then by the Great Depression, during which the home mission board had no funds for new projects.

When Andrew Thomson returned to China alone in 1929, he found that much of the Daokou mission compound had been destroyed by the military conflict that had triggered the mass missionary evacuation. In a letter written to the Toronto church office in 1932, he pled for support for hospital services, hinting that he would proceed on his own, if necessary: "I have been living in a desolate compound for more than three years. In that interval there have been six scares from military occupation. Once, at midnight, I had a parlay with a general and his bodyguard of fifteen men who had come over the wall, two of whom stood with drawn revolvers. Finally I forced them to leave."[22]

After painting a picture of the ongoing "threat of brigandage" and occupation by soldiers at Daokou, Thomson set out his proposal. He would use existing buildings and the services of a local Chinese doctor, H.T. Chang, rather than wait for the United Church to find support for a new hospital building and Canadian staff: "There is no hope of Canadians being allocated to [Daokou] for some time to come. Dr. Chang's coming here will mean [in addition to his medical expertise] companionship. Every last building we have will be occupied by the hospital. It is surely better than having most of the buildings idle as they have been for some years. [This plan] almost certainly ensures [the compound] against military occupation and is a big protection against bandits."[23]

Andrew Thomson requested a total of five hundred dollars to support his proposal. If not, "My wife and I will pay whatever is required to make [the hospital] go; it will not cost the Mission anything."[24] While it is not clear whether the United Church supported his plans, "some generous friends in Canada came to [their] assistance."[25] In his 1933 annual report, Thomson wrote that vacant buildings formerly used as a boys' school were altered "at small expense" to provide men's and women's wards and an outpatient department. In addition to supporting the services of Dr. H.T. Chang, Thomson was able to secure the services of nurses and "assistants," nearly all of whom were trained at Canadian mission institutions (in Henan and Shandong).[26]

The Daokou hospital opened on 21 November 1933. Andrew Thomson wrote a letter to his older children living in Toronto, his wife and three younger children having joined him the year before. It was "a big day for us," he wrote. "Our new hospital was officially opened, and now the Red Cross flag waves over the front gate! Over the gate-house I put up the regular church cross, and the ceremony dedication was carried on under its shadow … There was not room on the four walls of the guest room inside the main gate to hang all the silk banners and congratulatory scrolls [received from community members]."[27]

In response to the speeches offered by local magistrates, Andrew Thomson replied that he "hoped those who were there today would feel that this was not [his] hospital, nor merely that of the mission, but that it was a community affair."[28] His stated aim was for the Chinese to "organize among themselves a committee for cooperation" as a way to become invested in the hospital as their own.

A year later, Thomson reported that over seven hundred refugees had received treatment at the hospital and that they had offered to "receive and care for" all expectant mothers in the forty refugee camps on the edge of the flooded areas: "These camps were overcrowded: the people slept in their clothes, on straw and on the ground with no provision for privacy. The transition from such quarters to clean beds, with skilled care from nurses and doctor, a bright and warm ward and nourishing food, nicely served, was beyond anything they had heard or dreamed of. Fifty-two such maternal cases were cared for and not one baby was lost."[29]

In his 1936 report, Andrew Thomson noted that, in its three years of operation, the tiny Daokou hospital had given "6,698 first treatments, 10,947 repeat treatments, and [had] cared for 509 in-patients" as well as giving "free asylum" to expectant mothers from the nearby flooded areas.[30] The hospital did not turn anyone away because of lack of ability to pay for treatment. The entire cost was $5,000, with $1,700 being contributed by the North China mission hospital at Weihui. When Weihui was no longer able to provide supportive funds, Dr. Chang "gallantly offered to continue the hospital at his own financial risk."[31]

While Andrew and Margaret Thomson were establishing the modest hospital, Betty Thomson was honing her skills as a nurse and hospital administrator in Canada. Although there is no evidence to suggest that Andrew and Margaret hoped their daughter would work at Daokou, their hospital endeavours would have affected Betty's perspective on the relative value of pursuing a nursing career in Canada. In 1938, when Dr. McClure told Betty Thomson and Dorothy and Mary Boyd of the serious need for nursing work in China, and when Betty Thomson read newspaper reports of internees and orphans, she knew these were not exaggerations.

Margaret Thomson: The Irony of Separation

Margaret Thomson was no less effective in her chosen work than her husband. Steeped in an understanding of her role in missions as "women's work for women,"[32] Thomson's response to the needs of the women and children she met drew largely on her perspective as a mother. For example, when in 1915 her fifth child, Andrew McClure Thomson, died of dysentery at age four months, Margaret Thomson shared her grief with a woman from a small village who had come to speak with her after a meeting. This woman, Mrs. Kwoa, had just lost a baby the month before and admitted that she was having trouble sleeping at home "because of the presence of evil spirits."[33] She was curious about the Thomsons' religion; Margaret Thomson shared how her faith helped her deal with her own loss. Mrs. Kwoa eventually became the first woman to be baptized in that village.

In 1934 Margaret Thomson responded to the severe flooding of the Yellow River by arranging for one hundred women and children to spend the winter in an empty, two-story house on the mission compound. She and the women spread straw on the floor and covered it with matting; in that way there was sleeping accommodation for all.[34] While proud of her husband's work, Margaret Thomson saw her role in China as more than supporting his endeavours: she had her own work to do. Not that she saw missionary work as all serious and solemn. Apparently she had a "wacky sense of humour," collecting poems and jokes in a small black-covered notebook. One of these read: "A little girl was asked by the teacher to tell the story of Creation. She said, 'God created Adam. Then he looked at Adam and said "I think I can do better than that." So, he created Eve.'"[35] Thomson's determination and self-sufficiency was a good match for her husband's.

Margaret and Andrew Thomson were separated for a total of about five years between 1929 and 1942: eighteen months between 1929 and 1931, twelve months between 1936 and 1937, and two and a half years between December 1938 and his repatriation to Canada in the summer of 1942.[36] Thus, from the time Betty Thomson was eighteen, one or both of her parents were absent during some of her most critical decision-making periods, be it to enter nurse's training, postgraduate education, missionary nursing, marriage, or to evacuate China during the heightened war against Japan. Like her mother, Betty was accustomed to making decisions on her own.

Becoming Missionaries: An Elite Calling

The six mishkid nurses who returned to China between 1923 and 1939 comprised an unusual group. Whether intended or not, their return to China as missionary nurses provided opportunity to extend their Chinese childhood, potentially even replicating it for their own children, since five of them married China missionaries. While they would not have considered themselves as such, mishkid nurses comprised an elite group of women who were set apart from both ordinary nurses and ordinary missionary kids in important ways. Compared with the general population of Canadian women entering nurse's training, these mishkids had been exposed firsthand to the effects of natural disasters, poverty, and armed conflict. They knew the difference that good nursing care could make to individuals and communities, and they had been reared in a community where nurses were highly respected. They also knew that if they wanted to return to China as adults, they had to "earn" their entrance by offering recognized skills. Not every mishkid who wished to return to China as a missionary was allowed to do so. For example, Marion Menzies, who attended boarding school at Weihui and Kobe with Dorothy and Mary Boyd, was disqualified from becoming a missionary because she was considered to be overweight. Although Menzies would later be temporarily allowed into China as a United Nations Relief and Rehabilitation Administration worker in 1945, she would always regret being barred from returning earlier:

My personal disappointment came later that early summer of 1938. The WMS of the United Church, which had accepted me as a potential candidate, called me to take my physical examination by their lady doctor. Several women from the [Deaconess] Training School [in Toronto] went together to be examined by Dr. Edna Guest. I remember she had several of us naked at the same time. This was to ensure that we weren't overly modest and shocked by bare bodies. To my personal sorrow I was turned down. Dr. Guest explained that my stoutness was due to glandular imbalance and that an overseas appointment would exaggerate it. I tried to tell her that I was used to Chinese-grown vegetables and foods, but to no avail. I was devastated by the rejection.[37]

While Andrew and Margaret Thomson were delighted with Betty Thomson's decision to return to China, they were also anxious that she succeed; their daughter's success or failure would reflect on them as parents *and* missionaries. Success in this case did not necessarily mean success as a nurse—married nurses, after all, were expected to quit their jobs. Rather, success meant marrying a fine Christian man and participating together in meaningful Christian service. In a letter written to Betty Thomson some-time in 1938, Margaret Thomson informed her daughter that she would be meeting "refined and cultured" English people in the China missionary community.[38] She hinted that if Betty wanted to marry someone as sophis-ticated as Eric Liddell, for example, she would need to pay close attention to her comportment. Anxious that Betty should not appear "rough and un-refined" in her first formal speech to the members of the Woman's Mis-sionary Society in Canada in 1938, Margaret wrote out a sample speech for her "just to give you an idea of what you might say."[39] Margaret thought it was important for her daughter to go all out for this speech, making a "big effort" and taking care to get the words correct: "you'll always be glad afterwards if you do."[40] Margaret Thomson had an extra reason for want-ing Betty to do well: the Toronto audience comprised Margaret's peers. The speech that she wrote for Betty read in part:

Madame President and friends,
[...] I was told recently of someone who made a speech and when he had finished one of his Listeners said "There were three things wrong with your speech. (1) You read it (2) You did not read it well (3) It was not worth read-ing. I just wish to thank the members of the Missionary Society—for making it possible for us to go to Honan [Henan], and to assure you that we count it a priviledge [sic] to be allowed to have a share in the work among as courage-ous a people as the Chinese. We shall try to be worthy representatives of you in that land.[41]

Although we do not know Betty Thomson's response to her mother's let-ter—or whether she used the speech that her mother penned—the speech gives insights into the ideals of missionary work and what missionaries be-lieved the home congregants expected of them. It also reveals the purpose and power of the written letter in China missionary relationships. Just as letters had been the lifeblood of Betty Thomson's relationship with her par-ents during her years at boarding school, so also they were central to their relationship during her teenage years in Toronto when first her father, then both parents, were working in China. Margaret Thomson's directives to her daughter reveal something of the nature of their relationship; both love and instruction were dispensed freely, even if unbidden.

Margaret Thomson's 1938 letter also makes clear the family expectations. In addition to hoping Betty would marry well, Margaret wanted her daugh-ter to care for her during her declining years. "Of course if you marry an English man or a Scotchman," Margaret Thomson wrote, "you'll find it hard to do that [i.e., to live the 'last ten years of my life with me'], won't you!"[42]

As it turned out, Betty fulfilled both of her mother's wishes, expressed so bluntly in this letter: she married an English missionary *and* lived near her mother for the last 28 years of her mother's life. In fact, Margaret Thomson died in Betty and Godfrey Gale's Toronto suburb of Weston, in 1973.[43]

Summary

In 1888, China Inland Mission pioneer Hudson Taylor urged missionaries to come to China because a million a month were dying without God.[44] Fifty years later, mishkid Dr. Bob McClure urged Canadian nurses to come to China because thousands in Henan were dying without nursing care. Mishkids who responded to the call for nurses did so in the spirit of altruistic service that characterized their parents' brand of missions, but not with the same evangelical zeal. Indeed, by the 1930s, Canadian missionary nurses in Henan had shifted their focus from the evangelistic aims of the early pioneer nurses to a greater interest in—and alliance with—the broader professional aims of high quality nursing education and service (e.g., establishing a national Nurses Association of China and standardizing nurses' education across China).[45] To the mishkid nurses, nursing was a practical service—and their ticket to return to the land of their birth. They understood the stakes: missionary work was risky. But nowhere else did they experience the same sense of purpose and belonging.

There is no indication that Betty Thomson or any of the mishkid nurses went into nurse's training with the idea of returning to China as a missionary nurse. Thomson was aware of the need for nurses in China—her father had singlehandedly set up a small hospital in Daokou—but seemed content in the work she had in front of her at the Toronto General Hospital. She worked for six years at the TGH: three years as a student nurse, for which she won accolades and awards, and three years as a graduate nurse and university student, for which she won the attentions of the esteemed Jean Gunn. It was an impassioned, kitchen-table plea from Bob McClure that set her back on the missionary trail. Missionary nursing offered Betty Thomson, Dorothy Boyd, and Mary Boyd the opportunity to do something meaningful for the land of their birth, but it also promised something that even Toronto could not offer—a vibrant social community of like-minded youth. More to the point, having been disappointed with the character of the men she dated in Toronto, Betty Thomson recognized China as a place to find a husband who was also a soulmate. Following her friend Florence Mackenzie's footsteps to the TGH nursing school and back to China, Betty secretly sought what Florence had already found—a refined and dedicated missionary with whom she could start a new life.

Going to China as a missionary nurse was risky, but not without its rewards. From a professional point of view, nursing offered young single women a chance to prove their mettle as caregivers to the sick and injured. Going to a war zone only increased the significant admiration being paid missionary nurses by their nursing peers and mentors. From a religious point of view, missionary work offered young single women a chance to express their faith as an act of charitable and compassionate service. The United Church of Canada ethos embraced the notion of social justice among those whose need was most desperate. By returning to China—a land long equated with danger in the annals of Canadian missions—mishkids were held up as role models and the embodiment of Christian ideals. Finally, from a personal (familial) point of view, returning to China provided these young women with an opportunity to meet eligible bachelors with values likely to align with that of the Canadian missionary subculture. That China was dangerous increased its appeal as a fascinating, fulfilling, and respected vocation—and increased the mishkid nurses' appeal as marriageable women.

The "New" Missionaries (1939–1940)

By six-thirty Betty was all gussied up, frizzed, perfumed like downtown Toronto.

—Mary Boyd Stanley, letter

By the time Betty Thomson, Dorothy Boyd, and Mary Boyd decided to return to China, North China missionaries had been in Henan for fifty years. They would be returning to a well-established missionary community—not quite the rugged, remote, and rural setting their parents had committed to decades earlier. Nor would they be expected to make the lifelong commitment that their parents had made. While earlier missionaries had furloughs home every seven years, Betty, Dorothy, and Mary would be taking advantage of a recruitment scheme that allowed them to sign a much shorter (three-year) contract with the United Church of Canada Woman's Missionary Society. Never before had becoming a missionary nurse been so attractive: in return for a relatively short time commitment, these three mishkid nurses could expect to find meaningful work, excitement, and, if they were lucky, a suitable husband in China. For religious women of marrying age, there were few places in the world with as many desirable, eligible bachelors as the China mission field.

As part of the second generation of missionaries, mishkid nurses had a different idea of missionary work than their parents. Mishkids were an optimistic group, ready to "demonstrate that through the love of God and the power of faith, the nature of man and the quality of life could be changed."[1] Bob McClure, who with Jean Menzies was the first North China mishkid to return to Henan as a missionary, was considered restless, intolerant of the status quo, and eager for change. The first generation of missionaries came to China with evangelism as their primary task—that is, sharing a Christian gospel that emphasized people's separation from God through sin, Jesus Christ's sacrificial death that paid the penalty for all human sin, and the consequent requirement for humans to confess their sins (and their belief in Christ's sacrifice as pertaining to *them*) in order to be divinely forgiven and

restored to a full relationship with God. In other words, the first generation of missionaries aimed to save "lost souls" by leading people to become
Christ's followers, to convert to Christianity. In contrast, this new generation of missionaries was more inclined toward a social gospel—a larger vision of using Christian principles to combat injustice, suffering, and poverty
in society. The social gospel intersected well with the professional aims of
modern nursing in Canada and America in the postwar period of the 1920s
and '30s. The second generation of missionaries wanted to see practical results. In fact, the majority of mishkids who returned to China were nurses
or, like Bob McClure, physicians. McClure neatly identified the reason for
such a pragmatic approach to missions: medical missionaries *knew* when
they were functioning well; evangelists "merely hoped."[2] By the time the
mishkid nurses returned to China, medical missions had surpassed evangelism as a raison d'être for the North China Mission. This is perhaps best
described by Bob McClure's biographer Munroe Scott, in his description
of younger missionaries like Bob: "Although sheltered by British power
they were critical of exploitative colonialism and were sympathetic to Chinese nationalism; they tended to be theologically liberal and tolerant; they
tended to be puritans who regarded drinking, smoking and womanizing as
outright works for the devil; they were radicals who could bring themselves
to believe that schools and hospitals were as important as churches."[3]

The new generation of missionaries was a flamboyant one, eager to live
fully. Dancing was a regular past time. Sharing a Coca-Cola at a café, eating a meal of Peking duck at a restaurant, or attending the theatre were as
common as sightseeing when these missionaries found themselves in larger
cosmopolitan cities like Beijing. While frugality was a highly regarded virtue, frivolity was not unheard of: Bob McClure and Canadian nurse Coral
Brodie bought a couple of ex-racing ponies. Their rationale? They were "los-
ers and therefore cheap."[4] Thus, while the opportunity to assist the Chinese
during times of difficulty undoubtedly influenced Betty Thomson, Dorothy
Boyd, and Mary Boyd's decision to return to China, the fact that even wartime China could offer a vibrant social community was not lost on them.

Upon arriving in China in April 1939, Betty Thomson, Dorothy Boyd,
and Mary Boyd commenced language study at the College of Chinese
Studies in Beijing. They had a lot of work to catch up on: their particular
course had started the previous September. Perhaps not surprisingly, the
wealth of social distractions made it difficult to study. "Incidentally," Betty
Thomson wrote to her mother on 4 June 1939 after six pages describing her
socializing, "I often study, even when I don't happen to mention it!!"[5]

The tone of Betty Thomson's earliest letters to her mother and siblings in
Canada after arriving in China in 1939 capture the air of excitement that she

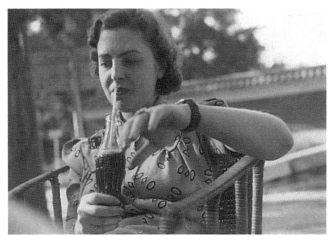

Fig. 3.1 Mary Boyd, Beijing, 1939

felt in renewing old acquaintances, shopping, dining, and going to concerts. Her letters are chatty, filled with names—many of them associated with the North China Mission ("Guess who arrived from Honan [Henan] yesterday? Mr. King!! My it's fun seeing all the folks one after another, arriving here.").[6] It was a heady, happy time—with opportunities to date and party in ways unheard of by the older missionary generation. The letters give little evidence that Betty Thomson was concerned about the war in other regions of China. In addition to language classes, she spent her time mingling in the "radio room" ("it was lots of fun; Bill Braestid improves on acquaintance"), leading chapel services ("we each have a 'go' at it") and playing tennis with Dorothy Boyd ("Dot has the greatest serve. It's grand being beaten in tennis. Nothing makes me madder than to be able to win easily.")[7]

This is not to say that everything was comfortable for the students. The war-related high cost of food contributed to the poor quality of the college meals, and the accommodations were stark. Still, Betty Thomson was pragmatic: "I have just been trying to convince Mary [Boyd] that what she found in her room was not a lug-bug [?] but a beetle! She has it in a box—and is firmly convinced that she will report it to Dr. Petters. I didn't work in the TGH for six years and emerge without knowing what those little insects look like."[8]

Beetles notwithstanding, there is little doubt that the period of language study was a fulfilling one—not least of all because of the affirmation that it was, indeed, a fertile ground for single missionary men and women to find marriage partners. Within months of their arrival, both Betty Thomson and Mary Boyd would be engaged to China missionaries. Although it was Mary who eventually married John Stanley, it was Betty who first caught his eye.

Betty Thomson first mentioned John Stanley in her weekly letter home on 28 May 1939. She wrote of going out for "duck dinner" with a group of thirteen, including John Stanley, adding in parentheses, "(will explain later)." John Stanley was the son of missionaries in Jinan; he had been studying Chinese for the previous two years with hopes of becoming a librarian at Yenching University in Beijing. A couple of days after they first met, John showed up at the library where Betty was and, after studying together for a couple of hours, he "asked me to go to a concert with him on Monday night." After Betty "had [her] hair done—and nearly passed out with the heat," she and John went to dinner and the concert. Afterwards she and two other couples went to John Stanley's home—the "cutest Chinese place he's rented"—where they listened to "*grand* music" and ate nuts "until we nearly burst open."[9] Five days later Betty Thomson and a few friends threw "a little impromptu party" at John Stanley's residence: "We found some music on the radio—so [Bill Matheson and I] rolled up the rug and 'went into our dance' ... with an audience all around ... (just young folks—don't be alarmed!)."[10] Despite such auspicious beginnings, nothing romantic developed ... or, if it did, there is no evidence of it. Within three months, Mary Boyd had fallen in love with John Stanley, and Betty Thomson was being courted by another missionary bachelor—London Missionary Society physician Dr. Godfrey Gale.

Evacuating Japanese-Occupied Regions

Betty Thomson, Dorothy Boyd, and Mary Boyd expected to spend the summer of 1939 completing their preparations for their new positions at the North China Mission hospitals in Henan. By June 1939 they had finished their written Chinese exams and were studying for their oral exams, to be completed by July. Because of the oppressive heat during summertime, the new recruits were to continue their language study via private lessons at Beidaihe. Betty Thomson had fond memories of Beidaihe. When she heard she was returning there in June 1939, she could hardly contain her excitement, writing to her mother in Canada: "Just think! Next week we'll be in Pei Tai Ho [Beidaihe]. Imagine that??? I can hardly believe my senses ... but Mary and Dot [Boyd] say it is true, so I guess it is."[11]

Beidaihe had become an essential part of the missionary experience—something the missionaries had come to view as both a reward for, and a reprieve from, the trials of mission work. The mishkid nurses did not question their privileged position in Beidaihe—where, for example, a Chinese "cook, a boy and an amah" went to the cottages there three days ahead of them to help prepare for their arrival.[12] This magical place had been the highlight of their childhood; now, by virtue of being missionaries themselves, Betty Thomson, Dorothy Boyd, and Mary Boyd could claim its magic as their own.

Betty Thomson travelled with Mary Boyd to Beidaihe via Tianjin, where they caught up with Florence Liddell. Because Eric Liddell could not take vacation until August, Florence made plans for her and her two daughters to stay with Betty at Beidaihe for part of June and July. Dorothy and Mary Boyd would stay with their parents. For Betty, life could not be better. In a letter to her mother she exclaimed, "Guess what! Eric and Flo's holidays will not be until August, so Flo and the kids are coming to Pei Tai Ho [Beidaihe] with us at Mae Lynns's!!! Whoops me lad!! Isn't it *wonderful*!!!"[13] With their unexpected reunion, Betty Thomson, Florence Liddell, and Mary Boyd acted more like giddy teenagers than sober missionary women. When a severe rainstorm interrupted their shopping plans, the three women went anyways, carrying "streamer rugs over our heads!"[14] The friends lost no time taking advantage of the rich social life at Beidaihe. Group dinners, beach picnics, and tennis matches filled their days. Betty Thomson's letters are filled with youthful joy—silliness even. In one particularly candid letter, she complained about a woman who insisted that the ladies' tennis tournament they were organizing be held at a court close to her residence: "We had made two trips over [to East Cliff] already to arrange the game—but the Mother of one of the 'ladies' burst out indignantly, 'The idea! Why should her darling child have to go all the way to West End to play! Why she'd be too tired to hit a ball—etc, etc! It didn't seem to register on her brain (if she had one) that we had to come the same distance—!"[15] Both literally and figuratively, Beidaihe was a long way from Henan.

While Betty Thomson, Dorothy Boyd, and Mary Boyd were renewing old acquaintances at Beidaihe (and developing significant new ones, as will be seen), missionaries at the North China Mission sites in Henan were urgently responding to severe flooding there. The summer rains came earlier than expected to Henan, and by July 1939 the Yellow River had flooded its banks. At the mission site at Huaiqing, walls and buildings collapsed, cellars filled with water, and gardens were destroyed. At Weihui, residents were forced to travel by boat in the city. As if flooding were not enough of a concern, the Japanese military presence in Henan was becoming more adversarial, inciting a public mood of distrust and anger towards the foreign missionaries by claiming that they, the Japanese, as fellow Asians, were committed to a common goal of economic vitality and stability in the East, whereas British (and Canadian) foreigners were there for selfish gain. As North China missionaries gauged a proper response to the local tensions, they sent out word that this was not a good time to send in the three new

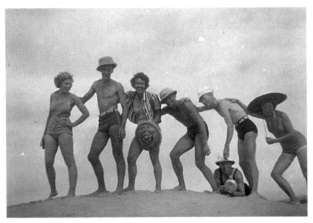

Fig. 3.2   Beidaihe, 1939

Canadian nurses presently at Beidaihe; the mishkid nurses would have to stay at Beidaihe while the crisis in Henan played itself out.

The three women could not have chosen a better place to be in limbo. With their immediate future uncertain, they took advantage of the opportunity to participate fully in the fun at Beidaihe. As it was, five mishkid nurses were at Beidaihe that summer: Betty Thomson, Dorothy Boyd, Mary Boyd, Florence Liddell—and Georgina Menzies, who had just married Dr. John Lewis. In fact Rev. Andrew Thomson, Betty's father, had given the bride away since Georgina's father had died in Henan when she was a young girl. "Georgie" Lewis, as she was known, was five years older than Betty. She had just completed seven years of missionary nursing at the North China Mission at Anyang. Georgie and John had come to Beidaihe as part of their honeymoon. This was the first time that Betty Thomson and Georgina Lewis had had an opportunity to really get to know each other. "I had no idea Georgie was so much fun!" exclaimed Betty in a letter home.[16]

Georgina Lewis's mother, the formidable missionary widow Mrs. Davina Menzies, was also at Beidaihe. Concerned that her new son-in-law would no longer have work at Shaanxi, Davina Menzies took it upon herself to write to the United Church of Canada mission headquarters to see if they would accept her new son-in-law at Anyang: "It makes me wish Honan [Henan] could secure Dr. John Lewis for a few months until his field is open again. I know at Changte [Anyang] it has been said if we only could get Dr. Lewis and keep Georgina. But of course at present I fancy we are still uncertain of returning inland ourselves."[17] As one of the longest-serving North China missionaries, and the wife of the mission's "martyred" pioneer, Davina Menzies had a certain amount of influence that she was quite willing to use if it would benefit her or her family. In this case, however, her request would become moot: shortly after, the Anyang mission was also evacuated.

On the same day that Davina Menzies wrote her appeal to the United Church—15 August 1939—Betty Thomson wrote her family that she "just had [her] first typhus injection."[18] Despite the uncertainty in Henan, the mission was preparing the three nurses to start their new positions there. "It looks as if we really were intending to go 'in' sometime, doesn't it?" Betty Thomson wrote, hinting that she, too, was nervous about the idea.[19] But it was not to be. While the North China missionaries relaxed and cemented social bonds during the carefree, privileged summer at Beidaihe, the crisis playing out in Henan would result in a missionary evacuation that would last for six years. In fact, none of the mishkid nurses would ever return to Henan.

Closure of the Anyang Mission Site

On 30 August 1939, the Japanese military gathered together the Chinese staff of the Canadian mission hospital at Anyang. Standing before them in the mission chapel, the Japanese authorities described a list of offences allegedly perpetrated by the Canadians and warned that the Chinese should no longer associate with these foreigners. They threatened the staff with this warning: those who did not leave by noon the next day would have their arms or legs cut off. Word passed around the mission compound quickly, and everyone took the threat seriously. Anticipating the imminent closure of the fifty-year-old mission site, missionaries immediately began distributing mission equipment and supplies to the departing staff. Within hours of the Japanese announcement, student nurses received their class records and extra books, graduate nurses received instruments and an obstetrical bundle, sewing women received a sewing machine, cooks received the kitchen equipment, and goatherds received live goats. At 9:00 p.m. on that same day, the missionaries and all the Chinese members of the mission celebrated the Lord's Supper together and then said a hasty farewell.[20]

By noon the next day, only six Canadian missionaries remained at the two mission compounds in Anyang. Missionary nurse Clara Preston, Rev. Don Faris, and Dr. Isabelle MacTavish were the only ones left at the West compound. Bill Mitchell, Grace Sykes, and Rev. J.C. Mathieson were ten minutes away at the East compound. Deciding that they were not going to be forced out by the Japanese, the missionaries stayed at their respective compounds for three weeks, keeping in contact with each other by telephone. By refusing to leave, the Canadians held out hope that the Japanese would allow them to remain in China. A Japanese guard stayed at the compound gate to ensure that the Chinese staff did not return. However, after three weeks, someone set the gates of both compounds on fire. Preston, MacTavish, and Mitchell were able to put out the East compound fire by creating a makeshift brigade, but the West compound had no running water.[21]

Tired and anxious, the missionaries' resolve began to falter. It broke altogether on the night of 16 September 1939, when nine grenades (of which four exploded) were thrown over the East compound wall. A poster pasted to the compound gate showed a prostrate foreigner with blood running from his neck. It read: "Englishmen, within three days if you are not away from this place, there will certainly be danger on your lives."[22] This was the end: it made no sense to stay. Clara Preston and Grace Sykes took a train to Beijing. There Preston went to the Peking Union Medical College for a month's work and observation of the wards. Eventually she would be transferred to Tianjin, where Dorothy and Mary Boyd would join her to work among refugees escaping both flooding and Japanese aggression. Grace Sykes returned to Canada on furlough.

Closure of the Weihui Mission Site

At Weihui, things remained relatively quiet until 4 September 1939. On that day the staff was called to the hospital where Mr. Chang, head of the local Anti-British Committee, ordered the missionaries to leave at once and not return. Canadian nurse Margaret Gay later recalled "a white-faced frightened looking little Chinese man" telling the staff that the hospital was to be closed without delay, and that patients, employees, and foreigners had to leave on pain of death.[23] One of the Chinese doctors, probably Dr. Duan Mei-qing,[24] pointed out that this would cause great personal loss since the workers' homes were in the compound and forty patients were still in the hospital. Dr. Duan consulted with the missionaries, and it was agreed that he would take over responsibility for the hospital. On 5 October 1939, the missionaries at Weihui received word that they must leave by 12 October or "drastic action" would be taken on the 13th. They left in small parties and eventually reunited in Tianjin.[25]

Closure of the Huaiqing Mission Site

On 6 October 1939, the Japanese started to occupy the Huaiqing compound. Eighty soldiers entered the compound requesting "tea and a rest."[26] That evening the Japanese Propaganda Department asked for billets for six hundred Japanese soldiers, who remained for three days. On 19 October, the Japanese asked Dr. Chang to co-operate with them in "taking over the hospital after the foreigners had been driven out."[27] Dr. Chang told the Canadians of the Japanese plans to take over. It was decided that everyone must evacuate. Dr. Chang was the first to leave, escaping with his family in wheelbarrows at midnight on 24 October.[28] The Changs arrived safely in Xian, having "gone across the country in several kinds of conveyances, walking a good part of the way."[29] On 26 October the first Canadian party made their escape from Huaiqing; Canadian nurse Margaret Gay—who had gone to Huaiqing from Weihui to nurse another missionary through a bout of typhoid—was among this group of exiles.[30]

Although it had seemed obvious to the Canadian missionaries that the threats to them and their Chinese colleagues necessitated their evacuation from Henan, doubt plagued them once they reunited in Tianjin. Rev. G.K. King asked in a report of the October events, "Were we right in leaving the property and work in this way?"[31] With the exception of Betty's father, Andrew Thomson—who, after a brief reunion with Betty at Beidaihe in August 1939, returned to Daokou for another year—all of the North China missionaries were evacuated from Henan by October 1939. It was the third mass exodus in the North China Mission's history.[32]

The Courtship of Andrew Thomson's Daughter

While missionaries at the North China Mission sites in Henan were contemplating the meaning of increased Japanese aggression in the summer of 1939, Betty Thomson and the other stranded missionaries were enjoying their "exile" at Beidaihe. Its natural beauty formed the perfect backdrop for renewing and strengthening missionary relationships. Moreover, its sandy beaches, crashing waves, and moonlit nights were ideal for spawning romantic developments. It was here that Betty Thomson met her future husband, Dr. Godfrey Gale.

Godfrey Livingstone Gale was also a child of missionaries. Rev. and Mrs. Kendall Gale had served in Madagascar with the London Missionary Society, an assignment that had earned Godfrey's father the moniker "Gale of Madagascar."[33] By this time Reverend Gale was deceased, and the widowed Mrs. Gale was living in England.[34] Godfrey was working as a physician at the Shandong Christian University Medical School (Qilu) in Jinan with the London Missionary Society. According to Betty Thomson's recollection fifty years later, she and Godfrey Gale met the first night he arrived in Beidaihe.[35] They were at a dinner party with approximately twenty other missionaries, seated at two round tables. Betty Thomson and Godfrey

Gale sat back to back at the adjoining tables. After dinner the tables were moved aside to allow the young people to dance. Betty remembered dancing with Godfrey; she also danced with other missionary men. Afterwards both Godfrey Gale and fellow LMS missionary Kenneth McAll walked Betty home. According to Betty's diary, the date of their meeting was 20 August 1939. Her diary entry reveals the intersecting tensions and excitement of romance, nursing, and missionary life on the edge of war: "Terrible war news—seem to be on verge of a War again. [Illegible—Mission?] refugees from Tientsin [Tianjin] arrived. Stuckley party on Lotus Hills—met Ken McCall [*sic*] and Godfrey Gaile [*sic*]. Dancing at 'the corner.' Ken like Eric Liddell. A *grand* evening."[36] It was only days later that Betty started to pay attention to Godfrey Gale's charms—a good thing, as it turns out, since he would return to Jinan on 6 September; they had less than a week to fall in love.

On 27 August 1939, a Sunday, Betty Thomson's diary entry reads: "Godfrey Gail [*sic*] preached. A very nice looking man—red hair."[37] On 30 August Betty joined the LMS missionaries, including Godfrey, for a breakfast picnic. On 2 September Godfrey and Betty were meant to have their first date. They had planned to have "elevenses" on Lotus Hills but Betty skipped out because of pouring rain.[38] In her diary Betty noted only: "Picnic with Bill—elevenses with Godfrey—tea at MacHatties all cancelled. More rain! (Heard next day Godfrey did go to Hills after all for 11's's)."[39] According to Mary Boyd's recollection forty years later, Godrey and Betty's date was rescheduled for that evening:

[Beidaihe] in late summer of 1939. Beidaihe on its ear because Limey Gale had a date for dinner at the Lotus Hills Cafe with one Canadienne Thompson [*sic*] that Saturday night. It was all over West End for days, over Rocky Point, even to East Cliff and such civilized peoples. No Canadiennes (none of the three) were on the beach that morning. Betty was bending her hair all afternoon. By six-thirty Betty was all gussied up, frizzed, perfumed like downtown Toronto. Come six-thirty, Betty's on the front porch swing. Mrs. Clark is fussing around madhouse. All sorts of Canadiennes are swarming around. But when then? Godfrey from English Beach rides his bicycle along the highway right behind the Clark house at six twenty-five—headed into the setting sun a mile a minute for the cafe to get there on time. A squinch of tyres, a scatter of gravel at the back gate, and he's gone in a cloud of "lust." At church the next day, with one voice the duet came out (during the clatter of the collection coppers): "And just where were you last night?!?" Everyone heard it, in glee. But it only happened once. In one lesson it was learned that modern packaging and wrapping requires pick up and delivery.[40]

On Sunday, 3 September, Godfrey paid a visit to Betty and her father on the pretext of bringing war news from Europe. On Monday Godfrey and Betty walked up to watch the sunset from Lotus Hills. On Tuesday they took a picnic walk to the Hills. By Wednesday, a week after their first get-together, the two were inseparable, knowing that Godfrey would be returning to Jinan later that day. Godfrey came over for lunch; the pair went swimming together; they saw Mary and Dorothy Boyd off to the train station. Andrew Thomson, who had joined his daughter at Beidaihe a few weeks earlier, was clearly in favour of the courtship. Sensitive to this being "Godfrey's last evening there," Andrew gave permission to the couple to have one last, private picnic at Lotus Hills.[41] Afterwards Godfrey joined Betty and her father to listen to a radio broadcast before travelling together to the train station, where Godfrey caught the 11:30 p.m. train to Jinan. "I still *hate* outgoing trains!" proclaimed Betty in a letter to her mother shortly after.[42] In her diary Betty Thomson coyly noted, "Saw Godfrey off. He told me. Remember??"[43] Whatever Godfrey told Betty on 6 September 1939, it was enough to seal their relationship. Betty left for Beijing five days later, finally en route to the North China Mission.

Godfrey Gale returned to his work as a medical missionary at Qilu Hospital at the Shandong Christian University in Jinan. In an eight-page, handwritten letter to "my dear Betty" on 11 September 1939, Godfrey made his admiration (and, more subtly, his hopes) clear: "You are constantly in my thoughts and each time I think of you I murmur to myself 'bless you' because you really are a great kid and I miss you. It seemed lonely somehow coming back to live by myself in this big house."[44] After a six-page description of his long journey from Tianjin to Jinan through Japanese-occupied territory, via rickshaw, sailboat, and train, Godfrey provided a contrasting, attractive portrait of the colonial domesticity that awaited him—one which Betty would undoubtedly find charming: "My boy and amah gave me a great welcome. They had got the house absolutely spotlessly clean, had polished all the brasses, washed all the curtains, cut fresh flowers for the vases."[45]

Godfrey Gale was an astute and sincere suitor, appealing to Betty Thomson's adventurous, religious, domestic, familial, romantic, and professional selves. He acknowledged her familiarity with China, writing "you must experience sailing along the Grand Canal sometime, if you have not done it already." He also emphasized their mutual religious beliefs, writing "many times a day I thank God for you." In addition, Godfrey shared with Betty his professional world, subtly appealing to her nursing identity: "This morning I went around [Qilu] hospital looking up old friends and in the afternoon went to my Out Patients [Department] as usual. They have provided me with a Chinese assistant in the ENT [Ears, Nose and Throat Department] now and have promised me a second nurse for Out Patients—or rather, a nurse to help my coolie [*sic*] there, so we feel ourselves in clover." After admitting his hope that "the mail will bring a line from you before long," he politely asked Betty to "remember [him] very kindly to Mr. Thomson and to the Boyds" and wished her a good journey to Weihui.

Godfrey Gale's attentions paid off. The day that Betty Thomson left Beidaihe for Beijing, there was new "trouble" at Weihui, and the return of the mishkid nurses was delayed once more. The three mishkid nurses bided their time in Beijing, where Mary Boyd was undoubtedly pleased to spend more time with John Stanley. Within days the North China Mission conclusively decided not to send the new nurses to Henan. Betty Thomson, Dorothy Boyd, and Mary Boyd were offered nursing positions at Qilu hospital, where the North China Mission had had a small presence since 1918. On 19 September 1939 the request came from Jinan: "Three nurses welcome. Come immediately."[46] The next day John Stanley gave Mary Boyd his fraternity pin—a pre-engagement promise of commitment. Life for the mishkid nurses was set on a new track, where family relationships would take primacy over their commitment to the United Church Woman's Missionary Society.

On 27 September 1939 Betty Thomson arrived in Jinan. It is not clear when Mary and Dorothy arrived; within weeks they were all re-directed to other mission sites. Shortly afterwards the request came from Qilu University—undoubtedly supported by Dr. Godfrey Gale—asking the North China Mission to allow Betty Thomson to take over as Supervisor of the Operating Room while a member of the Qilu nursing staff was on furlough. Although Thomson reported herself as willing to "work either in [Jinan] or West China," she wrote her employer, the Woman's Missionary Society, that the position at the University Hospital "appealed to her very much."[47] The North China Mission Council approved her relocation to Qilu University, appointing her in December 1939.[48]

Otherwise Engaged

Known today as Shandong University, Qilu University was founded in 1917 as the Shandong Christian University. Envisioned as a "union" university of Baptist and Presbyterian educational endeavours, Qilu brought together the American Presbyterian College (est. 1864 at Tengchou, Shandong), the English Baptist High School and Theological School (est. 1885 at Qingzhou), and three arms of the Baptist and Presbyterian Union Educational Scheme (est. 1904)—the Arts and Science College at Weixian, the Theo-

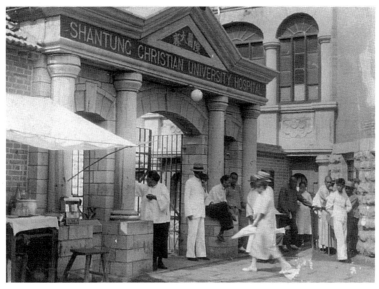

Fig. 3.3   Shandong Christian University gate

logical College at Qingzhou, and the Medical College at Jinan. Canadian missionaries first became involved with Qilu University in 1918 when Dr. William McClure was asked to assist with the Medical College. McClure moved to Jinan, where he taught until his retirement in 1938. In 1925 the university received a Canadian charter, formalizing the relationship between the United Church of Canada Mission and the United Church of Canada Woman's Missionary Society. In 1931 the university was registered by the Ministry of Education of the Chinese Government.[49]

When Godfrey Gale arrived at Qilu in 1937, there were forty-four faculty members in the Department of Medicine, including thirty Chinese nationals and fourteen foreign missionaries. In addition to United Church missionaries, Qilu faculty included missionaries from the United States (Presbyterian Mission North and South, Methodist Episcopal North Women's Missionary Society, American Board Mission) and Great Britain (Baptist Missionary Society, English Presbyterian Mission, London Missionary Society, Methodist Missionary Society, Methodist Women's Missionary Society, Society for the Propagation of the Gospel). Qilu boasted 1,600 Chinese graduates, most of whom were practising in different parts of China as teachers (690), doctors (370), and pastors, evangelists, or social workers (350).[50]

The United Church of Canada North China Mission's decision to become formally involved with Qilu University grew out of a desire to become more engaged with medical education. Given the opportunity to join the work either at Qilu or at the Peking Union Medical College in Beijing, Canadian missionaries chose Qilu in part because courses there were conducted in Chinese rather than English. By the 1930s a number of Canadians were working at Qilu, including nurse Coral Brodie, Rev. R.A. and Mrs. Mitchell, Dr. E.B. and Margaret Struthers, and Dr. William and Margaret McClure.

At the outbreak of the Sino-Japanese War in 1937, the Nationalist government urged all educational institutions to move to parts of China not occupied by the Japanese.[51] The West China Union University in Sichuan invited Qilu faculty and students to come to their institution. The West China Union University was also an inter-denominational institution supported in part by the United Church of Canada. In response to the invitation, the three upper classes of the medical college and four staff members started on the fifteen-hundred-kilometre overland journey to West China in the fall of 1937. Over the next few months most of the Chinese staff and students left for West China. The Qilu Hospital remained open but was seriously understaffed. When North China missionary Dr. Isabelle MacTavish was later seconded to Qilu University rather than the West China Union University, she decided that she was "glad indeed to go there, as there was quite a bit in the situation that seemed to me to make a strong appeal. The attempt to hold the university and hospital in our own part of China did not seem hopeless and I was glad to be one of the number to make the attempt."[52]

The Qilu University occupied a large area to the south of Jinan city proper, as well as an area outside the city walls. Beyond the university were mountains. Inside the city walls there were several staff houses and "a very fine hospital equal in standard and in some ways ahead of anything we had known in Britain."[53] The original Qilu Hospital was built at Jinan in 1915. In 1935 it had 110 beds and was purported to be "the best equipped in North China."[54] New premises erected in 1935 added 60 beds and a spacious outpatient department. In 1937 plans were under way to expand the hospital to 240 beds, with outpatient accommodation, an isolation building, and increased housing facilities for resident doctors and nurses. In the 1935–36 reporting year, a total of 2,806 patients were admitted, while an additional 84,252 persons were treated as outpatients. Furthermore, Qilu staff and students cared for 19,500 flood refugees accommodated in twenty-seven camps around Jinan.

In December 1939 Betty Thomson joined Coral Brodie as the second North China missionary nurse at Qilu. Brodie, who had originally come to China in 1923 with her good friend Jean Menzies, had been "temporarily" seconded to Qilu in 1927 after the North China Mission in Henan was evacuated due to civil unrest.[55] By the time Thomson arrived, Brodie had been at Qilu for eleven years. Thomson joined Brodie in one of the missionary houses on Qilu campus. Godfrey Gale wasted no time getting in touch. He dispatched a handwritten note addressed to "Miss E. Thomson, c/o Miss Brodie" which read: "Dear Betty, Welcome to Cheeloo [Qilu]! Glad you have come at last. I want to hear all about this amazing trip of yours. I'll try to slip up to Miss Brodie's [house] about a quarter to six-ish this evening. Cheers, Godfrey."[56]

Godfrey Gale proposed to Betty Thomson on Christmas Eve 1939; she accepted immediately. In her diary Betty exclaimed, "Engaged to my man!!"[57] The next day she wrote her mother about the engagement, noting "I said yes so fast! I feel as though I would burst with happiness!"[58] Her parents were hoping for such news. In a letter written to his wife five days before his daughter's engagement, Andrew Thomson gave this endorsement of her beau: "You would rejoice to know Godfrey Gale. I wrote Elizabeth [Betty] that if in the good Providence of God they should become man and wife I would be very glad. In the few short meetings I had with him I got the idea that he was both a man of high Christian principles and a man of no inconsiderable intelligence and culture."[59] Nine months later, Andrew Thomson would travel to Jinan to give the bride away. Margaret Thomson, however, would not meet her son-in-law for another six years—after their release from the internment camp in 1945.

Betty Thomson and Godfrey Gale decided to keep the engagement a secret at Qilu until letters could be dispatched to their parents in Toronto, Canada; Daokou, China; and Birmingham, England. In a letter written to her mother on 3 February 1940, Betty gushed with enthusiasm about her fiancé, her comments appealing to the class values of her mother: "Godfrey is so *grand*! He's more and more wonderful and I just ache with happiness! … *You'll* just *love* him, I know. He's so cultured and gentlemanly … and musical! He plays marvellously—and can hum parts from the Great Masters."[60] Not only was Godfrey Gale English *and* a China missionary, as a physician he was also a member of one of the most esteemed professions in the West. Considering Margaret Thomson's admiration of English and Scottish refinement and culture, her approval of the match can hardly be in doubt.

The Tricky Game of Resignation

Because the United Church of Canada's Woman's Missionary Society (WMS) only hired single women, nurses like Betty Thomson who married China missionaries were required to resign their positions and be transferred to their husbands' mission boards. Resignation was a daunting task; the WMS did not take kindly to missionaries breaking their contracts. And this was not a good time to resign: the WMS had recently lost both Coral Brodie and Jeannette Ratcliffe; Brodie had suffered a stroke on the night Betty and Godfrey were engaged, and Ratcliffe travelled to Jinan to care for Brodie and eventually accompany her back to Canada. Mishkid nurses now made up the majority of North China missionary nurses left in China.

Betty Thomson announced her engagement to the United Church in a letter dated 18 January 1940. The letter was addressed to Field Secretary Rev. G.K. King, a man she and her parents knew very well:

> If it isn't one thing it's another—and you are probably wondering why in the world I'm bothering you again so soon after you got me all nicely settled in Tsinan [Jinan]. This is really a "friendly" letter—not relating to business but the contents are very important notwithstanding. I am writing to announce my engagement to Dr. Godfrey Gale of the L.M. Society [...] I am sorry Dad isn't here so that he could do this [announcement] for us—but we can't wait any longer. The L.M.S annual meetings are in February and Godfrey wants to tell them about it then—and I can't let his Mission know before mine! (We have Dad's permission, of course.) Isn't it exciting? I am most terrifically [*sic*] happy—and am living above the clouds.[61]

Betty Thomson's euphoria at her engagement was tempered by her recognition that she now faced a tricky game of mission politics. Desiring to continue her job at Qilu hospital, she was struck by the irony that, as a married woman she would be required to resign from the WMS and then apply to the LMS to become a fully supported missionary nurse—only to keep the exact same position she already held as the Superintendent of the Operating Theatre at Qilu Hospital. Both the resignation and the application carried professional risks: to resign from the WMS meant breaking her contract and leaving the North China Mission desperately short of nurses; to apply to the LMS meant risking rejection due to a potential health threat—for Thomson had had a positive tuberculin test in her youth,[62] and "spots" on her lungs had been discovered on a chest X-ray in Canada in 1938.[63] In giving up her WMS position, she risked not being allowed to work with the LMS either.

In a letter to her mother written on 3 February 1940, Betty Thomson revealed some of her anxiety. Noting that the LMS secretary had requested both a "certificate of character" and a medical certificate, Betty worried that the LMS might reject her application based on her health history. Furthermore, according to Godfrey Gale, the LMS would "not formally acknowledge our engagement or approve of us marrying until we can prove the spots [on her chest X-ray] are harmless."[64] On 11 February 1940 Betty Thomson wrote to Mrs. Hugh Taylor at the Toronto head office with a proposal either to break the contract early ("this September half of my contract will be up") or to allow her to complete part of her three-year contract as a married woman:

> You will be surprised to see a second letter from me, so shortly after my first, but I am busily "scheming schemes" these days and want to tell you what they are [...] If it is felt at home that it is too soon for me to be released entirely [by the wedding date in September], would you consider allowing me to marry this Fall, and at the same time allow me to remain on full-time duty until next March? [That would] give the mission and hospital ample time to fill the vacancy on the staff which Miss Brodie's illness has necessitated.[65]

While social convention expected parental approval of the couple's engagement, exemplified by Betty Thomson's note, "We have dad's permission, of course," on a practical level it was not required. Conversely, the mission boards held authority not only over Thomson's employment, but by extension over her freedom to marry. Recognizing that the alternative was to delay the marriage until her WMS contract was completed, Thomson appealed to Ruth Taylor's sympathies as a family friend: "The world is so upset—and no one knows just what is around the corner for any of us that it seems a great pity to spend these next two years apart—when we might be together. I am sure we would both give better and happier service to our Chinese friends and patients if we had our own home to come to at the end of the day's work."[66]

Betty Thomson continued to look for ways to remedy her situation. She dispatched a letter to her mother in Toronto, asking to have their Toronto physician "Scottie" send a record of her last chest X-ray to Qilu immediately. At Qilu, her physician could compare the X-rays to see if there were any changes in the past two years. Noting that her Qilu physician was planning to send the most recent X-rays to the Peking Union Medical College in Beijing for a second opinion, Thomson exclaimed, "Isn't this a fine mess? Remember the stew I was in two years ago at this time? Please hurry 'Scottie' and the x-rays up."[67] The whole situation was exasperating to Thomson, who wrote, "After all, by marrying a missionary I am not leaving the Field at all [...] Especially since I'm not in [Henan]—and the [Qilu] hospital here don't [*sic*] care whether I'm single or married ... so why should [the LMS]??"[68]

Added to her anxiety about her future with the LMS was Betty Thomson's frustration at her job as Superintendent of the Operating Theatre at Qilu.

In a rare display of anger in a letter to her mother, she expressed resentment at one of the other missionary nurses at Qilu:

> I'm still superintending the nurses—and probably will all week again. Really Mother, it's just stupid—and I get so wild at Miss Evans for not doing it. I can hardly contain myself. She's been here for over *ten years*—knows all the departments—the language and the nurses, the customs, the tricks etc. and etc. And yet she leaves me to it all. [...] I've never met anyone who can antagonize me quicker.[69]

Finding herself in charge of operating theatres in two buildings within weeks of her arrival at Qilu was disquieting, and Betty Thomson directed her exasperation at Miss Evans whom Betty perceived as an experienced nurse who was unwilling to help:

> She takes no interest in anything except her own department—which is Hospital Supplies [...] The first morning when Miss Alderson was away I went to her for advice. She was handing out supplies—she stopped long enough to smile disinterestedly and say "I'm sorry, I'm afraid you'll have to figure that out yourself. I haven't time." Haven't time!! I have the O.R.'s—both buildings (116–118 patients) and all that goes with them on my inexperienced hands—while she hands out supplies. Honestly, I nearly committed murder![70]

According to Betty Thomson, Miss Evans was a rather formidable colleague—not only to her, but also to Miss Alderson and Miss Brodie who had "the same troubles with her." To Thomson, Miss Evans was "very attractive to look at when she's all dressed up—and nice, too. But when she gets into [her nursing] uniform—Wow!"[71] From Thomson's perspective, missionary work was a choice, not an obligation: "After all, I don't have to do this, anymore than she does." Putting up with cantankerous colleagues seemed a waste of precious energy. She consoled herself with the notion that Miss Evans was, as a single woman, pitiable: "However, poor thing, she hasn't got Godfrey—and I really pity her."[72]

Betty Thomson felt proud that she was able to "control" her temper despite feeling "consumed" and "burning up" with anger towards Miss Evans.[73] The following month she was even more relieved that she had held her tongue with Miss Evans. After "ten days of wordless warfare" between the two nurses, she approached Miss Evans and apologized for her feelings towards her:

> [I] asked her to please try to make a fresh start and also, to tell me what her reasons were for acting the way she had been. It wasn't all humble pie on

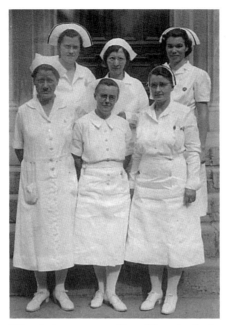

Fig. 3.4   Qilu missionary nurses (Betty Thomson, back row, right)

my part—because she had been to blame for most of it—and I told her so. And she said—to my utter surprise—that she thought *I* wanted the job [of O.R. Superintendent] and resented her interference!!! We just roared when we found out each other's feelings and thoughts.[74]

By May 1940 Betty Thomson had still not heard from the WMS. In the meantime the London office of the LMS requested a formal interview with her in order to approve her marriage to Godfrey Gale and subsequent transfer to the LMS mission. Annoyed and intimidated by the prospect, Betty admitted to her mother, "I'm kind of scared! What if they don't approve?? Godfrey was a bit mad—but they can't make exceptions for him naturally. *Do* you suppose they'll give me a Bible quizz [*sic*]?? Like in Tom Sawyer—('who were the first two disciples?' 'David and Goliath!')."[75] Until now, Thomson had never doubted her ability to meet the goals she set for herself. Now it seemed to her that her very future was on the line—and that it might take no more than a lack of Sunday school knowledge to thwart her desired course.

When Thomson finally obtained permission from the WMS to break her contract, she saw it as a cause for celebration. So did her father, who had recently arrived from Daokou. Andrew Thomson, Betty's "dearest, generousest" father, gave her a cheque for the exorbitant sum of one thousand dollars to "celebrate the good news of my release from the Mission."[76] To their credit, the WMS supported Betty Thomson's decision, acknowledging that the situation in China had changed since her initial commitment:

> It was felt by the [WMS] Executive that while the arrangement had been for three years, still the present upset condition in [Henan] has changed the situation entirely and we did not feel justified in asking Miss Thomson to complete her three years of service ... We are very sorry to lose Miss Thomson but, of course, our loss will be someone else's gain [i.e., the LMS] and she is not lost to Christian work in China.[77]

In the months leading up to the wedding, Betty Thomson and Godfrey Gale worked to prepare his home for her arrival. They celebrated Godfrey's twenty-seventh birthday by moving Coral Brodie's furniture into "our" house, and then planted artichokes in the garden. Because the North China Mission stations had closed, an Interim Committee comprised of Rev. G.K. and Mrs. King, Mr. and Mrs. Forbes, and Mr. Norman Knight moved to Jinan in May 1940 to await the outcome of the latest evacuation. In the meantime, Canadian missionary nurses Mary Boyd, Dorothy Boyd, Clara Preston, and Margaret Gay had been sent to Tianjin to work in the refugee camps. By springtime, Dorothy Boyd and Margaret Gay had been seconded to the West China Mission at Sichuan, while Mary Boyd was seconded to the Canadian Anglican mission just south of the Yellow River from the North China Mission—this small mission station was still in operation, with Canadian missionary nurse Susie Kelsey in charge of nursing services. Eventually Mary Boyd and Susie Kelsey would end up imprisoned together at the Weixian Camp—something they could not foresee when they started working together in early 1940.

Betty Thomson and Mary Boyd met up again at Beidaihe for the annual summer vacation in 1940. Much had changed since their idyllic summer the previous year; both were now engaged. Betty Thomson and Godfrey Gale had set their wedding date for 14 September; Mary Boyd and John Stanley had tentative plans to marry the following spring. Dr. Isabelle MacTavish hosted a wedding shower for Godfrey and Betty. Among the guests was eleven-year-old Mavis Knight, who helped bring in "a terrific pile of gifts."[78] Mavis (Knight) Weatherhead recalls Betty Thomson caring for her that summer when she was "floored with raging fevers and sore joints"—confirmed later in Beijing as rheumatic fever.[79] According to her recollection:

> Every morning I used to spike a fever of 104 or more. Then around 10 or so when the fever broke and I'd start to perspire, I'd call out to Mom that I was

"sprinkling." Then she was able to give me the daily bed bath. Mother came down with a severe ear infection and needed some nursing care [for] herself as well as for me. So Betty came to the rescue. I remember Betty saying I should pray that Mom's hearing would return because right then, she was quite deaf. Naughty kid that I was I just had to test out the truth of that statement. So when Mother turned to leave my room, I reamed off a few choice, and totally forbidden Chinese words. Yes—Mother was deaf all right. But if she had heard me, I would have received something extra with my morning bath![80]

For Betty Thomson, the summer was magical. At the shower, attended by women from the North China Mission and London Missionary Society, friends gave gifts of coffee sets and teacloths and table runners, along with gifts of music and poetry ("nearly everyone had written one—and they were a scream").[81] At one point Andrew Thomson, Godfrey Gale, Mary's fiancé John Stanley, and his father interrupted the women's party and sang a song about "Betty and her Gale." These experiences of creating community through song, drama, and art were central to the missionary experience, and would reappear in the internment camps.

A Jinan Wedding

Missionaries marrying in China underwent two ceremonies—a civil ceremony at the British Consulate in Tianjin, and a religious service at a church. Betty Thomson and Godfrey Gale's civil service was scheduled for 29 August 1940, and the church service for 14 September. The only member of Betty's family to attend would be her father, Andrew Thomson. Her mother and siblings shipped a wedding gift—a trunk filled with linens and clothing. Betty was overwhelmed by the letters and gifts that came pouring in. She was grateful for the attention of the missionary "ladies [who were] trying to make up for [her mother's] absence," but she missed her mother: "I'd give everything to have you here; there are so many things I'd like to talk to you about which are impossible by letter."[82] On the morning of 29 August, however, Betty Thomson became ill with a high fever and violent cramps; the civil service was cancelled. Although they were able to reschedule the service to 4 September, for Betty Thomson the civil service was incidental; it was the church service that mattered.

On the eve of her daughter's wedding, Margaret Thomson penned a letter stating, "You are so much in my thoughts today. As I write beside the fire it is just 8:20 pm and that means that it is almost 9 o'clock Saturday morning with you—and your wedding day has dawned!"[83] Although it would be weeks before Betty would receive the letter, it was important to Margaret to write precisely on the day of the wedding. As was the Thomson family tradition, Betty's mother's letter was a form of blessing extended to her daughter on a milestone day:

> A new life is beginning for you—a life which will be full of joy and richer than the old life—and I know that you will not only be happy yourself, but will do all you can to make the Chinese whom you will live among, happy— and how they do need friends who can give them the secret of lasting happiness. Tomorrow we are going to set the alarm at four o'clock so that we shall be awake and thinking of you while the ceremony is taking place. That will draw us closer and will be the next best thing to being with you in the flesh.[84]

On Saturday, 14 September 1940, at 5:00 p.m., Dr. Godfrey Livingstone Gale and Miss Elizabeth (Betty) Durie Thomson were married in the magnificent Kumler Memorial Chapel of Qilu University in Jinan, Shandong province. It was a grand event. According to newspaper reports, the church was laced with "dahlias shading from white through pink to deep red, with masses of pink asters and michaelmas daisies to give colour to the grey stone rail and steps."[85] Betty was dressed in a "charmingly simple gown of white georgette with high draped neck, long sleeves and a short train." Her maid of honour wore a floor-length dress of blue-green taffeta, while the two flower girls wore "high-waisted pink net" dresses with blue-green sashes. The men wore tuxedos; Godfrey Gale wore a top hat. Godfrey later wrote his new mother-in-law that her daughter "looked perfectly lovely in her wedding dress, so tall and straight and graceful, and that she carried off the whole ceremony and the reception with beautiful grace and charm. I never saw her look so beautiful."[86]

Betty Thomson's father conducted the service, with the participation of a number of prominent missionary men: Rev. H.P. Lair, Associate President of Qilu University, and Rev. Arnold Bryson of the London Missionary Society helped to conduct the service, and Rev. G.M. Ross of the Qilu School of Theology gave Betty away. Professor (later Sir) Stanley Prescott, President of Qilu Hospital, was the best man, and Mary Boyd was the maid of honour. In the absence of Margaret Thomson, Canadian missionary Margaret Struthers hosted the party. The wedding ceremony was captured on 8 mm film—an extravagance at the time. Were it not for the presence of traditionally clad Chinese, the black-and-white film footage captures what could easily pass for a European setting—with Western-style brick buildings, motor cars, tuxedos, silver settings and fine china, stained glass windows, and wedding cake. Although the war with Japan was escalating and many of the wedding guests were themselves exiles from their mission sta-

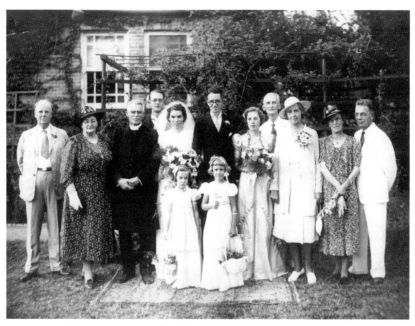

Fig. 3.5   Betty and Godfrey Gale's wedding, September 1940

tions, there is no evidence that anyone felt incongruence between the Gales' lifetime commitment to China's impoverished and sick, and an opulent Western wedding. Perhaps this wedding was an expression of hope for the future, not only for Betty Thomson, but for the many who poured their efforts into creating a dream-come-true wedding for a young woman whose mother and siblings were unable to attend. Perhaps it was a reflection of the high status of physicians and their wives. Or perhaps in the broader inter-war context, weddings of any kind were a welcome distraction and a place to pour one's anxious energy. Still, the image is striking. In the semi-colonized cosmopolitan cities of China, Western luxury and Chinese poverty had co-existed for half a century.

Betty Thomson's younger brother Murray, then eighteen, created a satiric two-page newsletter entitled "The Tsinan Tchit Tchat" that he dedicated to his sister's wedding. In a column with the caption "Kumlar Klue to Kalamity: Ancient Chapel Said Scene of Disaster Few Witnesses on Hand to View R.N. Tragedy," Murray Thomson wrote: "A gallant but gullible gal walked slowly to her doom here today led on by her unsuspecting father. She was a buxom belle from the beautiful smoke-filled city of Toronto in the far off Americas. She was a brother [sic] of the world recognized leader in wartology, M. McCheyne Thomson, her first name being Lizziedumb."[87]

Murray Thomson's newspaper is interesting on a number of levels. It provided a lighthearted medium to pass along family news, such as "Mother of Lizziedumb Reveals Qualities as Leader in Bible Soc. And wms." Additionally, it provided intimate insights into the lived experience of separation. For example, in an article entitled "Bost's Behavior Boorish: Honks Like a Madman but Speaks no Word," Murray described the behaviour of the church elder assigned to bring Mrs. Thomson and her children to church on Sundays in Toronto: "J.T. Bost, United Church Elder, continues to behave a beast as he picks up 'friends' with muttered grunts on way to church. Mrs. Margaret S. Sr. and Baby are usual victims and resentment is remarkable."[88] In this particular edition of "The Tsinan Tchit Tchat," Murray Thomson left two empty spaces for the rest of his family to send a message to the bride and groom. In one Betty Thomson's younger siblings wrote, in bold letters, "Howdy Dad!!! To the best dad in the world!" In the other they wrote, "Congratulations! Betty and Godfrey!! On Blessed Event # 1—Sept 14, 1940!!" They also teasingly added, "On Blessed Event # 2—July ?, 1941." One can imagine the giggling that went on with the second inscription. The cultural norms of sexual abstinence before marriage and of pregnancy soon after marriage were the subjects of whispered conversations, and therefore perfect fodder for sibling repartee. And, in the case of Betty Thomson Gale, they were very accurate: Margaret Mackay Gale was born ten months after the wedding, on 17 July 1941.

Summary

Gendered expectations for Canadian nurses were conflicting. On the one hand, young women were expected to be married and start families. On the other hand, nurses were expected to be both young and unmarried. Long-serving missionary nurses at the North China Mission were all unmarried.[89] In terms of marriage hopes, China offered more than Betty Thomson and Mary Boyd could imagine. Both Beijing and Beidaihe were rich beyond measure with social opportunities for missionaries. For Thomson and Boyd, Chinese language studies and nursing plans faded into the background as they came face to face with a wealth of potential suitors, settling remarkably quickly on two young men, both of whom were mishkids themselves. Godfrey Gale exceeded Margaret and Andrew Thomson's hope for their daughter: not only was he Christian and a missionary, he was also a gentle, intelligent, and refined young Englishman. To read Betty Thomson's letters from her first six months in China, one would not know that she was living in a country at war. Happily exiled at Beidaihe for the summer, she blocked out the reality of the war at their doorsteps, content to immerse herself into the joy of the moment. Or at least this is the image she portrayed in letters to her mother. From her diary it is clear that she kept abreast of the war news, joining Godfrey in his nightly habit of listening to the 9:15 p.m. news by radio.

To whatever extent Betty Thomson felt fearful of the drama unfolding in Henan and elsewhere in China and around the world, and of the resultant uncertainty about her nursing future, she did not reveal this in her letters. Whatever her expectations had been as a missionary nurse in China, it seems unlikely that she had expected quite as much fun, romance, and celebration as she experienced in her first sixteen months as a new missionary recruit. While she and the other mishkids provided some nursing service—Betty Thomson at Qilu, Dorothy Boyd at Tianjin, and Mary Boyd at Sanqui—Thomson's letters home suggest a preoccupation with a rich social life that blossomed around the edges of the war zone. Through her diary and letters we can trace the lives of some of the other mishkid nurses—especially Mary Boyd, Georgie Menzies Lewis, and Florence Mackenzie Liddell; by Betty's accounts their lives were unfolding in a similar, and intersecting, fashion.

Had Betty Thomson not been reared in China, and had her parents not faced innumerable crises as a direct result of their own missionary work, her relative inattention to the socio-political reality of China during this period might be interpreted as naïveté. Instead, given her later habit of focusing on the here and now as a strategy for survival, it is more likely that Thomson's emphasis on the social life in China in her letters to her mother reflected her awareness of what most interested—and frightened—her mother. As will become more apparent in the following chapters, Thomson emphasized in her writing gender norms expected of Christian women, but also embodied traits associated with masculinity. Like her father, she had a sense of daring confidence in her own assessment of, and solutions to, desperate situations. Although quite courageous and self-assured, she nevertheless exemplified conventional feminine traits displayed by her mother, including an ability to nurture a sense of family life that was not dependent on physical proximity, or even a shared physical space. It became Thomson's habit in China to internalize her fears—to push away thoughts of how the war, the Japanese, flooding, and communicable disease might directly affect her. Her ability to compartmentalize fears, make confident decisions, and create a sense of home in any setting would serve her well when the Japanese invasion finally penetrated the protected missionary enclave at Qilu in 1941.

Heeding and Ignoring Consular Advice
(1941)

"Accounts almost ready" is code for "situation critical, consul advises prepare to evacuate."

—Note in Andrew Thomson's diary, 1939,
in Murray Thomson, *A Daring Confidence*

Anno Domini 1941 was a watershed year for the mishkid nurses. For three
of them, Betty Thomson Gale, Mary Boyd Stanley, and Georgina Menzies
Lewis, it marked a year of both motherhood and internment—two events
that would remain central to their identities and experiences as missionary
nurses in China. It was also a watershed year in North China missionary
history. In January 1941 all six China mishkid nurses were still in China;
by May, three had evacuated. After the Japanese attack on Pearl Harbor in
December 1941 Betty Gale, Mary Stanley, and Georgina Lewis were placed
under house arrest, as was Canadian missionary nurse Susie Kelsey, with
whom Mary had worked in 1940.

Why did some Canadian nurses choose to evacuate China while others stayed? All had consular warning to leave; all had mission support to
travel back to Canada. None of the four who stayed was living or working
in the same community—each came to the decision to stay independently
of the others. This is a central question, yet it is difficult to pinpoint a common factor. One might presume, for example, that since three of the four
who stayed were mishkids this identity had the greatest bearing on their
decision. But this was not so: three of the missionary nurses who evacuated were also mishkids—that is, Dorothy Boyd, Jean Menzies Stockley,
and Florence Mackenzie Liddell. Or one might presume that being married to China missionaries might have influenced the decision since it was
only women and children who were evacuating. Again, not so: although five
of the six mishkid nurses were married to China missionaries, only Florence Liddell and Jean Stockley chose to evacuate with their children, leaving their husbands in China. Or perhaps it was the expectant mothers who
evacuated China? But in fact, Florence Liddell, Betty Gale, Mary Stanley,
and Georgina Lewis were all expecting babies in 1941, and the latter three

stayed. Finally, perhaps the decision was based on whether one had parents or other family living in China. Yet again, the results were mixed: Mary and Dorothy Boyd's parents were living in West China in 1941 but Dorothy left with her parents for Canada while Mary remained. Similarly, Jean and Georgina's mother Davina Menzies was living in China, yet Jean Stockley evacuated while Georgina Lewis stayed.

It appears then that while family ties to China weighed into the decision-making process, they were not predictive of the outcome. Ultimately the decision came down to the individual nurse—her character, her sense of well-being, and her belief in what was best for her and key persons in her life. Those who came to believe that their decision was based on what God was telling them to do found ways to accept the outcome—even if, as for Betty Gale, it meant four years of internment and her husband Godfrey's resultant illness and incapacitation; or, as for Florence Liddell, it meant four years of separation from her husband Eric before his tragic death at Weixian Camp.

As for Dorothy Boyd, the only single mishkid nurse as of 1941, as committed as she was to China missions, her ties to China had been severed with the 1939 closure of the North China Mission hospitals. While evacuation to Sichuan, to work at the United Church mission hospitals there, allowed her to continue the work she came to China for, neither she nor the other two North China Mission nurses who were seconded to West China were happy there. Not only was this the territory of other missionary nurses (who seemed to look upon their upcountry colleagues with snobbish disdain), it was also fully engaged with the war. Since Japan had already taken over northern China, the battles there had settled down. Not so in western China, where the next four years would be characterized by daily air raids and an increasing shortage of supplies. Eventually all three Canadian nurses at the West China mission, including Dorothy Boyd, would return to Canada.

What about Betty Gale, then? While her missionary upbringing and marriage factored largely in her decision to stay in Occupied China, there was one additional factor that set her apart from her peers: her father Andrew Thomson's decision to remain there, too. Although Andrew Thomson actually encouraged his daughter to evacuate, she had inherited his determination, stubborn confidence, and belief in the value of missions. Betty Gale wanted to be like her father in many ways, with one crucial exception: she did not want to rear *her* child in the absence of a father.

Wartime Conditions at Qilu Campus

Canadian missionaries who chose to work in Japanese-occupied China were aware at some level of the risk involved and already had acquired some useful skills. Andrew Thomson, for example, was well versed in the art of ciphered evacuation warnings as early as 1939. During this period North China missionaries used coded messages to relay information to and from the British consulates in Beijing and Tianjin. According to a memoir written by his son, Andrew Thomson recorded three of these in his diary:

"Accounts almost ready": Situation critical, consul advises prepare to evacuate.

"Paint available": Consul advises evacuate at once by rail.

"Enamel available": Look to your safety in the Chinese lines; danger of internment.[1]

In October 1940, in response to the escalating conflict between Japanese and Chinese troops, the Canadian Department of External Affairs issued an advisory for all Canadian women and children to evacuate from occupied regions of China. While aware of the evacuation order, Betty Gale's overriding consideration in the fall of 1940 was her new marriage.

Betty Gale was captivated by the man she had married. In a letter to her mother, written five days after their 14 September wedding, she wrote, "Oh Mother, its glorious being married to Godfrey! He's so super and considerate and loving, and a real Christian gentleman."[2] To Betty, Godfrey Gale was the embodiment of every important quality in a husband. When it came to religious sensitivities, she felt a sense of awe toward her husband: "I feel so far behind Godfrey spiritually, but hope with his help, to grow better each day."[3] The couple started their married lives together by incorporating religious practices: "We take turns with everything—with a reading and prayer—and it seems to give the right start to our day [...] I love to hear him pray—for he speaks [to God] as to a friend." To Betty Gale, her husband's name fit him very well: the name Godfrey, her Aunt Virginia told her, meant "at peace with God."

After a honeymoon at the oceanside city of Qingdao, Betty and Godfrey Gale returned to their missionary work at the Qilu Hospital. Betty's letters to her mother were still optimistic, including passages about the loveliness of their home. However, the excitement was tempered by a sense of foreboding. In an October 1940 letter Betty wrote, "Everything is topsy-turvy,"

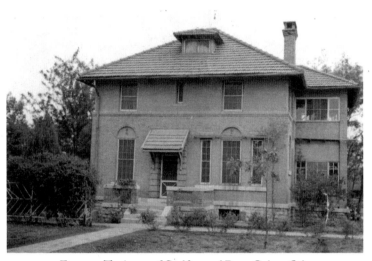

Fig. 4.1   The home of Godfrey and Betty Gale at Qilu

and yet, "I marvel at our peace."[4] In addition to the constant rumours of advancing Japanese armies were new rumours that the London Missionary Society was unable to send out any money from England to their missionaries due to war-related mail interruptions. Anticipating the worst, she wrote: "Godfrey and I made plans yesterday for what we think is bound to come."[5] Of most immediate concern was the potential lack of access to their mission salaries. The couple arranged for their salary cheques to be sent directly to Betty's mother in Canada to "store up for when we come home," to which she added, "(which may be very soon …)."[6] In the meantime, the Gales resolved to live "very economically" in China.

Despite the tightening restrictions at Qilu, Betty Gale still had a romanticized view of life in China, thinking of Jinan as "so perfect a place to live, and work, and have our children."[7] Although contraception was not a topic of conversation for polite society, her letters suggest that she and her husband were taking some measures to plan when their first child would be born—preferably October, "when we'd be safely back from [Beidaihe] and the weather would still be nice."[8] The good news came earlier than expected. On 25 December 1940—exactly a year to the day after writing her parents of her engagement—Betty was again writing her mother of a milestone event: "The next red-letter day will be July 21st 1941—and we don't care if it's a boy, girl, or twins!"[9] Betty was thrilled; at age thirty, she was already older than most first-time mothers of that era. She immediately set about plans for the child. If it was a girl, she would be named Margaret after both Godfrey's and Betty's mothers. Her middle name would be Mackay—the maiden name of Betty's mother.

This is not to say that Betty Gale had no reservations. To her friend Gwen Grimbly in Canada she wrote, "you are probably thinking, 'what a time, and place, to have a baby'!! And in some ways it isn't a very bright prospect for our little one. If we had deliberately planned for 'it'—we would be feeling a little conscious-stricken to-day, but we didn't and 'he' is coming in spite of us—so we feel that the whole matter has been taken out of our hands."[10] On the one hand, Betty turned to her faith to sustain her, writing, "if anyone should have faith and trust in God, it certainly should be I—for these last two and a half years have been just filled to the brim with happiness—and everything has seemed to be planned and prepared for me."[11] On the other hand, she was "afeerd" at the news of war, and at the prospect of staying in China, writing, "my faith wavers a bit, sometimes!"[12] Setting her anxieties aside, Betty determined to prepare for the new baby with joyous anticipation. "My only fear," she quipped, "is that he may not have red hair!"[13]

"Paint Available": Evacuation Orders

To Betty Gale, fear was an acceptable response to the growing threat of war, provided it was tempered by rational thinking and did not give way to hysteria. Her internal struggle is seen less in her cheery letters to her mother, than in a 5 February 1941 letter to Gwen Grimbly. Grimbly and her family lived across from the Thomsons' house at 33 Rose Park Drive in Toronto. The two women had been friends for a long time before Gwen, too, became a nurse.[14] In her letter Betty writes, "Gwennie, isn't the news horrible these days? I just feel heartsick for our English friends here—especially my husband."[15] The German *Luftwaffe* had begun bombing England on 7 September 1940, and for fifty-seven nights in a row there were air raids on London. The Blitz continued relentlessly for eight months on additional targets, including Birmingham, where Godfrey's mother and sister were living.

The missionaries at Qilu listened to international radio broadcasts for war news, something Betty Gale found increasingly difficult, knowing she was "able to do nothing."[16] Moreover, Godfrey Gale felt a sense of responsibility to his homeland. He was feeling "keener everyday" to return to England. Betty surmised that, if the Qilu mission were to close, Godfrey would be "off like an arrow from a bow."[17] It is unlikely that the prospect of going to England was very appealing to Betty, given the wartime conditions and her unfamiliarity with the country. However, she did write to Gwen: "I'd go, too, but they [the English officials] would not let me in."[18] It was, as she knew, a moot point: "Of course, we can't get away now, from this place," she wrote, "as ships [to England] are almost non-existent."[19]

Although there were passenger ships sailing across the Pacific and Atlantic, taking one was risky. The Gales knew, for example, that LMS physician Dr. Dorothy Galbraith had been aboard the *Western Prince* on 16 December 1940, en route from Canada to England, when it was torpedoed by a German U-boat in the Atlantic. Although sixteen lives were lost, Galbraith and 153 others were rescued at sea after five hours by British sailors—"a miracle beyond hope that we were found."[20] Sailing the high seas during wartime could be a perilous venture, something the Gales were keenly aware of when the time came for women and children to evacuate China.

On 3 February 1941 the North China Mission secretary Rev. G.K. King wrote a letter to the United Church of Canada Woman's Missionary Society describing the imminent departure of long-serving Canadian missionary Miss Margaret Brown. "She is quite perturbed over the growing tenseness of the political situation and has secured sailings for March," he wrote.[21] Upholding an accepted view of women as the weaker sex requiring protection, King believed that other missionary women should consider leaving, too. He dispatched messages to North China missionary nurses working in outlying regions, requesting that they head into the larger cities—like Jinan, Tianjin, or Beijing—where they would be less isolated and presumably safer. Anticipating possible evacuation from China, a number of missionaries left baggage in King's care in Tianjin, "to be forwarded to Canada in case the situation seemed ominous."[22]

Rev. G.K. King's concerns about missionary evacuation extended to Canadian women like Betty Gale who, although no longer employed by the mission, were still considered part of the North China Mission community. Without any clear direction from the United Church mission office in Canada, King felt that the onus of making a decision regarding evacuation was left on him, a role he resented. Although he would soon feel a greater sense of urgency to evacuate missionary women and children, in early February 1941 King guessed that "we may weather the storm—or at least that however threatening the weather appears, there is nothing so far to indicate that we must of necessity be engulfed."[23] A month later he changed his mind.

On 7 March 1941 King reported to the WMS secretary in Toronto that Betty Gale was booked on the "N.Y.K. Liner to Canada" via Kobe, Japan, to depart on 12 March.[24] Betty Gale had decided to evacuate.

Jean Stockley, the First to Leave

Although Betty Gale initially agreed to have a passage booked for her to return to Canada, she kept changing her mind. Her friend Florence Liddell was also trying to decide whether to leave China. At first, Betty concluded that she should return to Canada because it would be a safer place to deliver a baby. But she wasn't sure.

Married Canadian mishkids Jean Stockley, Florence Liddell, Georgina Lewis, and Mary Boyd (now Stanley) faced similar issues to Betty Gale when deciding whether or not to evacuate. Jean Stockley was the first to leave, sometime in early 1941. She had been living with her husband and children in Xian where they had been caring for twelve Chinese children—former pupils of the North China Mission school—who had fled Henan in 1939. By March 1941, Stockley and her children were reportedly living in the South of England. The United Church of Canada indicated: "We only hear occasionally now, but we trust and know He is able and faithful that hath promised, and will keep them."[25] Jean's husband, Dr. Handley Stockley, remained in Xian where, by 3 December 1941, he was reportedly still caring for the Chinese refugees whom he was reluctant to leave because they were so young and there was "no other plan for caring for them."[26]

While it is not clear whether Handley Stockley was placed under house arrest on 8 December 1941, he was still in China in February 1942, when he sent out a radiogram to his wife, Jean, informing her that all was well with him, with Jean's sister Georgina, and with their mother Davina Menzies. He also reported that Georgina Lewis had delivered a baby girl on 26 January 1942.[27] There is no record of Handley Stockley being interned. This suggests either that he escaped to West China—something that a number of people from Xian managed to do—or that, if he *was* placed under house arrest, he was among those repatriated in the summer of 1942.

Florence Liddell Goes Home

Florence Liddell was the next to leave China, in February 1941. She had been living in Tianjin the previous October when the Canadian Department of External Affairs issued a strong advisory for woman and children to leave Occupied China.[28] However, unlike the United Church of Canada mission board, the London Missionary Society for whom the Liddells worked was not requiring evacuation. The official LMS position was that "the present situation does not warrant any general withdrawal of LMS missionaries from North China."[29] The LMS recommended that missionaries maintain their present work "until conditions render this impossible."[30] Because the larger cities like Tianjin, Jinan, and Beijing were considered relatively safe, Florence Liddell and the children stayed at Tianjin while Eric worked at the LMS mission station in the more remote area of Xiaochang, his childhood home.

Within months, however, Eric Liddell and fellow LMS missionaries Ken and Frances McAll were eventually urged to leave Xiaochang by their Chinese colleagues, who "unanimously agreed" that local Japanese aggression against the Chinese was being aggravated by the presence of foreigners.[31] When Eric rejoined Florence in Tianjin, she gave him the news that she was expecting another child. Although they had decided to accept the LMS recommendation to stay in China, now the circumstances had changed. Betty Gale and Florence Liddell found themselves in similar situations: both were married to LMS missionaries who planned to stay in China, and both were in the early stages of pregnancy. They kept tabs on each other's deliberations. According to one of Eric Liddell's biographers: "Flo's best friend, Betty Thomson, was now back in China, married to Dr. Godfrey Gale and expecting her first baby in mid-summer. In February the Gales had requested passage for Betty, but later reconsidered. Betty packed and repacked three times before they finally decided they would stay together in China. Everyone balanced the difficulty of separation against the safety of those they loved most."[32]

To stay meant increased risk; to depart guaranteed loneliness. After weighing the alternatives, Florence and Eric Liddell decided she and their two daughters should return to Canada to live with her parents, who had recently gone on furlough in Toronto.[33] Eric, they trusted, would join them within the next year or two. Heather Liddell was only four years old when she left China with her mother. Sixty-six years later, her memories of the departure "are only baby memories of a loving, twinkly eyed nature mixed with a feeling of great loss."[34] To Heather, her mother was "my great heroine for all the wonderful happy childhood years she gave us even as she must have been suffering greatly."[35]

Dorothy Boyd Marries in Canada

Dorothy Boyd was working at the United Church of Canada West China Mission in Sichuan when she, too, was faced with the decision of whether or not to leave China. Unlike the other mishkid nurses, however, Boyd was not considered to be in danger. In fact she and other North China missionaries had been evacuated to West China precisely *because* it was perceived as a safe haven: nurses Clara Preston and Margaret Gay were there, as well as Boyd's parents, H.A. and Jessie Boyd. In reality, however, life in West China was exceptionally difficult. There were constant air raids by the Japanese, extreme supply shortages, and generally a low level of morale. By January 1941 all three North China nurses were struggling with their new appointment. According to a letter written by West China Mission Field Secretary Adelaide Harrison to the WMS headquarters in Toronto: "Misses Preston and Gay are finding our hospitals vastly different from [Henan …] Here after three and a half years of war, transportation difficulties, [and] soaring prices, our hospital supplies are almost down to rock bottom, which makes effective medical work, particularly in the nursing department, very difficult."[36] Margaret Gay and Dorothy Boyd tendered their resignations in the same month. On 6 May 1941, Dorothy Boyd wrote a letter to the Woman's Missionary Society stating: "For personal and family reasons I find that I shall have to put in my resignation to the WMS and go home in June when my parents sail. My father has already fixed [a] sailing date for me on the Pres. Coolidge leaving Hongkong on the 14th of June, and I have booked a seat on the CNAC plane leaving Chungking [Chongqing] on June 6."[37]

Dorothy Boyd's resignation came as a complete surprise to the WMS. She apologized for "spring[ing] this thing so suddenly" on the WMS but insisted, "I did not know myself until yesterday."[38] While it is possible that Boyd came to the decision to leave China quite hurriedly, she was not completely forthcoming with her employer. Within two months of returning to Canada, Dorothy Boyd married Canadian Phillip Johnston—holding the hasty ceremony in the Thomson family home at 33 Rose Park Drive in Toronto.[39]

Thus, within the first half of 1941, three mishkid nurses had decided to evacuate China—albeit for different reasons. For Jean Stockley and Florence Liddell, the well-being of their children seems to have been the primary reason. To these women, Canada represented safety, but choosing to leave meant becoming single mothers for the foreseeable future. It is little wonder that they deliberated for so long. In contrast, Dorothy Boyd made an apparently hasty decision to return to Canada. Unlike the married nurses, she did not have to consider the effect of her decision on a husband or children. However, unlike the married women, Boyd was expected to remain at her post, having been transferred to the "safe" part of China and still being under contract with the WMS. Perhaps this is why she was not completely honest about her reasons for leaving. It was more acceptable to suggest that her father had made the decision for her than to say plainly that she wanted to return home to a boyfriend. Betty Gale, Mary Stanley, and Georgina Lewis had no such pressure. Having already resigned from the WMS, they were free to decide for themselves what to do.

Left Behind: Decisions to Remain in China

When Betty Gale cancelled her sailing on a ship destined for Canada in February 1941, she knew that Florence Liddell had decided to return, and she likely also knew that Mary Stanley and Georgina Lewis had decided to stay. Mary Stanley's new in-laws worked at Qilu, and Betty Gale mentioned them frequently in her diary; she would often visit the Stanleys for lunch. Georgina Lewis would often visit Qilu, and Betty Gale knew that Georgina had just given birth.

Despite living in separate regions under different missions, the mishkid nurses kept fairly close tabs on each other. Although Mary Stanley, Georgina Lewis, and Betty Gale came independently to their decisions to stay in China, as will be seen, each had the counsel of older missionary relatives, and each was influenced by what she thought would be best for her young family.

Mary Boyd's Hasty Wedding

Mary Stanley and her husband, John, and son were living with some of John's relatives, the Wilders, in Beijing in the summer of 1941 with vague plans to return to the United States on a repatriation ship. Mary Stanley had just given birth to their son, Charles Alfred, in June 1941, and they hoped to return to the US with the Wilders. A lot had happened in Mary Stanley's life in the previous year: she had worked at St. Paul's Hospital at Sanqui with Canadian nurse Susie Kelsey, spent the summer recovering from typhus, been the maid of honour at Betty Gale's wedding at Tianjin, returned to work at Sanqui, evacuated to Beijing, married John Stanley, moved in with John's aunt and uncle, and had a baby. Like her sister Dorothy Boyd, Mary had moved from Qilu to Tianjin to work with refugees before being seconded to another Canadian mission hospital. Unlike Dorothy, however, Mary was not deemed suitable for the work in West China. First of all, she was engaged, meaning that her days with the United Church Woman's Missionary Society were limited. Second, G.K. King did not have a high opinion of her suitability. Noting that Mary was "temporary, engaged, and not looking forward to remaining with us," King suggested that Mary was not well suited for work in West China.[40] In his opinion, the most urgent need in West China was someone to head up the training schools for Chinese nurses. Her "lack of language, lack of local experience and her future plans and prospects," King wrote, "do not qualify Miss M. Boyd to undertake such work."[41] For her part, Mary Boyd was quite prepared to complete her three-year contract with the WMS at St. Paul's Hospital in Sanqui.[42]

In the fall of 1940, after having attended Betty and Godfrey Gale's wedding in mid-September, Mary Boyd described feeling "much more at home [at St. Paul's] than I did last spring: I knew the Hospital and the nurse and hoped to really contribute to the work of the church there this coming year."[43] Although the evidence suggests that Mary Boyd was more admired for her beauty than her nursing ability,[44] she nonetheless proved herself capable at Sanqui:

This fall [Susie Kelsey] as usual took in a new class of students: She hoped for a class of ten but in the end only two of the applicants met the requirements. However, two take as much teaching as ten. Miss Kelsey asked me to undertake the teaching of Practical Nursing and Snglish [sic] with this new class, thus leaving her time for classes with the more advanced students. Also, I was responsible in the Operating Room and Out Patients Clinic on alternate days, again leaving Miss Kelsey more time for the administrative work and the hundred and one other important things a Nursing Superintendent has to deal with in her daily round of duties.[45]

Mary Boyd had been back at St. Paul's for just a few months when G.K. King sent word to evacuate Henan. According to Boyd, she had been anticipating the advisory. When she received G.K. King's letter indicating that "the British Consul would like us to prepare to leave at once," Boyd had some difficulty deciding where to go. King advised that she head to Tianjin, Beijing, or Jinan.[46] Because her fiancé, John Stanley, was planning to stay at Beijing, she "naturally felt a pull North, too."[47] Boyd thought that, before making any definite plans, she should travel to Beijing to talk things over with John. Deciding it was "no time in the world's history [for them] to become widely separated and lead separate lives," she immediately tendered her resignation from the WMS.[48] Four days later Betty Gale received an invitation to Mary and John's wedding. The couple, it seems, was expecting a baby.

After two weeks of preparation, Mary Boyd wed John Stanley on 30 November 1940. Because of the short notice, none of Boyd's family was able to attend.[49] Betty Gale was her bridesmaid. John Stanley's father performed the wedding ceremony and Rev. Andrew Thomson gave the bride away. "Needless to say," Mary later wrote, "it was a very simple wedding."[50]

After the hastily arranged wedding, Mary Stanley wrote a letter of explanation to the WMS for her sudden resignation. Without giving any hint of her pregnancy, she wrote: "Apart neither of us were [sic] or could do our best work under the present uncertainties, and therefore were not being fair to our work, to each other, or to ourselves. Therefore the thing to do was to get married right away if at all possible and try to work things out together."[51] In the letter, she noted that she did not feel guilty about breaking her contract. Suggesting that she would have "felt more worried about that part" had the situation in China not been so unsettled, she reasoned that since "everyone more or less [was] uncertain about the future" she had legitimate grounds to resign.[52] Seven months later, Charles Alfred Stanley was born on 29 June 1941.[53]

It is difficult to overestimate the shame associated with unmarried pregnancy for women during this period of Canadian history—and not only for

missionary women, whose religious beliefs formed the core of their professional and personal identity, but for Canadian women in general. The social implications of a breach of societal sexual norms is exemplified in the
decisions of Canadian nurse Jean Ewen, who accompanied the famous Dr.
Norman Bethune to China in 1938. During her lifetime, Jean Ewen never
publically revealed the likely reason for her decision to depart China in
the summer of 1939: she was in the late stages of pregnancy. In September
1939, in Toronto, Ewen inexplicably married her brothers' friend—a man
she had just met. It was close to the time of her daughter's birth (that same
month), and it left unanswered questions and intriguing gaps in her various
memoirs about this period of her life.[54] Later, as journalists and historians
interested in the life and death of Norman Bethune plied Jean Ewen for
descriptions of her work in China, Ewen complied, but she kept any hint of
a China pregnancy carefully hidden from the public record.

Given the highly sensitive nature of such sexual "transgressions" at the
time, it would be unlikely that the written record would include any direct
reference to Mary Boyd's pregnancy as the reason for her hasty wedding.
Indeed, although the primary documents confirm the dates (and therefore
the timing) of the wedding and birth and supply general innuendoes, none
directly mentions the pregnancy itself. The matter of Mary Boyd's pregnancy is intriguing, not because it is surprising that a young couple (even
a "virtuous Christian" couple) would have sexual relations but because, if
Mary *was* pregnant, then the subsequent veil of silence that surrounded the
pregnancy provides some insight into the nature of the missionary commu-
nity-*as*-family. Just as Jean Ewen's brothers colluded to protect her honour
by helping to arrange her marriage to their American friend (a fellow vet-
eran of the Spanish Civil War), Mary Boyd's missionary community colluded to protect her honour by swiftly arranging a wedding complete with
all the sacred, legal, and familial angles covered. In so doing, they provided
an alternate, socially acceptable script to explain the hastiness of the nup-
tials. If Jean Ewen's pregnancy threatened to bring shame on her immediate
family, Mary Boyd's pregnancy—especially given that the father was *also* a
mishkid—threatened to bring shame on the China missionary community
as a whole. By the time Mary had given birth to a perfectly healthy baby
boy, the moral crisis had passed.

Mary Boyd Stanley: "We Didn't Guess Right"

After their marriage in November 1940, Mary and John Stanley committed
to stay in Beijing long enough for John to complete PhD studies at Yenching University. They recognized that any plans must be tentative. "If the

situation becomes so critical that we have to leave," Mary wrote, "I suppose [we will be in Canada] sooner. We must both have China blood right in us, I think, and are happy to live and work here in China, with the language and with the people as long as we can."[55]

Born Charles Johnson ("John") Stanley, John Stanley came from a long line of China missionaries. His great grandparents Charles Alfred and Ursula Stanley were among the first American missionary families to arrive in northern China, in 1862.[56] His father, Charles Alfred Stanley, was the Dean of the Theological School at Qilu.[57] John and Mary's son, Charles Alfred Stanley, then, was the fourth generation of "Charles Stanleys" to live on Chinese soil. Having decided to have their baby in China, Mary and John were living in Beijing in the summer of 1941 with John's Aunt Gertrude and Uncle George Wilders. After the birth, they decided to try to evacuate. According to a letter penned by Gertrude Wilders on 9 August 1941, they all "signed up for the next transportation of U.S. citizens, but have not much idea of when that will be."[58] They had vague plans to return to the United States together.

By November 1941 the Wilders and Stanleys were still in China; George Wilder was reluctant to leave. When a cable came from their mission board on 1 November 1941 "advising all who do not expect to stay thru, come what may, to leave at once," George Wilder was unmoved.[59] Although he did not desire to find himself in the middle of a warzone if the Japanese military advanced towards Beijing, neither did he want to leave prematurely. As he put it, he was "keenly aware" of "what serious results to our work and native colleagues might follow the departure of all missionaries from this compound, and we hesitate to take such a step until absolutely necessary, [even] when it may be too late to catch that last boat."[60] "Tomorrow," wrote George Wilder, "is in God's hands."[61]

By December 1941 Mary Stanley was expecting her second child.[62] On 7 December 1941 Gertrude Wilder wrote a letter stating, "Our hopes are that the worst is *not* going to happen and that it won't be too long before these very abnormal conditions begin to change. Of course they may worsen. A good many people think that nothing but a good drubbing will solve the situation out here."[63] George Wilder added, "The Consul General sends us an express letter saying there is a chance to sail in a few days for any who still contemplate evacuating. We are still unmoved and hope you do not worry too much."[64] The next day the Wilders and Stanleys were placed under house arrest in Beijing. Gertrude Wilder added a postscript to her 7 December letter: "They [the Japanese military] certainly were quick in the uptake. Pretty alert action, whatever one may say about their way of looking at things. We didn't guess right."[65]

Georgina Lewis: "Women Complying with Evacuation Order"

Two years after her marriage to Dr. John Lewis in 1939, Canadian missionary nurse Georgina Lewis was still very much connected to the North China mission that had employed her for seven years. Georgina was included in periodic reports on the movements of Henan missionaries. For example, on 7 March 1941, G.K. King noted that Davina Menzies was visiting her daughter at Chou T'sun, approximately two and a half hours by train from Jinan, following the birth of their son.[66] Perhaps this message had less to do with Georgina than her mother; Davina Menzies was a difficult person to keep track of.

On 13 March 1941 the Acting Under-Secretary of State for the Canadian Department of External Affairs in Ottawa acknowledged receipt of the following cable from the "Superintendent" of the North China Mission: "Women complying with evacuation order. Two men remaining in Cheeloo [Qilu]. Two waiting tentatively."[67] The two men remaining in Qilu were Andrew Thomson and D.K. Faris. The two waiting tentatively were G.K. King and R. Gordon Struthers. The rest of the cable, however, was incorrect: there were actually two WMS missionaries who were *not* complying with the evacuation order; one was Dr. Isabelle MacTavish,[68] and the other was Davina Menzies—who was ignoring urgings from the mission to leave. Seven months later G.K. King reported that he "just learned" that Davina Menzies planned to leave Shanghai on 6 October for Canada.[69] He was mistaken. Davina Menzies was again in Chou T'sun helping her daughter Georgina, who was now five months pregnant with her second child.[70] On 3 December G.K. King noted that Davina Menzies was "now in [Jinan] and is making no plans to move."[71] Furthermore, Georgina Lewis was expected to join her mother in Jinan later that week. Georgina was coming to consult professionally with friends, and to make arrangements for a visit with Dr. Gells, the specialist who had delivered her firstborn and was intending to deliver the second. But Georgina never made it to Jinan. Within four days of King's letter, the Japanese attacked Pearl Harbor and the missionaries were placed under house arrest. As it was, Georgina and John Lewis's second child Margaret Ann was born in internment, on 26 January 1942.

Betty Gale: "She Refused to Return"

Betty Gale proved as difficult to trace as Davina Menzies. On 7 March 1941 G.K. King reported that Betty Gale was planning to return to Canada from Kobe, Japan, on 12 March on the "N.Y.K Liner" back to North America.[72]

Betty's mother wrote a letter addressed to Andrew and Godfrey on 30 March exclaiming that "the big excitement [this week] was [the news] that Elizabeth is probably coming home in April. I know she will not come if conditions improve before they sail, but it is hardly likely that they will [improve] so soon as that. We shall be delighted to have her here of course, and to have a wee baby in this home again will be too wonderful for words."[73]

The following week Margaret Thomson wrote, "We are still wondering whether you are on the ocean, Elizabeth. No more letters have come from either you or Dad, but we think as so many others have said you were coming, that you must really be on the way. We are counting your landing in [Vancouver] on the 16th, and already we are planning for a [Henan] gathering here on the 25th, as Mrs. Leslie is coming to the city at that time and will be our guest."[74] The confusion continued when an April 1941 United Church mission report noted that "Mrs. G.L. Gale (nee Miss Elisabeth Thomson) and Miss Margaret Brown and Mrs. D.K. Faris reached Canada early this month."[75] The reports were wrong; Betty Gale was still at Qilu.

Betty Gale's diary entries between February 19 and 28 trace her momentous decision to stay in China:

> February 19: Messrs Knight, King and Struthers arrived today. They bring word that Can. Women and children are ordered home.
>
> February 20: Godf and Dad want me to go back to Canada—for "George's" [her unborn baby's] sake ... I could just *die* at the thought. Whatever shall I do? Matter now in Norman Knight's hands.
>
> February 21: Waiting to hear verdict. Visited folks for "advice." Still in a quandary.
>
> February 23: John Menzies Lewis born to-day! 6 lbs.
>
> February 24: Word from Don Faris. I have [a ship passage] booking for the 12th of March.
>
> February 25: Packed all day. Still dithering—to go—or not to go? That is the question!!
>
> February 26: To Stanleys for lunch. Have decided for myself—*not* to go!
>
> February 28: Miss Robins has my passage ... so my "bridges" are burned![76]

From her diary it is clear that Betty Gale sought out the advice of others, considered the implications of her decision on her unborn child, desired to respect the authority of the North China missionaries (despite no longer being under its auspices), and kept tabs of both Mary Stanley (via her in-laws) and Georgina Lewis (who gave birth at Qilu, by caesarean section). Most significantly, her diary demonstrates that she saw this as *her* decision to make. Years after her internment, Gale spoke to a friend about her pivotal decision to stay in China. Her friend's recollection of the discussion corresponds well with the diary entries:

> We were talking about the need for prayer and how God does answer prayer if we are open to His response. Betty said that her father definitely wanted her to go back to Canada where she would be safe and he had arranged for her travel. She started to pack her trunk but felt uneasy about leaving Godfrey. She unpacked and then started packing again etc. She was really confused and torn. Then that night, she decided to hand it over to God in prayer. She told Him that she could no longer see clearly what to do and left it in His hands. Betty said that when she woke up the next morning she was no longer confused and just knew that she should stay [...] so she unpacked her trunk. She also added that when Godfrey got so sick [with dysentery and later tuberculosis], she [felt] that he would not have lived if she hadn't been there to care for him. She knew that was why God had led her to stay in China.[77]

Two others later had similar recollections of Betty Gale's decision. Frances McAll, with whom Betty Gale was interned for four years, recalled that "after packing and unpacking, [Betty] reached the same decision [as me] and we decided then to stick together as far as possible for the mutual support we were going to need and for the sake of the babies we were both expecting."[78] Finally, according to Godfrey Gale, Betty simply "put her foot down and refused to return to Canada."[79]

Frances McAll would become a significant and lifelong friend of Betty Gale. Indeed, the McAlls and the Gales would develop a unique and enduring friendship, sharing parenthood and sleeping quarters through years of internment at three different camps between 1942 and 1945. Betty Gale met Ken McAll the same night she met Godfrey, in 1937 at Beidaihe. Godfrey and Ken were old friends "from school days" and had arrived together from England in 1937, the year of Japan's invasion of northern China.[80] After the requisite six months of language training in Beijing, Ken was sent to Xiaochang with fellow London Missionary Society colleague Eric Liddell, while Godfrey was posted to Jinan. Frances joined Ken two years later. They had met as medical students in Edinburgh. Frances had always wanted to be a missionary physician; she and Ken committed to work together in China as a medical missionary team after Frances graduated in 1939. Following a harrowing journey from Scotland (which included being stranded in India for six weeks and narrowly surviving a typhoon at sea), Frances arrived in Beijing in late 1939 to start language training. She and Ken married in Beijing in June 1940 before travelling together to Xiaochang to start their long-anticipated shared vocation. Their work was cut short when, in March 1941, the Xiaochang mission closed under pressure of the occupying Japanese. Frances was three months pregnant when they made what they thought would be a temporary move to Qilu, where they had been appointed medical officers to the staff and students of Shandong University—Ken for the men, and Frances for the women.[81] They were provided a small house to live in next door to the Gales. It was furnished with the basic necessities—they had left an elaborately furnished home behind at Xiaochang.[82] Recalling the early stage of her friendship with Betty at Qilu, Frances later noted, "Betty was older than I and much more experienced in the art of housekeeping. Her support over the next few months was something I could hardly have done without, though she actually had a way of supporting everyone within range. We were to get to know each other better than any of us suspected in those early days."[83]

Revised Expectations

On 7 April 1941 Margaret Thomson received word that her daughter was *not* coming back to Canada after all. She wrote Betty of her disappointment, but also quickly adapted her response to show support: "Two letters from Eliz. with the enclosed one from Godfrey, have just come, so our hopes are dashed to the ground! But I am very glad for *both* your sakes that you are not to be separated. It would have been very hard on you both."[84] Margaret Thomson, who knew the strain of separation from one's husband firsthand, took solace in the fact that at least her daughter would not be alone. In a letter written the next day, she recalled, "It was most interesting to see how the center of life has shifted for you, and I am so happy that it has. You remember how hard you found it to [say] good-bye the night you left Toronto. My heart ached for you that night and it was so hard to see you go off so alone. Yet after two years when the opportunity was given you to come back to the old home, you choose rather to remain in the new home. Life is strange, and it is wonderful how we mortals do change, and how a person who we have known a short time becomes more to us than the family we have lived in all our lives."[85] While putting on a brave front for her daughter, she was also a bit envious: with her husband still in China, it was Margaret Thomson who would face the war alone.

Although originally intended as a welcome back party for her daughter, Margaret Thomson decided to go ahead with the Henan Party planned for 25 April 1941. There were a number of Henan missionaries, including five who had just returned from China: Norman and Violet Knight,

Dr. and Mrs. Ross, and Margaret Brown—who all gave speeches about their experiences in Occupied China. Altogether the party was comprised of thirty-three adults and three children, all of them current or retired North China missionaries. Because people had heard reports that Betty Gale had returned home, Margaret Thomson found herself explaining and defending Betty's choice to stay: "Most people, while feeling sorry that they are not to see you, feel glad that you do not have to leave Godfrey."[86] Betty felt the same way. On 11 May she wrote her mother-in-law in England that she felt "so thankful I didn't leave last February" because she was enjoying her marriage to Godfrey.[87]

On 25 May 1941 Margaret Thomson wrote a birthday greeting to her daughter. "Remember how I used to say that I wanted you to live with me when I grew old? And now you are the daughter who is farthest from me. Yet I would not have it otherwise, for as Father said to me, 'what is best for you is best for me.' [...] May the dear baby be as great a comfort to you as you have been to me."[88] The tone of this letter is one of loneliness and resignation—a feeling of estrangement that was far from over.

On 3 July 1941 Betty Gale wrote her mother-in-law, "We are patiently waiting for our Big Event [the birth of their baby]—and find it a bit slow sometimes, as it is very hot. The average temperature of the last two of these three weeks has been 103 degrees [...] so we aren't exactly peppy."[89] Although missionaries would normally travel to Beidaihe to escape the summer heat, Betty's pregnancy kept the Gales close by medical care at Qilu. The "summer exodus" of the missionaries from Qilu meant that the Campus was becoming "more deserted every day."[90] Betty kept herself occupied by walking in the evenings with Frances McAll. Their due dates were so close that they were not sure who would "come off first."[91]

Both Betty's and Godfrey Gale's mothers were anxious for news about the arrival of their grandchild. On 9 July 1941 Margaret Thomson wrote: "We are expecting the cablegram very soon with the news of the arrival of—Jeremy John?"[92] Compared to the relatively stable life for Betty's family in Canada, life for Godfrey's family in England was difficult. Betty and Godfrey would receive reports of the air raids in Birmingham and, while they were "so thankful" that his family "escaped all harm," they worried.[93] Compared to England, even life in China seemed rather serene. As Betty wrote her mother-in-law: "Sometimes it doesn't seem right that we should be so peaceful here while you are going through such dreadful times."[94] Little wonder the London Missionary Society was disinclined to have their missionaries evacuate China—in some respects it was safer than England. Perhaps sensing a need for happy news, Betty informed her mother-in-law that, if they had a boy, his middle name would be Kendall, after Godfrey's father.

For both Betty Gale and her mother, letters to and from China had been a mainstay of their relationship. However, as mail service became increasingly disrupted and unreliable in 1941, Margaret Thomson turned to an alternative route to send messages to her daughter—through a radio broadcast out of California that could reach China. The broadcaster would read out messages that families sent to them by mail. The radio messages reached Jinan, but because the broadcasts occurred "at such a late hour" in China, a designated person would stay up to listen and pass the messages along.[95]

In the summer of 1941 Margaret Thomson kept Betty abreast of news of her friends Florence Liddell and Dorothy Boyd, both now living in Toronto. Florence Liddell, who was staying with her parents, would come to the Thomson home for tea. In July 1941 Margaret wrote with the scandalous news that Dorothy Boyd was in Toronto and planned to be married "as soon as her parents arrive."[96] Margaret made it clear that she did not support Dorothy's decision to quit China: not only had Dorothy reneged on her contract with the WMS, but doing so to marry a Canadian who had just enlisted in the military was both dishonourable and unnecessary:

> I am always sorry to hear of these war weddings, for it means a long separation, and the men go to such a different life that they will have very different ideas about most things when they meet again. I do hope Dot will be happy—it is a pity she did not complete her three-year contract. In the case of Mary and you, Elizabeth, it is different because you are both working still in China even though you are not under our Mission. It leaves a rather bad impression and I fear Dot may have a feeling of not having done the right thing, and it certainly will make the Ladies [of the WMS] hesitate to send any more girls out on short terms.[97]

Margaret Thomson did not find any redemptive qualities in Dorothy Boyd's plan. While her disapproval did not keep her from offering her home for the wedding, it did keep her from attending it.

Dorothy Boyd and Phillip Johnston were married in the living room of the Thomson family home at 33 Rose Park Drive. Margaret Thomson and her youngest daughter, Muriel, took a three-week vacation at a friend's home in nearby Haliburton. According to Margaret, "the Boyds came into this house when they reached [Toronto], and then when Dorothy's wedding was decided on so hurriedly, they had it here in the Living room … The Boyds were very grateful for the use of the house … When I came home I found such a beautiful purse and pair of gloves (all navy blue) that she had got for me [as a thank you]."[98] Margaret Thomson was delighted with the gloves, but felt sympathetic towards Mrs. Boyd. This all affirmed Margaret's growing conviction that *her* daughter had made the right decision by staying in China.

The Arrival of Margie

Shortly after Dorothy Boyd's wedding, Margaret Thomson received the cable she was waiting for. A baby girl, Margaret ("Margie") MacKay Gale, had been born to Betty and Godfrey on 17 July 1941. Betty, who had been anaesthetized with "a few whiffs of chloroform" during childbirth, awakened at 7:00 p.m. to the sound of "Margaret's powerful shouts resounding through the room!"[99] Margaret Thomson was delighted with her namesake: "We keep wondering about the wee girlie out in [Jinan] and longing to see her […] Dear me, it is quite a long line of Margarets. This is the fourth—I do not know for whom my mother was named or whether there was another Margaret before her."[100] In her diary Betty wrote, "Margaret is adorable. Very tired, but in the clouds!!"[101] In her journal she wrote, "She is here! Our beautiful little Margaret—a new heaven and a new earth opens for G. and me today."[102]

After two weeks in postpartum confinement at the Qilu Hospital, Betty took Margaret home in a rickshaw, accompanied by Canadian missionary Dr. R.G. Struthers on a bicycle. Waiting for them at home was Changta Sao, the amah they had secured to help care for Margaret, and Lan t'ing, the cook, "in their best clothes, beaming at us from the doorway. The furniture is shining, and the floors, flowers on the tables, curtains blowing in the breeze. Oh, it's good to be home!"[103] Betty was completely enraptured by her daughter, who had "beautiful clear grey eyes with long lashes; a cute nose and mouth—and a small pointed chin—or rather, two chins at present!"[104]

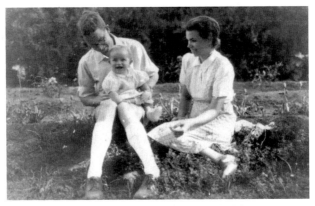

Fig. 4.2   Godfrey and Betty Gale with baby Margie, 1941

Ken and Frances McAll's baby, Elizabeth ("Eli") Joyce, arrived eleven days after Margaret—on 28 July 1941. "Changta Sao will be pleased to hear that their baby is *not* a boy," Betty wrote in her journal: "That would have been a fearful 'loss of face' for her, if M[cAll]'s had a boy—while we 'only' had a girl!"[105] On the day of Eli's birth, the Japanese froze all American and British assets in the country.[106]

"Drawing Near to the Edge of the Precipice"

Godfrey Gale had been expecting the United States and Britain to be drawn into a war with Japan since July 1941 when they had declared an oil embargo against Japan.[107] As he later recalled, "The British government had given us at least two definite warnings, when women and children and any men without definite work to do were urged to get away from occupied China."[108] During the anxious months leading up to Pearl Harbor, the missionaries at Qilu speculated about how the inevitable American or British declaration of war against Japan would affect them. Canadian missionaries had heard of atrocities committed by the Japanese in China, perhaps the best known of which was the "Rape of Nanking," when the Japanese military raped, looted, and executed civilians in the weeks following their occupation of Nanjing in late 1937. Canadian missionaries were familiar with the Japanese reputation for being ruthless and dangerous.

By 1941 the Gales and the McAlls had become keenly interested in the movements of the Japanese military. Missionaries could keep abreast of military activity via radio broadcasts, newspaper reports, and eyewitness accounts by missionaries and other expatriates all over China. Frances McAll recalled listening daily to a news broadcast "put out by an American broadcaster sponsored by Maxwell House coffee whose verbal offensive against Japan forced him to have to wear a bullet-proof vest."[109] "We often wondered," Frances added wryly, "just what was his life expectancy."[110] In Beijing Rev. G.K. King reported that "the Jap[anese] Troops' treatment of the civilian population was so bad that [the eyewitness] did not dare describe it lest he get someone in trouble through the censor."[111]

In addition to radio broadcasts, missionaries had access to the *North China Herald*, an English-language newspaper. From the beginning of the Sino-Japanese War in 1937, the *North China Herald* regularly reported updates on the whereabouts of Japanese and Chinese military forces, including which cities were held by which forces at particular times. For example, on 9 November 1938 the newspaper published a map of operations in China, noting that, since the last military operations map was published, "Japanese forces have captured Hsuchofu and reached the [Beijing-Hankou] Railway, and in the Yangtze they have occupied [Hankou], General Chiang Kai-shek withdrawing his troops from the Wuhan area west and southwest."[112] Missionaries, who were ostensibly neutral in matters of war, silently observed the increasingly aggressive tactics of the Japanese in acquiring Chinese territory. Although some expatriates accepted Japan's insistence that their motive was to improve the Chinese economy, by 1941 even these supporters voiced doubt at Japan's ability to "restore China to its former prosperity."[113]

Occasionally missionaries would send in special reports of their own to the *North China Herald*. In an article published on 5 February 1941, an anonymous "special writer" noted that, while "certain foreign business circles" would have "hailed with considerable satisfaction" the success of Japanese efforts in China, their failure was inevitable because of a "fault in the Japanese character"—namely, their attitude of superiority towards the Chinese.[114] Although missionaries were "neutral," some felt a sense of moral obligation to join Chinese in their "secret and passive resistance" against the Japanese.[115] In Frances McAll's words, "the Chinese in the occupied areas of China were unable to voice their opposition to the Japanese but it was clear that amongst thousands of foreigners in the country anti-Japanese feeling was mounting."[116] Ominously, on 19 February 1941, the *North China Herald* reported that "the only logical choice" for Japan would be to "go forward" in its quest for "supremacy in the Pacific."[117]

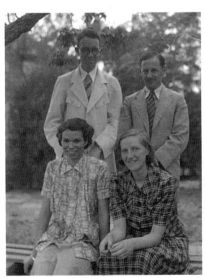

Fig. 4.3 Godfrey and Betty Gale (on left)
with Keith Graham and Frances McAll, at Qilu

Although "things seem[ed] very peaceful" for the Gales at Qilu in the fall of 1941, there was a sense among the missionaries that something was changing.[118] For one thing, the Japanese military was becoming increasingly restrictive of their movements. Although travel restrictions had been in place since 1 June 1941, when the Japanese army required foreigners to apply for Japanese-issued permits to travel around North China, now foreigners were being asked to obtain passes to move *within* Jinan itself.[119] "Really," Betty Gale complained to her mother-in-law, "the thought of walking on this earth without a pass, and a passport, and cholera vaccination certificates seems Heaven-like in itself."[120] Some Qilu wag composed a song about the new restrictions, to be sung to the tune of the African American spiritual "Ah got shoes, you got shoes, all God's children got shoes":

> Ah got a pass, you got a pass—
> All God's children got a pass—
> But when Ah gets to Hebben,
> Goin' to tear up dat pass
> And walk all ober God's Hebben.[121]

Back in Toronto Betty Gale's mother was somewhat aware of the tightening restrictions in China, not only because some of the weekly letters were not getting through, but also because of news from other missionaries. A letter from Eric Liddell to his wife Florence, for example, stated that he was "doubtful that Godfrey and Betty would get to [Beidaihe] as only those who had passes might travel on the trains."[122]

Margaret Thomson kept in close contact with Florence Liddell, updating Betty though chatty letters. When Florence delivered her third daughter, Nancy Maureen, on 17 September 1941 in Toronto, Margaret wrote to Betty about the response of Patricia Liddell, the oldest daughter. Patricia "was disappointed at first that the baby was a girl, but in her prayer one night last week she said 'And it is all right God that it is a girl' and the next night she said 'And I'm glad, God, that it is a girl.' So, the baby's stock is rising!"[123]

When baby Nancy Maureen Liddell was later baptised by Rev. H.A. Boyd in Toronto, Margaret Thomson hosted a post-baptismal party for thirty-five guests. Staying connected to the missionary community, it seems, was one way to counter any loneliness or anxiety she may have felt, with her husband, daughter, and granddaughter in Occupied China. "It was eleven when they left," Margaret wrote, "and were we all tired! I never saw it fail, that Mrs. A. [Armstrong?] arrived when the party was well over. Dr. A. is really a dear, and I know it is Mrs. A. who is to blame for their always being late."[124]

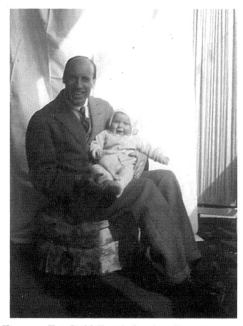

Fig. 4.4   Eric Liddell with daughter Patricia, c. 1939

Nursing at the Edge

While most of the correspondence between Betty Gale and her mother was filled with family news and social events, on 20 October 1941 Betty gave a rare account of some of her experiences with a group of Chinese children ("my club"). One day when the outpatient clinic was closed, Betty took some young students to the building where they played the piano and "insisted that I sing!! Awful din of laughter when I did!!!"[125] Apparently she had not expected such a large turnout: "huge crowd of children—far too many."[126] Betty Gale was not impressed with the students, referring to them as "filthy little beggars" who "practically all have colds—I caught a fine one, too!" These same "ragamuffins" gathered around her and a friend as they sat outside by "an ancient tombstone" to sketch the hills, and provided commentary on their work that wasn't "very flattering I must say."[127] Betty ended up giving two of her bobby pins to a girl who had become preoccupied with counting their number in Betty's hair. She went to bed early that night to prevent getting a cold.

By this time Betty Gale had returned to work; Changta Sao looked after Margaret. Gale had moved away from her position in the operating theatre to work in the "Private Patient Clinic" and was teaching nursing students.[128] She was one of seven Chinese and foreign nurses in leadership positions at Qilu who collectively oversaw the work of 60 staff nurses plus as many student nurses.[129] The number of student nurses had decreased in 1937 from 58 to 33: no new students were admitted because of the Japanese invasion of Manchuria. In fact, between 1937 and 1940 the total number of students at Qilu University had dropped from 651 to 77—33 of whom were nursing students.[130] However, by the fall of 1941, the Theological College had its full quota of students, and the Schools of Nursing, Pharmacy, and Hospital Technicians were "full to capacity."[131] Godfrey Gale had eight medical students—five men and three women; the first since 1937.

One evening in October 1941, Betty and Godfrey Gale invited two students over for dinner. Marilyn Sun and Pao Kuei Shih were roommates but were having difficulty getting along because Kuei Shih was a member of the student Bible study group (a "Groupie") while Marilyn was not. Marilyn was feeling rather resentful of her roommate. Betty Gale's strategy to reconcile the two was to "accidentally-on-purpose" set out a book full of pictures of the new "Moral re-Armament Magazine" and thereby "bring the talk around to the Group."[132] Betty explained to Marilyn that the group "wasn't anything different in religion; that she didn't need to change her already sound spiritual life if she came to our meetings, etc ... but that I hoped she would come, as we needed her help in our work with students who hadn't had her Christian background (her father is a Christian pastor at the 'Institute' here)."[133] While it is not clear whether the situation was resolved, it is interesting that Betty Gale felt obliged to help them sort through their religious differences, but even more so, that they trusted her to do so.

The students at Qilu were struggling with their own political concerns and factions, and they did not necessarily feel obliged to include the missionaries. In the summer of 1941 there was a sense of uneasiness among the staff nurses at Qilu Hospital, some of whom had become members of the University Communist Party, a secret organization that "would have been banned [by the Christian administration] had anyone known of its existence."[134] Nurses were being urged by communist colleagues to go on strike. While there had been reports of Chinese staff going on strike at hospitals elsewhere (for example, one hundred and fifty Chinese staff went on strike at Ste. Marie's Hospital in Shanghai in January), this is the first documented case of an attempt to strike at Qilu Hospital.[135] On 27 July 1941 the hospital nurses were warned by the communist group that "unless they stopped work their names would go on a black list to be remembered when the Communists eventually came to power."[136] Some of the nurses "belonging to a very strict and often despised Christian group calling them-

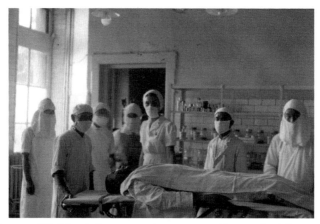

Fig. 4.5   Qilu Hospital operating theatre, c. 1940. Betty is third from right

selves 'The Little Flock'" refused to strike. Frances McAll had her baby in
the middle of this crisis but found that the nurse who cared for her "showed
no signs of the fact that she and about seven others were coping with the
whole hospital and facing a very threatening future."[137]

While there is no record of what became of the job action, it seems to
have been resolved by the time classes commenced in the fall. In early September, just as the nursing students were to resume classes, the "freezing"
order came from the Japanese, and "the country was flooded with rumors
of the status of the University and those connected with it."[138] Guards were
placed at the university and hospital gates. Although not all of the nursing
students showed up when classes started, a fair number did: twenty were in
their first year (pre-nursing), twenty-five in their second, ten in their third,
and twelve in their fourth, totalling sixty-seven nursing students. When
classes started on 9 September 1941, Godfrey Gale noted a spirit of goodwill and co-operation between the teachers and students. Betty Gale wrote:
"[It] is as though we realize this is our last chance with these students, as
though the seriousness of the world situation is drawing us all closer together and we feel subconsciously that we are drawing near to the edge of
the precipice."[139] As Godfrey later recalled, "there was a finer spirit among
us that Autumn than we had felt for many years." To him, this collegiality
was God's "granting of special grace, in unconscious preparation, as it were,
for what is to come."[140]

The Qilu University School of Nursing was based loosely on Florence
Nightingale's model established in the late nineteenth century.[141] During
the three-and-a-half-year program nursing students lived in residences by
the Qilu Hospital inside the city wall. They were provided room and board

(and possibly a stipend) during their training program. In addition to their hospital-based clinical training, the Qilu nursing students were expected to frequent the library for additional studying. The nursing library was comprised of recent professional publications and textbooks in both English and Chinese. This library included the complete series of the *China Nurse Journal* series, bound by year.

Nursing students at Qilu were monitored closely for any health concerns, and part of the role of the Director of Nursing Education was to oversee the health of her students. One reason for this concern was the high incidence of diseases like tuberculosis in nursing students in West China who had been part of the group of students that had evacuated Occupied China in 1937. At the St. Andrew's Hospital Training School for Nurses at Wusih, for example, the 1940 report noted that "the effects of the enforced evacuation of three years ago, with its travel, privation and crowding together of internees, are now seen in a higher incidence of pulmonary tuberculosis than that seen before the war."[142] As a result, 1940 applicants were accepted only after chest X-rays had shown clear lungs. In an effort to keep its students healthy, St. Andrews fed nursing students "bean curd milk" as a "mid-morning lunch," which reportedly "proved to be more than worth its cost in bringing about increase of weight and general vigour."[143]

At Qilu University, the Director of Nursing Education took responsibility to ensure that students received regular exercise and proper nutrition. This was monitored by a weekly weight chart and reinforced through "a scientific follow-up" on nutrition for those who were "either overweight or underweight."[144] To measure improvement of student health, nursing students were also submitted to a "posturegraph"—an X-ray (likely of the spine) taken before and after an exercise regime to see if there was any improvement. Finally, students were expected to submit footprints to check on the condition of their arches to "help those whose arches need strengthening" since "flat feet are quite common among Chinese girls."[145] For those deemed to require it, a "corrective" program was commenced. Each of the nursing students was also subject to regular physical examinations. In 1940 eight of the nursing students were found to have trachoma, a communicable eye disease that can cause blindness. An additional one-third had "Hong-kong Foot" (likely *tinea pedis*—a fungal infection).[146] In their quest to train nurses, the staff at Qilu felt a paternalistic responsibility for their students, and no one seemed to question the need for, or methods of, measuring and addressing health concerns.

After their pre-nursing year, students had to pass an entrance exam for admission into the nursing program. To graduate and receive their Nurses Association of China certification, they had to pass a one-day practical exam and three days' worth of written exams. In 1941 the clinical examination date was set for 8 December. Betty Gale was appointed as one of four examiners for the practical exams.

Last Chance for Evacuation

By the fall of 1941 the news of growing Japanese aggression in the Pacific was becoming increasingly worrisome. Finding the news "very bad these days" Betty Gale would simply "try not to hear what is happening."[147] She began avoiding radio broadcasts, leaving the room when Godfrey Gale and Andrew Thomson turned on the news. Instead, Betty busied herself with caring for Margie, working at the clinic and church, and reciprocating social engagements. Near the end of October, she wrote: "We work in the hospital, run clubs, help in the baby clinics, teach Sunday School, play tennis, and entertain friends [but keep wondering:] How much longer? What will happen? [What about] Margaret?"[148] To prepare for the possible outbreak of war, Betty started to collect warm clothing for the family, packing it into two suitcases. "If war breaks out soon," she wrote, "we must be ready." And yet, ready for what? She wondered what her packing priorities should be, given her small baby. Which clothes? Which medicines? Betty felt consumed by anxiety, going "over and over and over again" these things in her mind.[149]

In November 1941 Betty Gale was presented with a second opportunity to evacuate China. A "special evacuation boat" became available to foreigners living in Occupied China. The missionaries at Qilu were told that unless they availed themselves of this opportunity, "there might never come another chance."[150] Betty and Godfrey considered the idea but decided against it. The evacuees were only being guaranteed passage as far as Australia. They would have to figure out on their own how to get from Australia back to England or Canada. They decided that they "preferred to remain here in China among our friends even with the risk of being interned, rather than go to a strange land among strangers with the risk of even there being involved in war."[151] Ocean travel, they were well aware, was not safe either. For example, six months earlier a China missionary was evacuating from China to India on a British Royal Mail liner when the boat was "attacked by an enemy raider."[152] After two hours of intermittent firing, approximately three hundred passengers abandoned the ship in lifeboats, and they drifted for four days before being rescued by a British cargo ship. As it turned out, the Gales' instincts were correct. The evacuation boat they were offered in November 1941 was "caught on the high seas by the outbreak of war [and was] bombed by Japanese aircraft" near the Philippines.[153]

By the end of November Betty Gale was feeling "as Noah must have felt as the water kept rising and folks kept dying all around him and he remained safe and sound and happy."[154] Still, she said, "it wouldn't surprise us much if those [happy] days are almost over."[155] As winter approached they began to consider war "more and more likely" and all they could do was "to speculate what our own fate would be in that event, and to make such plans and preparations as we could."[156] Gale's greatest concern was having enough warm clothing. On 25 November she wrote to her family in Toronto:

> Rather expecting to go to sheltered (but cold) enclosures before long—we have been preparing our warmest clothes—and piling them in little piles. Margaret has a lovely se-mien bag to be tied into, complete with hood. Also a nice hot water bottle which we hope may be kept filled. I shall wear ski pants—three pairs of socks. Chinese shoes—three or four sweaters—fur coat and scarf for my head, and fur gloves. Godfrey umpteen socks, Chinese shoes and all his heaviest clothes. Dad will be a la Chinese—gown, shoes etc. fur cap for head, and fur mitts. In short we hope we shall be warmly clad (if and when). But won't we be a picture.[157]

The sense of uneasiness grew. On 4 December 1941, the United Church mission headquarters in Toronto sent the following cable to Rev G.K. King: "Due Difficulty Transmission Funds And Increasingly Critical Situation Strongly Advise Immediate Withdrawal Hodge MacTavish Faris Canada Others Proceed West."[158] Despite the urgency of this request, none of the North China missionaries left the occupied region. On 6 December 1941 G.K. King wrote to Taylor and Armstrong in Toronto a somewhat cryptic "Delay Transmission Funds."[159] The next day the Japanese military bombed Pearl Harbor. All missionaries remaining in Occupied China were placed under house arrest.

Summary

When later asked "why did [you] not leave China earlier when there was a chance to get out?" Godfrey Gale responded: "I felt, simply, that I had a job to do there in the Hospital and Medical School."[160] To understand Betty Gale's decision to go against consular advice by staying in China, it is important to recognize this key point: her husband was committed to staying in China regardless of whether his wife stayed with him. Whatever Betty's feelings about her duty to China, she was caught between the desire to provide her unborn child with a secure home and the desire to live with her husband. Thus, her decision ultimately came down to this: Was she willing to separate from Godfrey for the next few years, leaving him alone to face certain internment without her? Distilled to this essential question, it is perhaps easier to understand why, once Betty made up her mind to stay, she would no longer be swayed: she "put her foot down and refused to leave."[161] Once interned, Betty Gale would be offered three more opportunities to leave China. The only one she agreed to was also the only one that included Godfrey departing with her. Betty and Godfrey Gale would thereafter maintain: "we have never regretted our decision to stay."[162] As Betty wrote in her notebook at Pudong camp seven months *before* liberation: "This internment has been marvellous for me in some ways, and I'm very sure that God intended Margaret and me to stay here with Godf[rey]."[163]

Betty Gale was a remarkably independent-thinking, determined woman—traits inherited from and nurtured by her missionary parents. But these were also traits demonstrated by other Canadian missionary women, including the other mishkid nurses. In China, missionary women had the opportunity to push gender norms, exercising levels of agency not typical for Canadian women of this period. While mission authorities imparted advice and imposed rules and contracts, they seemed loathe to enforce them. When nurses told to leave, stayed, or when nurses told to stay, left, the most that missionary boards in the homeland or their representatives in the field could do was to express their disappointment and withdraw their support. Canadian missionary nurses whose lives had been invested in China understood this. They understood that they would always be part of the family, even if they disappointed their parents.

In contrast, Godfrey Gale's unpublished memoirs suggest that members of his church community in England were critical of the their decision to knowingly place themselves in harm's way by choosing not to avail themselves of the evacuation ships. Furthermore, Godfrey was criticized for remaining in China instead of assisting in the British war effort by joining the British National Service. After his release from internment, however, he gave a polite but unapologetic response to such criticism: he believed he could be of better service in China than elsewhere, "for I felt that service in the Medical School and Hospital was perhaps helping a little to bring in the Kingdom of God and the Brotherhood of all men"; and he therefore felt right to stay in China "as long as work was possible."[164] To those who criticized the London Missionary Society for not insisting that missionaries evacuate, Gale wrote: "Our Missionary Society said they were perfectly willing to consider any applications for permission to evacuate, and in fact urged us personally to consider the matter carefully"; therefore, "our decision to stay was made entirely on our own initiative and responsibility."[165]

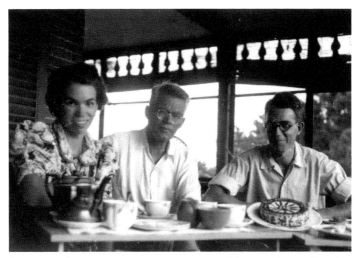

Fig. 4.6   Betty and Godfrey Gale with Andrew Thomson (middle), at Qilu

Ironically, the Canadian missionary nurses who chose to evacuate were judged more harshly by their peers in Canada than those who decided to stay.

Betty Gale's father, Andrew Thomson, also chose his own path. Thomson's missionary career was defined by his sense of autonomy. Driven by a deep sense of social obligation and a profound compassion, he worked in unconventional ways to attend to the needs he saw around him. He had ignored consular advice before, when deciding to return to Henan in 1939 after the other North China missionaries were evacuated from the region. Although Thomson encouraged his daughter to evacuate, even purchasing passage tickets, it seems likely that he also admired her decision to stay. Besides, with both her father and her husband at Jinan, Betty Gale would have two men to support her.

Were the decisions to stay in China based on naïveté? Certainly in the case of John and Mary Stanley and their relatives in Beijing, the Wilders, it seems that at least some missionaries believed they would be able to simply wait for "the last boat out." Missionaries believed in the value of their work, to be sure, and naturally equated evacuation with quitting or giving up. At Qilu, many of the remaining missionaries were hoping that the worst of the war would not come to "the quiet gentle backwater" where they were living.[166] Still, the Gales made preparations for internment, while others trusted that they would get out of China before any dire consequence befell them. Ultimately, however, missionary work was an act of faith, and missionaries accepted (and even delighted in) the risks that their work entailed.

Practising the Fine Art of House Arrest (1942)

We suddenly realize we are prisoners ... it's a strange, unhappy feeling.

—Betty Gale, "Journal," 10 December 1941

The morning of Sunday 7 December 1941 was clear, warm, and sunny. Godfrey Gale had turned down an early morning invitation to join friends in shooting ducks because he had "lecture notes to revise for the morrow."[1] Seventy missionaries remained on Qilu campus and, at midday, they heard some "pretty bad" news over the radio from Shanghai, which included: "Roosevelt's direct appeal to the Japanese Emperor to avert war; two heavily armed Japanese convoys headed for Bangkok; Thailand Prime Minister given full powers to deal with any national emergency; Thailand Government getting ready to leave Bangkok if necessary, and so on."[2] The nature of China's war with Japan was on the verge of changing. Betty wrote in the margins of her diary, in pencil: "Getting Suspicious!"[3] What would more international involvement in the war mean for the missionaries?

The Gales attended a 5:00 p.m. evening service that same day at the Kumler Chapel with Rev. Andrew Thomson presiding. In the middle of the church service the electric lights suddenly went out. Someone responded by bringing in candles in tall candlesticks and placing them on each side of Andrew Thomson at the pulpit. Betty Gale described the candles casting "flickering shadows on his face—and on the beautiful gray stonework in the Chapel."[4] Everyone sat close together in the pews, not only because of a sense of closeness "in spirit," but also because it was "bitterly cold." Betty Gale wondered, "Is it an omen?"[5] The Gales invited friends over for supper and "somehow it turned out to be the most hilarious supper and evening we had for a long time—a curious inexplicable hilarity."[6]

Americans would remember 7 December 1941 as a "date which will live in infamy."[7] The Japanese had launched surprise attacks on Hawaii, Guam, Malaya, the Philippines, and Wake Island. To American President Franklin D. Roosevelt, speaking to the American Congress the day after the attacks, the fact that the surprise offensive on Pearl Harbor occurred while the United States was in the midst of peace negotiations with Japan made it all the more deplorable. As Roosevelt urged the American public to "remember the character of the onslaught against us" when they took up arms against their new enemy,[8] the Canadian public also had to come to terms with an enemy now understood as deceptive, opportunistic, and sadistic.

Japanese Takeover

On Monday 8 December 1941 Betty Gale began her diary entry with these words: "M. weighs 16 lbs!! War declared this am by J[apan] and A[merica] and B[ritain]. Am packing up a few things just in case!!"[9] When she later reworked her memory into a journal she expanded the 8 December entry this way: "Margaret weighs 15 [sic] lbs to-day! Is that more important—that I write it down first, before saying that Japan declared War in the United States, and Britain, last night? It helps to keep me from panicking, in any case—thinking of those pounds. "War is declared to-day!" "Yes, I know, but Margie weighs 15 lbs."[10]

Earlier in the day, at 7:30 a.m., Betty Gale had made her way to the Qilu University Hospital to supervise the clinical examinations of the fourth year nursing students. Twelve nursing students were registered for their national examinations, beginning with practical examinations on 8 December and followed by three days of written examinations. There were four examiners, including Betty. Betty expected to be at the hospital most of the day. When she returned to the campus at 9:30 a.m. to feed and bathe Margie, she had every intention of going back to the hospital to continue the exams. "Needless to say," she later wrote, "I didn't go back to finish the exams and the other examiners thought all manner of awful things about me until they were summoned an hour later and heard the news, too."[11]

Godfrey Gale had gotten up late on 8 December. Tired after the company of the previous evening, he only had time for a "hurried half-hour's revision of lecture notes with my Chinese teacher before breakfast."[12] He lectured the medical students from 9:00 a.m. until 10:15 a.m. "with rather more than the usual sense of freedom," the subject being the spinal cord, membranes, and spinal nerves. When the students went to their dissecting, Godfrey was "surprised to see Japanese Gendarmes guarding the medical school gate and refusing to allow anyone either in or out."[13] The Japanese Gendarmerie was in charge of civilians.[14] Godfrey wondered if Betty was "caught with me on the Hospital premises—unable to go home to bath or feed Margaret."[15] Suddenly Godfrey received a telephone call from Andrew Thomson who was on the Qilu campus. According to Thomson, everything was quiet on the campus, with the Japanese Gendarmes now in command. All of the students had been sent to their rooms. "Betty," Godfrey noted, "had been the very last person to get onto the Campus! She had got to the [Qilu campus] gates on the way home at 0915 at the same time as the Gendarmes and had slipped through them unobserved!"[16]

At 12:20 p.m. Godfrey Gale received an urgent message that he was wanted by the Hospital Superintendent. Hurrying outside, he "found that a convoy was being formed of Japanese Gendarmes with fixed bayonets to escort us home for lunch, and after all we foreign doctors and nurses had been collected together we were solemnly marched through the streets, and out of the [Jinan] city gate onto the university campus, where we were dismissed to go to our various homes."[17] By the time Betty saw Godfrey pedalling up the road, Japanese soldiers were coming in and out of their house, where they confiscated the Gales' radio, took a "good look around at our possessions," and asked "thousands of questions."[18] All around campus, radios, binoculars, and cameras were confiscated. And the only car on campus—the one belonging to the Qilu University president—was commandeered.[19]

In their separate accounts of that day, Betty and Godfrey Gale expressed surprise and relief at the politeness of the soldiers, and that they were not immediately taken into captivity. "Had several groups of J's in," Betty noted in her diary, "they took our radio—alas!"[20] Godfrey had been concerned that "we men might have been taken right off to a concentration camp without even an opportunity to say goodbye or to pick up a toothbrush or pair of pyjamas."[21] In other words, it could have been much worse.

After eating lunch in their home, Betty and Godfrey Gale prepared for "what might be the worst contingency possible—that [they] would be sent to separate concentration camps."[22] Betty had already packed suitcases of warm clothing. Now Godfrey packed a knapsack and a small kit bag with a few "essentials" including a "Moffat New Testament and small Hymnbook, a book of prayers, two packs of cards, E.V. Lucas's booklet *The Open Road*, medical supplies, string, matches, notepaper etc."[23] Of particular interest is the Lucas book, subtitled "A Book for Wayfarers." Published in 1913, *The Open Road* is an ornate, gilt cloth-bound anthology for travellers with over two hundred poems including works by W.B. Yeats, Elizabeth Barrett Browning, Lord Byron, P.B. Shelley, and Rudyard Kipling. With sixteen colour plates of paintings by Claude Shepperton, this book "aims at nothing but providing companionship on the road for city-dwellers who make holiday. A garland fitted to urge people into the open air and, once there, to keep them glad they came."[24]

The pressing question was, what would a family need to survive a concentration camp? While both Betty and Godfrey Gale gathered medicines,

Betty also concentrated on the need for protection from exposure to cold weather. Godfrey focused on the need for books and games; intellectual engagement was essential to survival, too. Their prescience would prove accurate: the boredom of incarceration was later listed as one of the main difficulties of civilian internment, along with the more obvious difficulties of lack of food and medical care, loss of privacy, isolation, and illicit neglect.[25]

Peggy Pemberton-Carter, a China internee between 1943 and 1945, whose wartime journal was later reproduced as a book, offers an interesting comparison to the preparations made by the Gales.[26] When the thirty-eight-year-old wealthy socialite received a summons to appear at the Civil Assembly Centre in Shanghai for her impending internment in the Lunghua Camp in 1943, she had one month to shop for appropriate goods. Included in her baggage were saucepans, a kettle, enamel plate and mug, knives, forks, and spoons, a coffee pot, gardening tools, washboard, burrs, a dustpan, mop, readymade shelves, a bucket and "the bedroom utensil"—possibly a chamber pot of sorts.[27] Pemberton-Carter also bought a bolt of cotton for curtains, sunhat, gumboots, sleeping mat, fan and fly swatter, towels, sheets, garden seeds, quinine, aspirin, wire, rope, nails, pliers, wooden clogs, soap, salami sausages, shoelaces, insect powder, pins, needles and thread, and two tin openers. In addition, "since I hate to be hungry," she filled "every spare inch" with tins "of every kind" of food.[28] Once these items were packed into her trunks, there was little room for clothing. Her wardrobe was "consequently reduced to the bare minimum of slacks, shorts, shirts, raincoat, sweaters, heavy shoes and socks and fur jacket."[29]

In addition to practical supplies, Peggy Pemberton-Carter packed three Penguin anthologies of poetry, Shakespeare's *Tragedies*, a *Plain Man's Prayerbook*, H.G. Well's *Outline of History*, a Russian grammar, a shorthand primer, and some crossword puzzles—"which seems to be a selection that should do for most moods."[30] Although not everything she brought was of immediate value (she also packed a small sum of American Express cheques hidden in a box of talcum powder), Pemberton-Carter would discover that having such a variety of goods was useful for bartering for food as internment wore on. If the Gales' main fear was cold, illness, and boredom, Pemberton-Carter's main fear, it seems, was hunger.

As it turned out, Betty and Godfrey Gale would not need those packed suitcases for another eight months.

Closure of Qilu University: Tacit Resistance

Perhaps one of the most interesting characteristics of the early days of house arrest was the immediate, collaborative, tacit resistance of civilians against their captors. At Qilu, this was revealed in Betty Gale's bold entrance through the university gates behind the marching soldiers, but also in missionaries' stealing and hiding medical supplies, in medical staff and students' expunging evidence of ongoing classroom instruction, and in the emerging game of deceiving their Japanese guards. Resistance against the Japanese suddenly expanded from primarily a Chinese preoccupation to one for missionaries, too.

Within an hour of being reunited at their home at Qilu on 8 December 1941, Godfrey and Betty Gale and the other missionaries were summoned to the university administration building "to hear our fate."[31] They were told that the university was to close immediately. No new patients were to be admitted to the hospital, and as soon as existing patients were discharged, the hospital would be closed. Until then, the Japanese would form a "convoy guard" to escort doctors and nurses between the main campus and the hospital.[32] The missionaries were asked to register their names, and then return to their homes to prepare an inventory in triplicate of all their possessions and of all their money in the bank ("*that* won't take long," Betty quipped).[33] They also had to list the name of every book in the house ("that *will* take long").[34] For now the missionaries would be allowed to stay in their homes, which would also be searched.

Of immediate concern to the gendarmes was the confiscation of radios. Controlling communication was a key aspect of war. Effective immediately, no international post was allowed. First class mail within China was still allowed, although very little.[35] As the soldiers entered each home they first took a "flashlight photo" of each family standing behind their radio set, which was then "disconnected and carried off."[36] The soldiers also took eggs, soap, candles, and tea. Still, the politeness of the Japanese was disarming. One gendarme apologized to the Gales for "the accident" (Pearl Harbor), adding "I hope there will soon be peace."[37] Another apologized for inspecting the house. Eager to keep the Japanese soldiers happy, Hoong Run ("Red Jewel"), the Gales' house servant, whispered to Betty, "Give them salt; they like it!!"[38] The image of this teenage boy trembling beside them would become seared into Betty's memory.[39]

The Japanese also requested inventories for both personal and institutional properties, as well as reports on property and finances, "usually with a demand that the information be furnished at once without allowing time to collect material."[40] They demanded all keys to institutional buildings so that further access to these buildings was by special permission only. They also put up English notices around the campus stating that they had "no intention of ill treating or molesting us if we kept the peace and obeyed their orders."[41] There were four rules, the breaking of which would result in "severe punishment":

1 We must not go more than 6 kilometres from our homes
2 We must not stay away from our homes for more than 24 hours
3 We must not hold meetings of any kind without special permission
4 We must not transfer any property of any kind to third parties.[42]

In addition, servants were not allowed to leave the campus: missionaries would do the necessary household shopping themselves, accompanied by a guard. The missionaries were to carry a pass at all times, and "bow very respectfully every time we meet a 'J.'"[43] Although Betty Gale did not "see a need of a pass when we are always accompanied by a sentry," she wrote, "ours not to reason why—ours but to do—or die."[44]

Within a week of receiving her pass on 10 December 1941, Betty Gale was finding ways to "lose her Jap[anese] guard" when she went shopping.[45]

Last Days of Qilu Hospital

The months leading up to Pearl Harbor had foreshadowed the eventual closure of Qilu Hospital. The capacity of the institution and the endurance of the staff had been "taxed to the limit" for a while.[46] Thus, when the Japanese military closed Qilu campus on 8 December 1941 the running of the hospital was initially "not greatly disturbed."[47] With the exception of the X-ray department being sealed up and the order that a Japanese gendarme be in attendance "if we wanted to use any apparatus from the Massage and Electrotherapeutic Department," much remained the same at first. According to Godfrey Gale:

> All the nurses and Chinese staff were calm. All the Chinese, in fact, were overjoyed at the outbreak of war. They have the utmost faith in the fabulous power of the British Empire and the U.S.A. in the West. They look to us to release them from the grip of Japan and hail this as a big step towards their own deliverance. The result is that behind the backs of our guards, we are greeted on the streets with smiles and little courtesies and receive many messages of sympathy and little gifts.[48]

Doctors and nurses were escorted to and from their homes on Qilu campus and the hospital a few blocks away. Dr. Isabelle MacTavish found the ordeal humorous: "You would have been interested and perhaps amused to see me going from the campus to the hospital twice daily and back escorted by a Japanese guard with a rifle and bayonet."[49] Eventually the Japanese soldiers were replaced by Chinese troops under the supervision of two Japanese military police. According to MacTavish, "they got tired of escorting us, or perhaps felt they could trust us after awhile, so we just signed in and out at the campus and hospital gate on arriving and leaving."[50]

Despite assurances that the hospital would not close until all existing patients were discharged, on 10 December a "rumour got round that the Japanese military were going to take over the hospital at 10:30."[51] Not knowing what that might involve, the missionary medical staff "made a beeline for the Dispensary and got in supplies of necessary drugs, not only for ourselves, but for everyone in our community, leaving I.O.U. notes for what we had taken."[52] The problem now was getting the medical supplies out of the hospital. Godfrey Gale sent a Chinese labourer out to buy some meat and apples, and then he took a wastepaper basket, put the drugs and supplies in it, covered the contraband with the food, and "carried them home under my arm without anyone being any the wiser."[53]

At 11:00 a.m. the missionaries received word that all Chinese doctors, nurses, and labourers who lived on the hospital premises would be given one hour to get all their possessions out, after which the gates would be locked. "So, for the next hour absolute pandemonium reigned while they all rushed to get their things through and dumped in any convenient spot before the time was up. All the gates were then sealed except the one main gate that was carefully guarded."[54] When the gates were later manned by Chinese soldiers, Godfrey Gale reported that more things went through those gates than the personal property of people living there because the guards reportedly allowed their friends to slip out behind their backs carrying hospital property with them.[55]

The hospital remained open and on 11 December Godfrey Gale met with eight medical students to continue their anatomy lessons. Meanwhile, students at the Qilu campus were receiving conflicting orders from the Japanese: there seemed "to be no coordination between the various authorities who consider themselves responsible for us, and no definite plan."[56] At 5:30 p.m. all the "Campus Chinese" were called together where they were "harangued by a Japanese soldier who spoke very poor Chinese—so that everyone came away with a different idea of what he had said."[57] The Gales' three servants came to them in tears saying they had been ordered to clear out and not to take anything with them. Anticipating the loss of their amah, Changta Sao, their house servant, Hoong Run, and their cook, Lan Ting, Betty and Godfrey Gale took last-minute lessons in "breadmaking and how to work the incredibly difficult stove in the kitchen."[58] Lan Ting

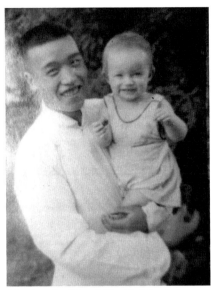

Fig. 5.1   Red Jewel (?) with Margie in 1942

also left Betty with a list of shops to go to for their food, and which vendors *not* to go to. "I feel hopelessly young and stupid and scared," wrote Betty on the eve of Lan Ting's departure.[59]

Although the hospital remained open, the university closed on 11 December, and all the students were dismissed. To Betty Gale, it was "a heartbreaking sight especially for those who helped establish it."[60] The students were told "not to mix with the foreigners—but many … slipped in quietly to say goodbye, and to hug Margie."[61] As the child of long-serving China missionaries, the meaning was not lost on Betty: "It has taken many years to build up [Qilu]—with a lot of money—and, even more, much love and understanding. Is it all to be thrown away?"[62]

The twelve senior nursing students whose practice examinations had been temporarily interrupted on 8 December were later awarded their nursing diplomas. Afterwards "the entire University community expressed great admiration for these twelve students who continued uninterruptedly their four days of [practical and written] examination in spite of unsettled conditions all around them [including] turning the hospital over to the Japanese."[63] Their papers were graded and sent to the Nurses Association of China headquarters. Passing these exams made students immediately eligible for the coveted NAC certificate.

When classes were ordered stopped, the senior nursing students had only two months left of their three-and-a-half-year program. Since they had each successfully passed the national examinations, it was decided that they had earned their diplomas. A few days after classes were halted at Qilu University, the students were sent home. Later the third year nursing students were accepted into the training school of the Kailan Mining Company Hospital in Tangshan for the completion of their studies. The second year students were given a record of the work they had completed. Nursing staff removed textbooks and journals from the library and hid them in "the far corners of the attic" of foreign residences for safekeeping from the Japanese invaders.[64]

Three days after the departure of the three members of the Gales' household staff, Changta Sao and Hoong Run returned. Betty Gale heard the back door open and someone running through the hall. She came out to the upstairs landing in time to see Hoong Run bounding up the stairs two steps at a time. "He is very excited and very much in earnest as he pleads with me to allow him to come back and work for us—and not to send him away again."[65] While Lan Ting did not come back ("he is old and terrified of the 'J'"), Betty was relieved to have the service and company of Hoong Run and Changta Sao.[66] Hoong Run had to learn to cook in Lan Ting's place. By Godfrey Gale's estimation the household had enough food and coal for about three months—"if we are careful."[67]

On 13 December 1941 the missionaries received their "first news of the outside world": the sinking of the British battleships *HMS Prince of Wales* and *HMS Repulse* off Malaya, the devastating attack on Pearl Harbor, and fighting in Thailand, Hong Kong, and Manila.[68] There was also news that the German attack on Moscow had been abandoned, and that the Chinese Eighth Route Army was fighting close to Jinan, attacking Japanese outposts and cutting railway lines. The loss of the two battleships and the destruction at Pearl Harbor were "hard to believe."[69]

Godfrey Gale continued his anatomy lectures with medical students until ordered to stop on 15 December 1941. The Japanese had not been aware that lessons were continuing until Dr. Gordon Struthers casually mentioned it to the Japanese commanding officer. Furious, the officer ordered all educational activities to cease at once "on pain of severe punishment."[70] Alerted that the soldiers were en route to the medical school, Godfrey and the medical students hurriedly placed the cadavers "back into formalin tanks," cleaned the dissecting tables, cleared the chalkboard, placed specimens and charts into cupboards, piled up benches against the wall, and left the building—all within ten minutes—thus effectively thwarting the soldiers.

On that same day Betty Gale and another missionary "decided to try the experiment of going down town to do some shopping" and so went to the campus gate where they "solemnly picked up a Japanese soldier complete with gun and sword" to accompany them.[71] As the women "marched round the shops," a "distinctly amused group of Chinese onlookers" followed at a safe distance.[72] All the shopkeepers were full of inquiries as to how the internees were all getting along. Taking advantage of the Japanese soldier's "obvious ignorance of Chinese," the shopkeepers told the women "over and over again" that "now we are all together in this war."[73] To emphasize their solidarity, Chinese merchants gave the missionary women specially reduced prices.

Such furtive acts of Chinese support would continue through the war, at Qilu as elsewhere. Canadian nurse Susie Kelsey, now under house arrest in Sanqui, Henan, was at first forbidden to step foot outside her house and lived mostly on presents of flour, eggs, fruits, and cakes from Chinese friends. "Always the Chinese tried to protect us," Kelsey later recalled. "They remembered how we sheltered them in the hospital compound when their enemy first looted the town."[74]

On 18 December the Japanese military visited Dr. R.G. Struthers to ask him three questions:

1 If the hospital were to remain open, would the staff be willing to stay on and work there?
2 If the hospital remained open, would Struthers be able to find money to run it?
3 If the hospital should not be allowed to run, would we be willing to be repatriated?[75]

Godfrey Gale's response on hearing the question of repatriation was simply: "It was an interesting suggestion!"[76] Three days later the military announced plans to take over the hospital. Gale noted a "general gloom settling" over the hospital as many nurses, technicians, and Chinese labourers began to leave, along with patients who had recovered enough to return home.[77]

The impending hospital closure seemed to act as an invitation to looting. On 23 December Godfrey Gale "spent a hectic morning" at the hospital checking lists of inventories because a "constant stream of things have been stolen and taken off by coolies [sic] and hospital workmen."[78] Godfrey believed that some of the valuable equipment in his Ear Nose and Throat Department had been stolen by his labourer—"who has ideas of setting up as a doctor now!"[79] The Japanese also took what they could. One physician "witnessed a steady depletion by the Japanese Military and others" of hospital equipment and supplies.[80] This included typewriters, telephones, tools, and machines from the university workshop and printing press, and the stock of paper and stationary. The Augustine Library was also sacked; even shelving disappeared.[81] At first the Japanese gave receipts for the equipment they took away, but later this formality was no longer observed. The missionaries were quietly enraged by the pilfering of the hospital and other supplies. As the author of the "1942 Qilu Hospital Report" acerbically reported, "our material equipment was subjected to a consistent program of appropriation on the part of the military."[82]

Finally, after five weeks of speculation, the Qilu Hospital was closed. The keys were handed over to Japanese army officers. According to one report, both provincial and city governments made repeated appeals to the Japanese to reopen the hospital.[83] When the Japanese refused this, the Jinan city administration reportedly funded the rebuilding and enlarging of one of its buildings as a new hospital. Although the implication was that Japan did not wish to allow a "foreign" hospital in Japanese-occupied China, the City Hospital was staffed almost entirely with ex-Qilu doctors, nurses, and other hospital personnel. Four missionary doctors also obtained permission to assist at the new hospital as a way to relieve the "distress" caused by the closure of the Qilu Hospital.[84] Most of the limited number of supplies and instruments that remained at Qilu were granted to the new City Hospital.

Unreliable Reports from China

While Betty and Godfrey Gale resigned themselves to their new restricted lives in Qilu, family and friends in Canada grew increasingly anxious about their fate and living conditions. Initial correspondence between missionary families and the United Church headquarters downplayed any danger. For example, in a January 1942 letter to Marion Faris, whose husband Don Faris was under house arrest with the Gales, Rev. A.E. Armstrong wrote of "our belief that British and American nationals in Japan, Korea and Japanese-occupied portions of China will suffer no other conveniences than that of being restricted to their own property" and would be "treated as well as possible by the Japanese."[85] By February however, Marion Faris was starting to feel nervous. "The situation at Singapore has been weighing a bit heavily on me," she wrote to A.E. Armstrong, referring to the Japanese attacks on Singapore five days earlier.[86] When Singapore surrendered to the Japanese amid rumours of atrocities perpetuated upon thousands of prisoners of war, families of the Chinese internees began to fear the worst.

Marion Faris, who was struggling to rear three young children on her own in Vancouver while her husband was in China, continued to write to A.E. Armstrong. She was anxious to get in touch with her husband. In

March she noted that reports of the missionaries being well treated did not "go down very easily with me."[87] Recalling that Don had once been "roughly handled" by a Japanese guard, she believed that the Japanese were "just aching to get their hands on the foreigners."[88] Now that they had them "totally within their power," Marion could not imagine that the Japanese military would "change their spots."[89]

The tone of this particular letter verges on the hysterical. Marion Faris had heard a rumour that the Qilu missionaries ("40 adults and 10 children") were being held prisoner in one, crowded building:

> I can well imagine those barbed wire barricades have been moved to enclose a space beyond which our people can't go. The sanitary facilities are apt to be very limited also for such a large number and the hot weather is not far away. The thermometer goes up to 118 degrees in the shade [in Jinan] on occasion. If our men had been free to do so, they would have got a much more definite word out to W. China re: their welfare.[90]

Although Faris realized that her "surmises may not be correct," she was also "under no illusions as to what the Jap[anese] Military are capable of doing." Furthermore, she could "well believe our people would be in real danger once the J[apanese] begin to suffer real reverses."[91] Faris believed that all the reassuring news from China was actually counterproductive. From her perspective, "our people need real prayer," but Canadian Christians would not pray if they were not informed of the real danger the missionaries were in. She was concerned that prayer "was not apt to come when churches at home feel that the missionaries are being well-treated."[92]

For his part, Rev. A.E. Armstrong was hardly reassuring. In a confidential letter responding to Marion Faris's concerns, he cited his own experience in the Far East in 1919, after the First World War, as reason to believe that atrocities could well be committed by the military without the Japanese government's awareness:

> It is quite natural that you would [be concerned] since you know what the Japanese military are capable of doing. You did not mention their [atrocious] treatment of the British and American [military personnel] at [the fall of] Hong Kong, and of course it must not be assumed that they would necessarily treat our people in the same way [...]. You may be right in your surmise [that reports suggesting all is well are incorrect] but I think we may still believe the cablegrams which have come from different quarters [...] which are to the effect that the Japanese are not ill-treating foreigners in their hands but are leaving them fairly free [... My opinion is] that the Japanese Military

are not much concerned about the very few foreign missionaries they have in their possession."[93]

Nor was A.E. Armstrong reassuring about Marion Faris's own safety in Vancouver. Faris had been contemplating a move to Vancouver Island for the summer because of the cheap rent there compared with Vancouver. With limited access to her husband's missionary income, she was hoping to save money before returning to Vancouver in the fall. Seemingly oblivious to the angst his message would bring, Armstrong agreed with her plans, noting that while houses were "scarce" in Vancouver, "there are probably some people moving out of Vancouver because of the possibility of [Japanese] Air raids and sabotage."[94]

Communicating with Canada

Without reliable news sources, family and friends in Canada tried to make sense of the circulating rumours. Later, as the war progressed, innovative methods of communication between Canada and China would be developed, including weekly radio broadcasts sent out from Los Angeles in which Canadian and American families could send messages that they hoped would be picked up in China and somehow relayed to internees. Furthermore, once the enemy aliens were organized into internment camps, the International Committee of the Red Cross would provide a "Service Civilian Internees" messaging system to send and receive short (and heavily censored) messages between China internees and their families in Canada. But in 1942 even the Canadian Department of National Defence did not have reliable means to obtain information from China. In a document entitled "Advice to the Relative of a Man who is Missing," the Department of National Defence reassured family members of missing military men that "endeavours to trace him [will] not cease."[95] While meant for military families, this document also provides insight into the difficulty obtaining reliable information related to civilian internees. That is, the government discouraged families from listening to radio broadcasts to obtain information about their loved ones:

> The moment reliable news is obtained from any of these sources [diplomatic channels and the International Red Cross Committee at Geneva] it is sent to the Service Department Concerned. They will pass the news on to you at once if they are satisfied that it is reliable. It would be cruel to raise false hopes, such as might be raised if you listened to one other possible channel of news, namely, the enemy's broadcasts. They are listened to by official listen-

ers, working continuously night and day. A few names of prisoners given my enemy announcers are carefully checked. They are often misleading, and this is not surprising, for the object of the inclusion of prisoners' names in these broadcasts is not to help the relatives of prisoners, but to induce Canadian listeners to hear some tale which otherwise they could not be made to hear. The only advantage of listening to these broadcasts is an advantage to the enemy.[96]

The message was clear for missionary and military families alike: communication between Canada and China was now a complex issue best left to the government. It had clear ramifications for national security.

In February 1942 G.K. King managed to get a letter out from Qilu to A.E. Armstrong at the United Church headquarters in Toronto. Because it would be hand-delivered by a Dr. Bell, G.K. King could be candid. In it he gave a general account of where the missionaries were living under house arrest; he also noted that Georgina Lewis had given birth to a baby girl. Furthermore G.K. King made it clear that the interned missionaries each remained in Occupied China of their own accord, "contrary to your express instructions," and therefore had to accept responsibility for the consequences. "They were loath to move," wrote King, "[but] I think they have no regrets ... of course that does not say that were the opportunity presented they would not now accept a transfer!"[97]

In the early days of house arrest letters like this one from G.K. King could be sent to Canada via Canadian missionaries living in Sichuan, which remained unoccupied. North China missionary nurse Clara Preston, for example, who had been seconded to the United Church West China Mission in Sichuan, passed along news to Canada from missionaries Isabelle Mac-Tavish and Eric Liddell who were under house arrest at Jinan and Tianjin respectively. In one of her letters MacTavish noted that "Betty, Godfrey, wee Margaret and Mr. Thomson, Gord [Dr. Struthers] are all well."[98] In a letter to Mrs. Taylor in Toronto on 2 February 1942, Clara Preston summarized some of the letters she was passing along to families of the missionaries—for example: "Eric's is a beautiful letter and I know it will mean much to Florence."[99]

On 1 March 1942 Eric Liddell sent a letter to Clara Preston which she typed out and sent to the United Church headquarters in Toronto, with a copy to his wife Florence. In it Liddell gave a general picture of his life under house arrest in Tianjin. Like the Qilu missionaries, those living in the cosmopolitan city of Tianjin heard on Monday 8 December that war had been declared. Guards were placed at the entrance to the British Concession[100] and those on the outside, like Eric Liddell, were unable to get any news from those under house arrest in the British concession. Liddell was living in the French Concession and had to report to the Japanese regarding possessions, property, and finance. Within a week all radios had to be reported. Meetings were banned, except a weekly prayer meeting—"on condition that it was not of a political nature."[101] The London Missionary Society hospital was allowed to continue and only had two or three visits from the Japanese military, who "seemed more interested in the drugs, operating room and instruments than anything else."[102] After Christmas all foreigners were to be moved into the British Concession except hospital staff. Eric Liddell also sent a message about Bertha Hodge, who was the only United Church of Canada missionary living in Tianjin. "Her house is now full," he wrote, "the missionaries of the M.E.M. [Methodist English Mission] at south gate moved in and are staying with her. They seem to be a very happy bunch together."[103]

In addition to sending letters via Sichuan during the early days of house arrest, missionaries were also able to get messages out by radiogram. Provided someone was listening on the receiving end and was willing to pass along messages, this worked well. The following message was received by the Official Listening Post at Ventura, California, in early February 1942, and was forwarded to Rev. E.G. Robb, a relative of Davina Robb Menzies, in Toronto: "Inform Jean all well. Quiet. Congratulations on your father's birthday. Margaret Ann [Lewis] born Choutsun January 26th. Mother [Davina Menzies] present. Georgina [Lewis] well. Mother now Tsinan [Jinan]. Your last letter September 1st. Am still writing weekly. Much love Jean, David, Tom, Dorothy. (sgd.) Handley Stockley, Sianfu [Xian]."

What is of particular interest in this letter from Handley Stockley to his wife, mishkid nurse Jean Stockley, is its note about Jean's father's birthday. Given that her father, James R. Menzies, had died in 1920, why would he be sending birthday congratulations? Even if it was the family's habit to note James's birthday as a form of remembrance, it still does not make sense—because James R. Menzies' birthdate was November 18. A more probable explanation is that Handley Stockley was sending a coded message to his wife. "Congratulations on your father's birthday" likely had a pre-determined meaning. One can only speculate on what that message was.

While missionaries residing in China's north were under house arrest, those in Shanghai were still free to move around. Canadian missionary Winifred Warren sent a letter from Shanghai to the Woman's Missionary Society headquarters in Toronto in March 1942 noting that she had sent a Christmas greeting by radio to Mr. Forbes in Vancouver. She also noted, in a more enigmatic way, that she had sent another letter "by our friend where co-worker Jean Sommerville is. She has now, I hear, reached Jean and I hope has found a way of sending word to you."[104] At that point enemy aliens living in Shanghai were free to move about, provided they were registered. To travel outside of Shanghai, however, would require a special pass. Winifred Warren passed along what she had heard about other Canadians who were under house arrest, including Bertha Hodge, the Kings, and those at Jinan. Like the other United Church missionaries, Warren also provided information about the Canadian nurses who were not, or no longer, directly associated with the North China Mission. She noted that Susie Kelsey was "in her own home" at Sanqui, for example, "with very friendly intercourse."[105] And she noted that Davina Menzies was back in Jinan on 27 February after spending a month with her daughter and new granddaughter.

Canadian missionary families pressed the home missions office for information about their loved ones; the news coming out of China was not reassuring. On 18 April 1942 Gerald Bell sent a letter from West China to Toronto, bringing A.E. Armstrong up to date with some fearsome reports. Bell wrote about the arrival in Sichuan of two orphaned English children. Their father had been a young English businessman in the Salt Revenue Service in Guiyang. Their mother, an American, had been born in China—possibly to missionary parents. They happened to be in Hong Kong at the time of the Japanese military attack there in December 1941. "At the time of the capture," Gerald Bell wrote, "she was among the unfortunate foreign women to suffer at the hands of Japanese soldiers. The husband was killed trying to defend her honour. And afterwards she was bayoneted to death. It is a terrible and very sad case."[106] Stories like these added to the Canadian missionaries' collective fear of the Japanese military—a fear that had started to develop years earlier.

Fear of the Japanese

Rumours and evidence of Japanese atrocities being committed in Japanese-occupied territory were not new to Canadians. For example, in 1938 the China Aid Council published a book entitled *War in China: What It Means to Canada*.[107] Geared towards a Canadian audience and containing graphic photos of victims of violence, it described "Japanese militarists" as having a "deliberate policy" of "fiendish crimes" including "robbery, murder and rape."[108] Furthermore, the Japanese were said to be "stooping to … unspeakable bestiality" in order to break the resistance of the Chinese people; "bayonet practice on living victims is only one form of savagery practiced in this campaign."[109]

Now, in March 1942, Rev. A.E. Armstrong was faced with a dilemma as the public spokesperson for the United Church mission board in the midst of fearful reports coming from China. While privately expressing his fears to Marion Faris, publically Armstrong suppressed them. Ignoring Faris's concern that an uninformed Canadian public would not effectively pray for the interned missionaries, he glossed over the internment crisis faced by the missionaries. In an article that he co-authored (published in *The United Church Observer* in March 1942), Armstrong downplayed the danger of internment, simply stating "all missionaries safe."[110] Official mission publications tended to emphasize stories of missionary faith and endurance when facing difficult circumstances. But there were no stories coming from the internees. Instead, Armstrong focused on the Chinese Christians who, "during these days of trial and testing," were reportedly displaying "fortitude, loyalty and Christian courage."[111] All that could be said about the missionaries was that they were "thought to be well and in their own homes."[112]

While mission correspondence in Canada from 1942 reveals a heightened sense of fear among those awaiting news from China, diaries and memoirs written by the internees themselves do not suggest the same level of fear. Godfrey Gale, who was surprised by the politeness of the Japanese, noted that the Japanese soldiers embodied a "curious mixture" of brutality and serenity.[113] On the one hand, in "battle or on punitive raids among the villages, one cannot imagine anyone more brutal and in fact, devilish." Yet, on the other hand, "they have with this a deep love of home and children and nature."[114] At the hospital, for example, off-duty Japanese soldiers gravitated towards the nurses and the children's wards. "The nurses," Gale wrote, "have the greatest difficulty in keeping them away."[115] On Christmas Eve, "every little patient had a Japanese soldier sitting by their bedside holding their hand."[116] To Gale, the best explanation for such gentle behaviour was that the soldiers missed their own wives and children: "they have told us that they get no leave home, and will not go back until the war is over."[117] Trying to make sense of the discrepancy between the brutality and gentleness of Japanese soldiers, Gale decided to believe that it was his experience of the Japanese as gentle, loving folk that represented "the real Japan."[118]

House Arrest: Unintended Internment Training Ground

Godfrey and Betty Gale lived under house arrest on the Qilu campus for eight months, from 8 December 1941 until 10 August 1942. During that time they each kept a diary and wrote letters. While each documented ways in which they adapted to the new and evolving circumstances under the Japanese, Godfrey emphasized more of the logistical and administrative difficulties while Betty emphasized how social relationships impacted their house arrest, and vice versa. Three of the most interesting aspects of this period are the ongoing acts of resistance, the deepened reliance on communal and intercessory prayer, and the slow shift toward increasingly interdependent (communal) living. Although the Japanese would not have intended it as such, this period of house arrest served as a training ground for internment, providing opportunity to hone survival skills that would serve the missionaries well in the months and years ahead.

Furtive Christianity

Betty and Godfrey Gale sensed that the relationships they forged with individual Japanese gendarmes and their commandants would be *the* key determining factor to how they were treated. While missionaries had no control over the political situation that turned them into enemy aliens, they recognized that individual Japanese could choose to exercise their authority through either civil or violent means. Because oversight of the civilian prisoners was generally administered by Japanese consular rather than military administration, civilians, as it turned out, generally received better treatment than military prisoners. However, the missionaries did not know what to expect. One area that the missionaries resisted (and resented) the most was restriction of their religious freedom. On the first Sunday after being placed under house arrest, the missionaries met for an evening service at St Paul's chapel, accompanied by five armed Japanese soldiers and an interpreter who "took down notes of all that was said and done."[119] Isabelle MacTavish "tried to get the guards to remove their caps" out of respect for Christian tradition, "but without success!"[120] Betty Gale noted in her diary that "we held our breath" during the sermon, "in case [the minister] said wrong things sometimes!"[121] The following Sunday a group of Japanese soldiers entered in the middle of a sermon given by Godfrey Gale. When he was done, the soldiers took a roll call of all who attended. The Japanese authorities then refused the missionaries permission to have a Christmas Day service or even Christmas parties. One day, three of the "finest Christian members on staff" were taken by the Japanese for questioning. After three months of "repeated grilling had failed to uncover any incriminating evidence," Dr. Yang, Mr. Lo, and Mr. Hu were released.[122] Although the missionaries desired religious freedom, they were also aware that Christians could become targets of Japanese aggression.

Since a Christmas service was not allowed, the Gales found their own, private way to celebrate the occasion. They lit a "roaring grate fire" in their living room and opened their own presents in front of a Christmas tree. Their room was strewn with strings of Christmas cards, streamers, and decorations—albeit on "a very simple scale, of course."[123] To Betty, Margie's first Christmas was lovely, "in spite of rain and cold and imprisonment."[124] To Godfrey, their imprisonment "only served to make our fellowship closer and more intimate, and in many ways we have never had a better Christmas."[125]

Bloody Bill

Most accounts from Qilu during this period commented on the unexpected politeness of the Japanese soldiers. They also consistently reported on the inhumane behaviour of their commandant—a man variously nicknamed "Bloody Bill," "Terrible Bill," "Pygmalion Bill," and "Gestapo Bill" (there is no surname recorded). On 31 December 1941 Godfrey Gale wrote that this man was "inhuman, a regular fiend without a spark of humanity or reasonableness in him"—after witnessing a confrontation between Bloody Bill and Dr. R. Gordon Struthers.[126] Convinced that Dr. Struthers had hidden large stores of money at the hospital, Bill "whipped out his sword at Struthers and towered over him threatening to cut off his head on the spot." When Struthers pointed out that all the money and food in the hospital was gone, Bill "called him a liar and knocked him about."[127] The situation was resolved when the Superintendent of Nurses went into the office and refused to leave until Bill had gone.

A few days later, Bloody Bill accused Dr. Smyly of hiding some funds at the Leper Hospital, which was nearby Qilu. Bill assaulted the doctor in front of his patients, "knocking him about and hitting him in the face because certain lepers had gone home against official orders."[128] He announced that if more patients left the hospital they would be shot, and Dr. Smyly severely punished. The following week Bill assaulted Rufus Dart, the hospital accountant, on two occasions, vaguely accusing him of doing something improper with the hospital finances. On the first occasion he struck Dart more than thirty times while Dr. Shields stood by helplessly watching. Insisting that Dart kneel, Bill "drew his sword and really might have killed him in his insane rage had not the Chinese interpreter interfered."[129] Rufus Dart "thought his last hour had come" but "says he felt quite calm and was not afraid to die."[130] The next day Dart was struck "more than a hundred times, knocked down many times, held down and had lighted matches put under his nose etc. all in an effort to get 'information' about the hospital finances." To Dr. Shields, waiting for Bill to come around each day was like "waiting for one's execution each morning."[131] He and the others felt on the verge of collapse. To Godfrey Gale, Bill was "an absolute devil."[132]

On one occasion, Bill showed up at the Gales' front door with a Japanese woman and child. Betty, who considered Bill "dangerous and quite schizophrenic" served tea, watching nervously as the trio made themselves at home, talking to Margie and playing the gramophone and piano before leaving without explanation. The medical missionaries determined among themselves that "Pygmalion Bill" was mentally unstable and "not quite normal." Dr. Scott referred to him as "Batty Boy."[133]

The Gales recorded three instances where Japanese officers entered women's homes with intentions of sexual assault. On the first an officer entered a cottage where three American missionaries lived alone. Passing two of them on the main floor he "clumped upstairs to find the third." Confronting what he thought was another Japanese officer at the top of the stairs, he "stops dead in his tracks, salutes smartly, turns on his heel—and goes clumping down again—his long sword banging on every step."[134] As it turns out, the figure on the top of the stairs was his own reflection in a long mirror. On another occasion the Commanding Officer—who was "quite drunk"—showed up at a missionary residence at 10:00 p.m., forced his way in and went upstairs looking for the room of a certain woman. Other missionaries heard the noise, locked her door and steered the man "meek as a lamb" downstairs and outside.[135]

On the third occasion Betty Gale was having coffee at the home of a single missionary woman, May Kay, when none other than "Bloody Bill" came "swaggering up the walk."[136] Apparently surprised to see that Kay had company, his smile "turn[ed] into a scowl" as Gale pointed to a chair and immediately set a cup of coffee in front of him. As the trio sat in strained silence, Betty Gale and May Kay drank "countless cups of coffee" waiting and wondering what to do. Although Bill spoke no English, they were not sure how much he understood. In a moment of inspiration, Gale picked up a pile of sewing patterns from a nearby table and began to show them to Kay as a way to camouflage their conversation:

B.G.: [holding up a pattern and pointing to it] Do you like this dress is your cook home?

M.K.: No, it looks too skimpy he's gone out.

B.G.: How about this skirt when will he be back?

M.K.: It has too many buttons when he is finished shopping what shall we do?

B.G.: Now here's a nice blouse shall I go for help?

M.K.: Has a horrible collar for heaven's sake don't go.

B.G.: Look at this cute hat keep giving him cookies and if he doesn't go soon let's make a bolt for it.[137]

When Bill stomped away a few minutes later, the women were relieved. And they had learned a lesson about the value of subversion techniques.

In the tense atmosphere of house arrest, the missionaries became highly adept at finding ways to resist their Japanese captors and defuse potentially explosive situations. In situations like the ones described above, the missionaries relied on exacting politeness as a form of resistance. In others they provided favours to the Japanese, recognizing that this was an investment in their own self-preservation. When Godfrey Gale was approached to treat medical conditions of ailing Japanese officers, for example, he saw it as an opportunity to curry favour for the missionary community at large—be it reduced violence or increased commodities like food or medical supplies. For example, on 5 January 1942 Gale was called to attend to the Japanese Commanding Officer who was suffering from "toxic" tonsillitis. After providing the man with Steptocide, Gale asked to be brought to the deserted Qilu Hospital to pick up necessary supplies.[138] While he noted only that he picked up ice and an ice-bag for the patient, Betty Gale added that her husband also "grabbed every instrument he could lay his hands on, and filled his pockets full! Also medicines! He even had things stashed away in his shirt!"[139] To Godfrey Gale, the recovery of the commanding officer was critical: when Betty asked him upon his return whether the officer was very ill and whether there was any chance he would not recover, Godfrey responded grimly, "He *must* get better—for all our sakes."[140] In her diary Betty wrote, "G.G. got called out at 10:30 pm to see the head 'J' here, who is very ill. Not home until 12:00! Hope he doesn't die."[141] Apparently he recovered.

Guilty School Boys

A few months into their internment at Qilu, Godfrey Gale was asked to take a look at the ear of a Japanese military surveyor. After treating him and writing a prescription, the man asked if the medicine could be found in the old Qilu Hospital—which it could. They found the medicine in the former Ear, Nose and Throat Department, now "filthy dirty, covered with dust, smelling foul and looking thoroughly desolate."[142] Suddenly the surveyor turned to Gale and said, "Just take anything you want." Picking up a dozen different kinds of instruments, Gale was told "with a smile" to "put them in my pocket as I went out of the Hospital gate!"[143]

Over time the missionaries became more adept at subversive techniques, and bolder in the process. On 23 May 1942, the day after missionaries had been informed that all Americans, Canadians, and twenty Englishmen and women were to be repatriated, one of the men "discovered" a "great treasure drove" of valuable Chinese antiques—seventy packing cases in all—hidden in the foreign children's school. (Undoubtedly the "discovery" was prompted by the impending evacuation of most foreigners from Qilu.) The items had been collected approximately twenty years earlier by Dr. James M. Menzies, a United Church of Canada missionary at the Anyang mission station who later became famous for his research on ancient oracle bones from the Yin Ruins. Among the collection were priceless bronzes, porcelains, oracle bones, and scrolls. The missionaries made plans to bury them in a safer place so that the Japanese would not find them. One spot was the dirt basement of the McAll home. Another was an old grave where the coffin had "sunk a long way down" leaving "lots of room for boxes of stuff to slide in on top."[144]

Looking like "guilty school boys," a group of missionary men, along with Betty Gale and Frances McAll, set out in the pouring rain after 9:00 p.m. and spent the next few hours carting the antiques to holes freshly dug in the McAll's basement and the old grave. To thwart the Japanese who might wonder about the now-fresh grave, the treasures were covered with a dead dog before the dirt was replaced. The group celebrated their "nerve wracking but highly successful" operation with giddy excitement over a cup of hot tea.[145]

Emboldened by the success of their rebellious act, Betty Gale and Frances McAll agreed to participate in a related plan the following evening. Asked to smuggle some of the ancient scrolls to Chinese friends living within the city walls of Jinan, the women made plans to conceal the contraband in their baby prams and walk to a designated spot (by this time they were allowed off campus without a guard). They placed the treasures in the well of their baby prams, covered them with mattresses, set babies Margie and Elizabeth on top and "set off gaily" to the Qilu gates.[146] Unfortunately the guards, perhaps sensing their nervousness, commanded them to lift the babies, taking no time to "uncover the loot."[147] Ordered to take the antiques to the Japanese Commandant's Office, the women agreed, but once they were out of view, they ran for home instead. "Never again," Betty Gale wrote, "never, never again."[148]

The missionaries were not the only ones on Qilu campus engaging in acts of resistance. During the early hours of 3 April 1942, Changta Sao, the Gales' amah, almost got caught by the Japanese while slipping through the barbed wire fence. The Chinese servants, it must be remembered, were also confined to the campus, rendering them similarly isolated. Betty Gale, having noticed a tear in Changta Sao's jacket, confronted her. Changta Sao immediately responded that she had slipped under the fence to buy cloth to make new slippers for Margie. Although Changta Sao held up cloth to support her claim, a more likely explanation was that she had slipped out to see her mother: she had torn her dress two months earlier climbing through a hole in the fence, and the Gales told her never to do it again because "if a sentry had seen her do it, he might have shot her without further question."[149] Smuggling people and goods through the Japanese-imposed barriers had become a way of life. Supporters inside and outside the campus walls found ways to smuggle goods and notes of encouragement to the missionaries. The missionaries drew on such demonstrations of solidarity to strengthen their resolve to endure their ordeal.

Hoong Run also demonstrated an act of resistance in support of the Gales—one that they later learned became a dangerous daily routine. On 21 February 1942 the Gales managed to purchase three goats, including a nanny called "Shasta," which provided them with a much-welcomed, daily eight pints of milk. When the Japanese sent word two months later that they had plans to confiscate all the goats the next day, Hoong Run came up with a plan to thwart them. After securing permission from the Gales to proceed with a secret but "really safe plan," the Gales awoke the next morning to find a large jug of milk on the table, but no sign of Shasta. Looking like a "cat who had swallowed a canary," Hoong Run continued to provide milk for the Gales for the remainder of their confinement at Qilu.[150] On the day of their departure, Hoong Run revealed his strategy: after smuggling the goat off the campus, he had a friend outside bring the goat to a designated spot along the fence very early every morning, at 4:00 a.m.—and Hoong Run milked the goat through the fence.[151]

Through their own and others' acts of resistance the Gales gained important tools for survival, and developing trust—with both friends and enemies—could make all the difference.

Training in Intercessory Prayer

As Christian missionaries reared in religious homes and schools, Godfrey and Betty Gale were acculturated into routines of daily prayer, Bible reading (also called "Quiet Time"), hymn singing, weekly church service attendance, and participation in church sacraments such as baptism and communion. Now confined to the campus and with their former roles as educators and practitioners replaced by more basic roles like gardening and gathering coal, the Gales found themselves more introspective and curious about the value of one of the most basic tenets of Christian faith—intercessory prayer. For Christian missionaries, as with all Christians, the practice of praying for others was considered central to the spiritual development and nurturance not only of the persons prayed for, but also of the persons praying. Finding themselves with more free time and less opportunity to physically assist those who needed medical care, a small group of missionaries decided to take more seriously the practice of regular, intercessory prayer.

By February 1942 the Japanese authorities had decreased some of the restrictions on group meetings. After church one week, the Gales invited a small circle of friends to come over after supper to read and discuss some Christian literature. Since "most of us were medicals," the group decided to read a recently published book *The Eternal Voice*, by a respected London minister.[152] In particular the group was interested in a chapter on "spiritual healing," which described non-physical methods of healing.[153] A week later Dr. Gault, one of the physicians, called the group together to pray for a friend in the United States who was sick with tuberculosis. After much discussion they decided to split into three groups and pray together for thirty minutes each Sunday in designated homes. Each group would pray for the same list of people. On 22 February 1942 Godfrey Gale wrote, "This experiment in intercessory prayer may have important results for us all."[154]

The Gales' group met at 8:30 a.m. on Sunday mornings. Among the people prayed for the first week were Dr. Gault's American friend, a Chinese baby on campus with pneumonia, Dr. Yang who was imprisoned in Jinan, "John in Singapore," and a Qilu missionary with tuberculosis.[155] The group also prayed for their Japanese captors. By 16 April Godfrey Gale reported that there were signs that the intercessory prayer was successful: "Bloody Bill" was becoming less aggressive—he had "gradually become more friendly and pleasant, more willing to agree to our requests, less likely to swear and storm, and more likely to listen to reason."[156] When Andrew Thomson, an ardent abstainer, suggested to Bill that he would "be much better if [he] didn't drink and went to bed earlier," Bill replied, "what you say is true."[157] This softening of his character, the Gales concluded, was in part influenced by the Christian attitude displayed by the missionaries towards him, and in part due to their intercessory prayer.

The intercessory prayer groups took their new role very seriously, keeping records of those prayed for and their progress. To these scientifically minded groups, part of the reason for this experiment was to "discover the conditions necessary for the spiritual healing of sickness—its scope and limitations."[158] In situations where they felt that recovery was not in the range of medical experience, the groups prayed "along other lines."[159] And they reported favourable results. In two instances—one American missionary and one Chinese woman—"recovery took place in what is usually a fatal condition—and we could not explain this fully on medical grounds."[160] In the case of the Chinese woman, moreover, her healing led to her and her husband's conversion to Christianity.

After a few months Godfrey Gale declared the experiment complete. He concluded that "the evidence points undoubtedly to the existence of great spiritual powers of which we have little conception and over which we have as yet very little control."[161] However, "it is this lack of control over these powers that prevents us from using prayer in any kind of scientific way, as a line of therapy."[162] To Gale, while prayer could have an influence on the mental and spiritual attitude of both patient and physician, "one cannot promise that [illness] will shorten in any appreciable way."[163] Miraculous cures were the exception, not the norm. Thus, while Godfrey was willing to keep an open mind about the possibility of direct healing through prayer, what was more important was prayer "that each sufferer should find God's will for himself—or herself—in the particular circumstances in which they are placed. For this is ultimately a higher objective than to seek simply for relief from physical disability."[164]

Intercessory prayer, then, would not be used as a form of medical treatment during internment. Rather, the Gales would continue to consider prayer as a valuable source of strength and comfort, one that would provide them with a sense of purpose in the internment camps.

Training in Communal Living

The third area of preparation for internment unwittingly provided by the experience of house arrest was the shift towards intensive communal living. Although the missionaries at Qilu were already familiar with being part of a community that supported (and irritated) one another, they also enjoyed a significant amount of personal autonomy. Most significantly, Godfrey and Betty Gale had their own home, which they ran according to their own tastes and preferences. The Gale family home was a symbol of their identity as a family. Their practices of decorating, child rearing, gardening, meal planning, religious development, and sexual intimacy were aspects of their lives that required neither community negotiation nor approval. While social gatherings had always been a significant part of missionary culture, individual missionaries could exercise a certain degree of independence in terms of who they associated with, how often, and under what circumstances.

When the missionaries were initially placed under house arrest, they expressed enormous relief over being allowed to stay in their own homes. While their public domains were affected by professional, social, and religious constraints, their private domains were, for the first few months, left largely undisturbed. Lines of division between Christian denominations remained, for example, as Anglican missionaries met at different locations from the LMS missionaries for church services. Over time, however, the need to work together blurred conventional distinctions based on nationality or denomination. After four months, the missionaries were required to abandon their private homes, crowding together into residences in one section of the campus. These months were an important time of training for the eventual lack of privacy, crowding, restricted food, and medical care, and for the interpersonal conflict and simple boredom that characterized civilian internment across China.[165]

A serious difficulty during these few months was the lack of funds. Bank accounts were frozen and, according to a Qilu University report, "Chinese who would willingly lend to us could not do so safely."[166] The most immediate and vital concern for the confined missionaries was the need for food and warmth. By the end of January the Gales were in danger of running out of coal. After taking coal from the hospital but feeling guilty about not asking for Japanese permission, they obtained consent to haul coal from the university men's dormitories. "We shifted about 8 tons in the small handcart," Godfrey Gale noted, "a filthy game but the hard work in itself is exhilarating."[167] By February 1942 most of the Gales' cash had run out. The missionaries made do with sharing food and other resources, but realized that they would have to augment their food sources. After living on millet, corn meal, bran, peanut butter, carrots, and cabbage, some of the missionaries crafted crude bows and arrows to hunt the rabbits that roamed the campus. And they started to dig a large communal garden—which eventually produced an abundance of vegetables and flowers. In March the Japanese authorities gave a small loan to the internees (250 yen per adult) after arrangements to secure further financial assistance through the Swiss Consulate "failed to secure the approval of the Japanese authorities in [Beijing]."[168] Three months later there was still no approval for Swiss financial aid.

Promises of Repatriation

Plans for the repatriation of enemy aliens at Qilu began to take shape towards the end of March 1942. It was a complicated process given the interruption of communication capacity. Various plans were relayed in telegrams from Tokyo to the Japanese Embassy in Beijing to the Qilu staff and other British and American residents in the Jinan area. The unofficial Swiss consular representative conveyed the information to and fro. According to the "Qilu University Report of 1942," the unnamed Swiss consular representative and "those who assisted" were able to secure "friendly contacts" with the Japanese officials. The author of the report credited the efforts of these individuals in "securing more favorable treatment than many other enemy nationals received in other cities."[169]

On 1 April 1942 the Japanese authorities informed the 70 missionaries that they would be leaving Qilu on 6 April for repatriation. Approximately 600 expatriates from China would depart Shanghai aboard the Italian steamer *Conte Verde* and sail as far as Lourenço Marques (Maputo), the capital of Mozambique. There they would meet up with 900 expatriates from Japan, sailing aboard the *Asama Maru*. These 1,500-odd passengers would transfer to the *Gripsholm*, an 18,000-ton vessel accommodating 1,584 passengers.[170] Repatriation would involve a voyage of some 29,000 kilometres that would take ten weeks.[171] In preparation they would have to evacuate their homes, sell off their furniture to the Japanese, and move in together into a row of five houses at the southwest corner of the campus. After considerable negotiation, the missionaries were able to secure fourteen houses.

Within a few days the Gales had "crammed" into Don Faris's house, along with Betty's father, Andrew Thomson, May Kay, the McAlls, and Welles Hubbard. In total there were ten living in the home, plus three in the nearby servant's quarters. The group christened their new home "the Mess" in honour of the chaotic atmosphere when they first arrived."[172] There was enough room for each family to have separate sleeping quarters but the children, Margie Gale and Eli McAll, shared a room. The group divided up vegetables from the garden into appropriate amounts for each newly appointed household. While Betty Gale was comfortable with the idea of sharing chores and food, she was less enamoured with the cooking. May Kay, for example, enjoyed serving alfalfa, soya beans, curds, and rough cereals—foods with "potent vitamins" that nonetheless caused Betty indigestion.[173]

Repatriation promises came and went. The groups kept themselves occupied by organizing their routines to include regular games (tennis and bridge), skits, art exhibitions, literary clubs, education of missionary children, music concerts, and tea parties. Godfrey Gale taught lessons in geography while Betty Gale taught art. Betty also busied herself knitting toy dogs, rabbits, mice, and a big doll for Margie and Eli's upcoming first birthdays in July. As it turned out, the elaborate party—complete with a princess theme and guests in costumes—would take place shortly after the departure of fifty-five of the seventy missionaries from Qilu campus on their way to repatriation ships in Shanghai. The party would give the remaining missionaries a necessary emotional lift. While Betty Gale had agonized over her original decision regarding whether to evacuate China in February 1941, when faced with the opportunity to leave China with her father on a repatriation ship for Canadians and Americans in July 1942, she had already firmly decided that she would not go without Godfrey. "I wouldn't leave G. for anything," she wrote, "we will see this through together—with Margie as our ballast."[174]

In a letter penned to her family two days before her father's departure in June 1942 (a letter Andrew Thomson would carry with him) Betty Gale wrote, "I have spent the day packing Dad's odds and ends—it's nice to think they will be unpacked in dear old "33" [Rose Park Drive] by you folks."[175] To Betty, who had prepared herself for imprisonment in a concentration camp, the "repatriation business" came as a surprise—"we can scarcely believe that it may really happen."[176] Although she admitted she would miss her father, it was Godfrey who wrote more directly about the loss of Andrew Thomson:

> The party for the first repatriation boat to Canada and the United States will be leaving in a few hours. Dad is very kindly taking a bundle of letters with him in the hope that they will get through. He has promised to post some of mine home to England. It will be a real wrench when we say goodbye to him on the platform tonight. It has been a great privilege having him live with us during these past eighteen months. He has been a tower of strength during many difficult decisions. He is a kind of Elder Statesman on the Campus—a person who can speak with authority from a rich experience … His keen scholarship, kindly spirit and humour have contributed not a little to the spirit here. He has helped us hold together to face the unaccustomed situations of the past six months. I think we are all hoping that we will be able to come back to [Qilu] when the period of reconstruction begins.[177]

After a week of tearful farewell parties, the Gales were given permission to accompany the departing missionaries to the train station to see them off. While Betty Gale was "glad for them" she felt "very sad for ourselves—and left behind."[178] It was "awful seeing them go," she noted in her diary, "we feel few now."[179] Betty hoped that she and Godfrey might be able to leave, too, but "the British plans are rather vague and the Government doesn't seem keen about arranging for ships."[180] She was also concerned that they may no longer be eligible to leave: "Of course we really can't blame [the British government] if they refuse for they gave us plenty of warnings and advice about leaving last year, and we didn't obey them."[181] This was the closest Betty Gale would come to suggesting that she might regret her decision. However, on the very same day that she penned these words, Godfrey penned a very different perspective in a letter to his mother in England: "Betty and I never regret for a moment our decision to remain here together."[182] It was not completely accurate, but it was a script that eventually neither would depart from.

In June 1942 Andrew Thomson was one of approximately 1,500 civilian internees who boarded the Japanese ship *Tatutu Maru* in Shanghai, bound for Lourenço Marques. There they met up with the Swedish ship *Gripsholm*, carrying Japanese prisoners from Europe. The prisoners were exchanged,

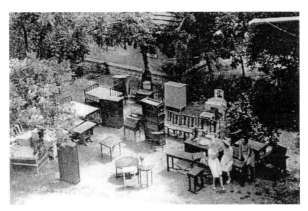

Fig. 5.2   Missionary belongings being sold in 1942

and Thomson sailed on the *Gripsholm* back to North America, arriving in Montreal on 25 August 1942.[183]

On 13 July 1942 those left behind in Qilu received word that they, too, would take a train to Shanghai and board a repatriation boat bound for North America. The general feeling on campus was, surprisingly, one of exhaustion and depression: "a combination of intolerable heat—and the everlasting suspense of not knowing what is going to happen—or *when*."[184] Word finally arrived on 6 August that the group would be evacuated four days later, on 10 August. Ordered by the Japanese to sell their furniture to the Chinese, the missionaries brought their larger items to the front lawn that very day. On 7 August dozens of Japanese arrived early to "slash all our prices in half."[185] When the Chinese arrived, "it was "bedlam!!! It is wild, but in an incredibly short time everything has disappeared. We find we have made very little money out of the sale."[186] The Japanese, as it turns out, took all the money that should have gone to the missionaries. But anticipating their imminent repatriation, none of this seemed to matter—the missionaries took it all as "a huge joke."[187] As Betty Gale wrote: "Who cares? In three days we will be ON OUR WAY HOME!"[188]

On 8 August Georgina and John Lewis arrived from Chou Tsan with their two children; they were to be repatriated, too.[189] On the evening of 10 August, Hoong Run prepared the last meal for his employers. It was, as Betty described it, "a madhouse scene."[190] Throughout the day dozens of Chinese had hovered around them, "waiting to grab the tables, chairs, and our beds and dishes as soon as we finished using them." When they sat down for dinner, Chinese persons whom they did not know "stood right behind our chairs—and as we finished each course, the plates would be snatched away by sleight of hand, it seemed."[191] When Godfrey got up to get something, his chair immediately vanished, leaving him to finish his meal standing up.

After dinner Hoong Run and Changta Sao accompanied the Gales and their belongings as they walked for the last time to the Qilu campus gates. After giving Margie a final hug, the pair stood, as Betty later wrote, "waving us off—with tears running down their cheeks. They were running down mine, too."[192] (Hoong Run would stay in touch with the Gales by letter over the coming years).[193] A tremendous crowd was at the train station to see them off and to wish them "*i lu p'ing an*" (peace, or light, on our way). In an ironic display of respect for the Qilu University president, the Japanese sent a car to pick him up and chauffer him to the railway station as a show of "honor as befitted his rank."[194] It was the president's own car—the one the Japanese had commandeered eight months earlier. While the local press corps snapped photographs, old students, teachers, and friends quietly shook hands with the Gales before slipping away. The four-decade legacy of both Shandong Christian University and the Thomson family missions in northern China had come to an unceremonious end.

Summary

After months of anxious speculation, Godfrey and Betty Gale were placed under house arrest at Qilu University Campus in Jinan, along with seventy other missionaries. Their first response was relief, in part because the Japanese soldiers were unexpectedly polite, but also because the men were not immediately carted off to separate concentration camps, as they had feared. Being allowed to stay in their own home, the Gales adjusted remarkably quickly to the new circumstances, finding innovative ways to meet their needs for food, clothing, shelter, and companionship.

Their loss of freedom was gradual—imperceptible even. At the very beginning they lost the right to move around freely off campus, requiring Japanese passes and escorts even to walk to the hospital nearby, but this requirement was later slackened. They also lost three of their Chinese house staff, only to gain them back again a few days later. They lost the freedom to celebrate Christmas in church, but were able to celebrate it at home. They were no longer allowed to teach, but they managed to fit in a few more lectures and final examinations before this was stopped. The hospital was closed and looted, but some of the physicians were allowed to continue work at other nearby hospitals. In other words, initially the internees were actually permitted more than they expected, and they felt less anxious about their treatment under the Japanese. By the time they were forced to sell their belongings to the benefit of the Japanese at the end of their house arrest, they were not even upset, having so detached themselves from their belongings and their sense of civilian rights.

The worst experience during the period of house arrest was the lunatic and cruel behaviour of the Japanese Commandant, "Bloody Bill." Few escaped his erratic behaviour, and many had reason to be terrified of him. The Gales found their own ways to deal with Bill, from Betty's thwarting of Bill's advances towards one of the missionary women, to their intercessory prayer on his behalf. Bloody Bill's tempered behaviour over time affirmed their belief in the value of tact, and of prayer.

Through Betty Gale's experiences during the early part of her new identity as an "enemy alien," we see, really for the last time, her relationships with the Chinese people. Like her missionary parents, Gale distinguished between different classes of Chinese and acted differently towards each group. To members of the labouring classes—usually men who carried heavy loads or pulled missionaries in rickshaws—she was courteous but not sociable. She did not learn their names but, like those around her, categorized them simply as "coolies." Aside from shopkeepers and certain other workers, most of the Chinese she related to were Christian. Gale regularly interacted with younger Chinese girls, creating a "club" for them and welcoming them to her home. Her exasperation towards their noisiness or annoying behaviour seems not unlike the way a young Canadian adult might have responded to a group of boisterous Sunday School children in Canada. To her nursing students, too, Betty Gale assumed an air of authority and professionalism not unlike what one would have expected between a nursing instructor and students at a training school in Canada. She took an interest in their lives, intervening in their conflicts and inviting them to socialize at her home. Still, it is not clear whether some of Gale's Chinese guests were nursing colleagues; there is no indication that she enjoyed a strong friendship with any Chinese nurse in particular—or that any of them sought friendship with her. Although China was her adopted home, Gale identified herself quite clearly as a Westerner, and she sought most of her friendships among other foreigners.

Of all the Chinese she related to, Betty Gale was closest to her household workers—amahs, cooks, and house servants. Her childhood familiarity with having household staff undoubtedly influenced the easy relationship she seemed to develop with Hoong Run and Changta Sao in particular. Gale felt genuine affection and appreciation for these two, and the feeling appears to have been mutual—as particularly demonstrated by the risks they took on the Gales' behalf: returning to their home after being banished from campus and furtively obtaining goat's milk and other supplies during the months of house arrest.

Although the missionaries experienced loss of freedom, privacy, and belongings, they also found that they could be resourceful in previously untapped ways. Betty Gale was bolder than she thought, attempting to smuggle valuables off campus after furtive attempts to safeguard valuables on campus had been successful. She learned that she could share a home with others and put up with inconveniences like different cooking styles. And she learned that having a baby to care for was more a source of comfort than of strain. Most important of all, Gale learned that she made the right decision by staying in China. At some level, the idea of being interned was a challenge to her, one not so different from that of being a China missionary in the first place. She wanted to see if she could handle it. Believing that her trial was now over, Betty Gale boarded the train to Shanghai with the confidence that she had endured her ordeal in a way that she, her husband, her parents, and her daughter might be proud of.

Adjusting to Columbia Country Club and Yangzhou Camp B (1943)

Japanese Authorities have been forced to group British and Allied Subjects in special centres to prevent espionage in occupied China. To allow families to remain together they have created civil assembly centres as distinct from internment camps where individual members of families would be separated.

—Telegram from the High Commissioner of Canada in the United Kingdom to the Secretary of State for External Affairs in Canada, 2 April 1943

The internees [of Yangzhou Camps] give the impression of being lost and forgotten in an interior city of limited resources.

—Confidential dispatch from the High Commissioner of Canada in the United Kingdom, 14 September 1943

On 10 August 1942 Betty Gale and Georgina Lewis set off with their families and the remaining dozen or so Qilu missionaries on a train filled with expatriate evacuees from all over north China. They were bound for Shanghai. For Betty Gale, one exciting thought edged out all others: they were going home! Anticipating a thirty-hour journey before boarding the repatriation ship *Kamakura Maru* bound for Europe and Canada, the Gales were unconcerned about their lack of money and relatively few belongings. Betty Gale felt unencumbered—free even. Even when the train journey took a nightmarish turn, the Gales kept their spirits up, imagining the reunion with family after an additional two months at sea on the repatriation ship. It was not to be. Within hours of their arrival at the "temporary" shelter at Shanghai, they and most of the other Qilu missionaries discovered that their names had been removed from the ship reservation list: expatriates living in Shanghai had wrangled away the reserved spots for all but seven of the seventy-seven missionaries who had just left northern China. This had been the last opportunity to evacuate China. Together with 350 other internees, the Gales found themselves jammed for seven months into a once-exclusive British country club meant to accommodate thirty-five. The following year, on 11 March 1943, the Gales were transferred to Yangzhou (Yangchow) Camp B. They soothed themselves with the thought that they had at least avoided the notorious Pudong (Pootung) Camp, set in a condemned industrial district across the Huangpu River in Shanghai. Six months later, however, on 30 September 1943, they were transferred to Pudong. John and Georgina Lewis were transferred from the Columbia Country Club to Ash Camp for the duration of the war. John and Mary Stanley remained under house arrest in Beijing until being transferred to Weixian (Weihsien) Camp in northern China until the end of the war. Georgina Lewis's and Betty Gale's internment, therefore, overlapped for only a few months in Shanghai.

This chapter is divided into two parts: Columbia Country Club (August 1942 to March 1943) and Yangzhou Camp B (March 1943 to September 1943). Drawing mostly on Betty Gale's journal, diary, notebook, and correspondence during this period, it traces Betty's internal struggle to accept and adapt to her unexpected identity as civilian internee.[1]

Columbia Country Club, Shanghai

Although Betty Gale felt weary beyond words when charcoal-burning buses dropped off the last load of northern evacuees at their temporary shelter in Shanghai at 3:15 a.m. on 12 August 1942, she was buoyed by the hospitable reception staged by members of the Shanghai British Residents Association—a local organization that had been organizing relief efforts in Shanghai since the war began. The surprise of genteel, late-night pots of tea and buns were a welcome contrast to the stifling heat, violent bouts of gastric illness, and subsequent quarantine they had experienced on the train. As it happened, a few hours into the train ride, five Qilu missionaries in the Gale's coach were struck with severe and protracted vomiting and diarrhoea. Fearing cholera, the Japanese authorities demanded that the coach be put under strict quarantine. Despite the 41°C temperature, the passengers were forbidden from opening the windows, lest the Chinese guerrillas shoot at the train—a bizarre explanation. Furthermore, the Gales had run out of fluids for Margie; two flasks had broken. The quarantined coach was detached from the rest of the train and, after the passengers were sprayed from head to foot with antiseptic from a flimsy plastic insecticide sprayer, it was pronounced clean.

Having lost their connection with the rest of the train, the abandoned passengers were eventually taken across the Yangtze River by ferry, put on a fresh train, and then taken by bus to Shanghai. Three of ill missionaries were taken to a local hospital, where they were diagnosed with food poisoning. At the Columbia Country Club (ccc), Betty and Godfrey Gale were pointed to camping cots in separate areas filled with sleeping internees. Fully clothed, Betty fell into a deep sleep, certain that the worst was over. At breakfast the next morning Betty was informed that they (and the Lewises) had been removed from the evacuation list. "Told this a.m. that only 7 of our party of 77 can go," she noted in her diary. "Spent day trying to rest."[2]

Unlike the long-anticipated prospect of confinement under the Japanese in the months leading up to Pearl Harbor, the Gales entered the next phase of their internment in a state of shock and disbelief. Although there is no record of Georgina and John Lewis's reaction to the news, one can assume it was similar to the Gales'. When Betty Gale first glimpsed their crowded, cacophonic surroundings at the ccc, she had no idea that they would be there for seven months, let alone that they would be internees in progressively decrepit camps over the next three years. The discovery that British residents of Shanghai—many of them thought to be wealthy and/ or well-connected to the local British Embassy—had appropriated most of the missionaries' reserved berths pitched Betty into an emotional crisis. As Godfrey understood it, the British Resident's Association had "wangled their friends into our places."[3] While it is not clear whether or to what the extent the new passengers contrived their way onto the *Kamakura Maru*, at least some were British officials who were granted passage at the last minute by a "special exchange agreement."[4] Out of the 350 expatriate internees who had travelled with the Gales from northern China, only 120 would get on the boat—seven of whom were from Qilu.

Those who had their places taken were outraged. Canadian Desmond Powers recalled travelling with the Gales from Tianjin to Shanghai with the same plan—to catch the repatriation ship home. In Powers's view, the berths were "snatched by Shanghai taipans."[5] Nicknaming the repatriation ship "Wangle Maru," Betty Gale struggled to come to terms with the unfairness of the situation. In a hastily-written letter to her parents on the day of the *Kamakura Maru*'s departure, the emotionally charged Betty fumed:

Only 7 out of the 77 [Jinan] folks [can] go ... and a similar percentage of folks from [Tianjin], [Beijing], etc. Apparently the Swiss Representatives had everything fixed up—and didn't even know of the changes—which were made by the Jap[anese] and the S'hai [Shanghai] Council. The S'hai people were annoyed because so many of the "country" folk were getting away, and they couldn't, that they got the "J[apanese]" to cross out 500 of us—and replace the number with people from here![6]

For both Betty and Godfrey Gale, having been required to hastily sell their belongings and leave their Qilu homes only to be thrown indefinitely into an overcrowded building fifteen hundred kilometres away was galling. Although they were relatively free to travel around Shanghai with Japanese permission, they had no money and few contacts there. To Betty, if only the Japanese had "been decent about it and let us know a few days before we left our homes, we wouldn't mind so much. But they didn't do that—and here we are, packed in like sardines and no prospects of leaving."[7] Observing a toddler with whom she shared a room, Betty saw her own fear reflected in the child's "terrified blue eyes."[8]

Adjusting to the ccc

Located at 301 Great Western Road in Shanghai, the Columbia Country Club had been a popular club for wealthy "Shanghailanders" of all nationalities. The well-furnished, two-storied clubhouse was built in a Spanish style with a red tiled roof. It sat on five acres and boasted an outdoor swimming pool and an indoor bowling alley. Starting at the time of the Gales' arrival, the ccc was used by the Japanese to house enemy aliens from outside of Shanghai awaiting repatriation. Of the approximately 350 expatriates who were stranded with the Gales when they lost their berths to influential Shanghailanders,[9] in Betty's estimation ninety percent were missionaries. The main difficulty was finding space for everyone. Approximately 150 women and children were placed on camping beds in upstairs bedrooms and hallways, and in the dining room, while 120 men were "packed head to tail" in the bowling alley and an additional 80 men were crowded into the bar. Betty and Margie shared a room with four other women and eight children. Men were only allowed upstairs at allotted times, leaving their wives to care for the children. Internees were summoned to meals by a gong; after waiting in long queues, they were served "decent" food in cafeteria style.

At first Betty Gale felt overwhelmed by the noise, stench of dirty diapers, lack of privacy, and separation from Godfrey. She spent much of the first few days on her bed, watching Margie play, noting "there is really no other place to go right now, as everything is so disorganized."[10] During mealtime beside the stagnant pool, a "plague" of large black and blue flies hovered over the plates, causing Betty and the other mothers to fan the flies away with one hand while shovelling food into their children's mouths with the other. When Margie became ill with dysentery, Betty had to care for her through long nights without Godfrey's help, and she began for the first time to doubt her decision not to evacuate sooner. At a low point—the day

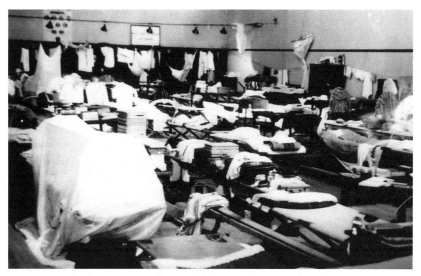

Fig. 6.1   CCC bowling alley being used as a dormitory in 1942

before the "Wangle Maru" set sail—Betty wondered: "Oh, should I have taken her home when the Canadians left?"[11]

This period of internment—or, perhaps more accurately, displacement—at the CCC set the tone for the rest of the Gales' internment years. As Betty Gale slowly accepted the reality that she would be confined in China "for the duration," she began to adapt to her new environment. Her key concerns were Margie's increased exposure to illness and injury, their separation from Godfrey at night time—particularly when Margie was ill—and their lack of money. In each of these areas Betty learned to become increasingly dependent on the generosity of others. She chose to be grateful for many small things: for stolen times of intimacy, for assistance in caring for Margie, for daily food and other necessities, and for distracting social activities in which to pour the endless days. As days stretched into months at the CCC and the internees settled into a routine of sorts, Betty came to recognize and appreciate the social and spiritual wealth available to her in this new community—and she also came to recognize, resent, and avoid those whose behaviour appeared selfish or demoralizing.

Although Betty Gale was candid about her frustrations, especially in letters to her parents, she was also determined to accept the situation she found herself in and to strive to see the good in it. She and her friend Frances McAll agreed that, although it was frustrating to lose their place on the *Maru*, the group at the CCC was ultimately better equipped to withstand the

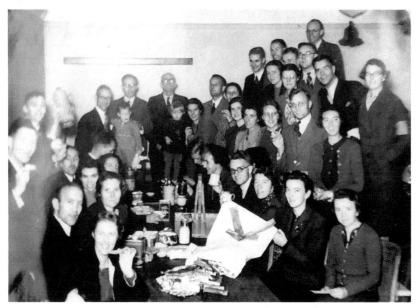

Fig. 6.2   Christmas at the ccc, 1942. Betty Gale at centre on the left.
Note the armband of suited man on the right

difficulties of internment since many were missionaries with practical skills as teachers, doctors, and nurses. Furthermore, although the lack of privacy and overcrowding was grating, they could appreciate the abundant hot water and sufficient heat—luxuries not available at Qilu. Also, the meals were tasty and were prepared and served by Chinese kitchen staff. Finally, Betty Gale had plenty of friends to spend time with, including fellow North China mishkid nurse Georgina Lewis, her husband Dr. John Lewis, and their two infant children.

In fact, internees at the ccc managed to develop such a relatively pleasant atmosphere that those who visited commented on it. For example, Canadian missionary Winifred Warren, who had been seconded to Shanghai from northern China the previous year, visited the ccc in December 1942 and noted that "some of us who live more apart rather envied their big-family celebration" of Christmas. The carol-singing, Christmas tree, and even a production of Handel's *Messiah* had been "so well planned."[12]

In contrast, Winifred Warren found the Chinese church services she was attending difficult to follow because they were conducted in an unfamiliar dialect. The irony is significant: as someone who would not be interned until the following March, Warren envied those who were trapped at the ccc because of the sense of community they enjoyed.

Before long the internees had organized themselves into groups to teach courses on everything from sewing and shorthand to medical ethics and anatomy and physiology lessons. They also conducted concerts and plays, and took turns babysitting each other's children. Betty Gale even surprised herself by agreeing to teach a ballroom dancing course with Godfrey to a class of fifty. She wrote, "I can imagine the incredulous looks on the faces of men I've danced with in Canada if they learned of this!"[13] Within weeks people had started to form habits as to which seats they would occupy in the communal hall and how they would spend the evenings there. Some parents read stories to their children. Behind them, a group of three "frail and sweet and gentle" unmarried elderly women visited with each other—prompting Betty to wonder if they would survive years of war. Beside these women was a young "thin wisp of a woman with pale red hair, and a tiny face, colourless and delicate" who would sit beside her blind husband every evening reading books to him "in a soft voice no one else can hear—he tilts his head towards her, clasps his hands and listens—and remains like that—a statue—as long as she continues. She is a marvel."[14] Although the separation of men and women rendered marital intimacy virtually impossible, Godfrey and Betty managed this too: recognizing the restrictions posed by internment, acquaintances and friends in Shanghai offered the Gales the use of their homes for occasional weekend outings while someone at the ccc babysat Margie. Betty discreetly likened these to a second honeymoon, from which she drew courage.

Although it is not clear how letters travelled from the ccc to Canada, they apparently had other means than routing their letters through contacts in Sichuan. In an October 1942 postcard addressed to her parents in Toronto, Betty Gale's tone was upbeat. Anticipating the mail delays home, she wished them a "Merry Merry Christmas" and reassured them that Margie is "lovely—fat and adorable" and no longer pale. Betty sprinkled her postcard with light-hearted descriptors of her roommates ("charming"), weekends away from the ccc ("glorious"), and weather ("lovely"). While she mentions briefly her work as a "marger" (meaning unclear) and Godfrey's busyness with studying, Betty's greatest concern, it seems, was to keep her parents from worrying about her. "Lots of gay times, too," she wrote, "games, chess, bridge, dancing, so don't worry about us!!!"[15] Betty was also aware that her parents were not her only audience: the letter is signed as examined by a censor.

Families of internees counted on church, government, and private sources to keep them abreast of the latest news of their loved ones. Between Pearl Harbor in 1941 and the Japanese surrender in 1945, there was little correspondence between missionaries and their mission boards, but any information that slipped through was shared widely. During the early part of the war radio messages (radiograms) were regularly sent out by short wave to California, from where they could be forwarded to family in Canada. As the war progressed, all correspondence was hampered; even if letters could be posted, there was a chance that the postal ship would not arrive safely at its destination. During the Gales' time at the ccc, the International Committee of the Red Cross (icrc) started to take over responsibility for getting messages to and from internees and their families in Canada. Both internees and their families were required to use special forms supplied by the icrc. They were limited to twenty-five words. Turnaround time could take a year or longer. Still, to the missionaries and their families, correspondence was invaluable.

In the meantime, the Qilu missionaries who left China on the repatriation ship became important sources of information on the well-being of those left behind. Although Canadians were eager to hear their stories, the missionaries were cautious to share too much; eight Canadian missionaries associated with the North China Mission were still in China on their way to internment camps, including Betty Gale, Mary Stanley, Georgina Lewis, Bertha Hodge, Winifred Warren, Rev. and Mrs. G.K. King, and Susie Kelsey. The Foreign Mission Board was also cautious, believing that the Chinese Christians might also be in danger. For example, there was a delay in Toronto getting the *Honan Quarterly Summer Issue* out to Sichuan in 1942 because the Foreign Mission Board "felt that there were some things that ought not to be made public."[16] Information about China was first screened by repatriated missionaries Andrew Thomson, Gordon Struthers, and Don Faris because they "were in a position to see the possible danger the Chinese Christians might be in if certain things in the original copy [of the Henan report] became public."[17]

At the ccc, Betty and Godfrey Gale grew very appreciative of the generous spirit that this unsettling experience brought out in many of those who still lived freely in Shanghai—both Chinese and foreign. In addition to irregular visits to acquaintances' homes in Shanghai, the Gales were treated on occasion to restaurant meals. In the early months before the Japanese closed all places of amusement, the Gales would take turns attending a large church service run in the Old Roxy Cinema by Chinese staff and students of Hangzhou College. While the Japanese restricted contact between the internees and their Chinese friends in Shanghai, some met the internees secretly at expatriate homes to talk and pray together. On one Sunday in February 1943, after a particularly inspiring church service, retreat, and prayer meeting, Betty wrote in her diary: "Begin to feel a new aim in Life and a strong desire to make real use of my life."[18]

Eventually internees were required to sign out and wear red armbands when they were away from the Country Club (inscribed with a "B" for British, an "A" for American, plus a personal number), but even then they enjoyed relative freedom to wander around Shanghai. Betty's greatest irritation lay not with the Japanese, but with members of the British expatriate elite still living in their luxurious homes in Shanghai. Undoubtedly still rankled by the appropriation of their *Maru* berths, her perception of influential British businessmen and their wives was further tainted by an unexpected visit to her room by four strange women who came to "see how the internees live."[19]

Walking into Gale's bedroom without warning, the socialites ("British, I'm ashamed to say") found Betty and her four roommates dressed only in their slips as they spent the morning sewing, tidying up, and watching their children play. Incensed by such callousness, Betty wrote: "The unutterable gall of them … we feel like animals in a zoo—and are furiously angry. One of them, a young girl, has the grace to look ashamed—but the others keep asking questions and poking about, not in the least put off by our noncommittal replies."[20] When some of the approximately eight thousand expatriates still living in Shanghai would later join the missionaries as internees, Betty would be especially wary of any suggestions of entitlement or superiority.

Shanghailanders

The Shanghailanders would play an important role in Betty Gale's early experiences in Shanghai and at Yangzhou Camp B. In one sense Gale was correct that the wealthy and influential British expatriates had retained some of the privileges associated with treaty port life in Shanghai. In her memoir about her time as a civilian internee, Peggy Pemberton-Carter described a life in pre-1941 China that defied the wartime conditions affecting much of the rest of China since the invasion of Japan in 1937. Pemberton-Carter had moved with her widowed mother from Paris to Shanghai during the First World War because they "could live in a style and fashion that had become increasingly difficult in Europe after 1918."[21] Expatriates living in Shanghai could still have "all of the pleasures that made the Edwardian era a halcyon period for those with money."[22] After her mother's death in 1938, Pemberton-Carter was totally without family obligations and responsibilities—and she was financially independent. Like other wealthy foreigners living in China's cosmopolitan treaty ports, she perceived Shanghai as the "Never-never Land of Extra-territoriality"—a place of complete freedom and protection, where British, American, and French authorities, backed up by gunboats anchored in the harbours, ensured the safety of their citizens.[23] In Shanghai it was possible to lead a life of high fashion, including theatre, extravagant dinners, and elegant homes, even after the Japanese invasion of northern China in 1937.

Despite the ever-increasing military activities of the Japanese, upper-class foreigners living in Shanghai did not perceive the possibility of real danger; they had no incentive to depart. As S.W. Jackson so eloquently noted, "Nobody wanted to believe that an era was at an end and Shanghai society continued to act as if it were rearranging the deck chairs on the Titanic despite the vessel's collision with the iceberg."[24] In March 1943 Peggy Pemberton-Carter became one among the thousands of enemy aliens interned in Shanghai.

A similar feeling of invulnerability persisted among upper-class foreigners living in Hong Kong despite a "nasty warning of what might happen" to them in June 1940, when Japanese were fighting against the Chinese at Kowloon, just across the peninsula from the island of Hong Kong.[25] So many Chinese were wounded that several schools in Kowloon were converted into hospitals, and the casualties were so high that the "smell of dead Chinese" drifting into Hong Kong was "unmistakable and unbearable."[26] This incident prompted the Hong Kong Colonial Government to demand that all (British) women and children leave the colony immediately. Ironically, after a period of relative peace, husbands began holding mass meetings to demand their wives' return. They complained about discrimination in allowing so many other women to stay in Hong Kong—women who had "enlisted almost overnight as auxiliary nurses, air raid wardens, stenographers and cipher clerks" in order to stay there."[27]

"Our Security Has Gone"

Although this period of internment was characterized by relative peacefulness, occasional crises reminded Betty Gale that she was, indeed, imprisoned and they awoke in her a sense of fear. At one point the internees received news that the Japanese had unexpectedly seized and jailed four hundred expatriate men in Shanghai. The men had been dragged from their beds and incarcerated in the notorious Bridge House jail—a place known for its torture of prisoners. On hearing this news Gale noted that "life has suddenly turned horribly black and cold and we all feel old and shaken ... we do not know what has happened to them—or who might be taken next."[28] This was a stark reminder of the danger hovering at their doorstep; they were in enemy territory. Fearing that Godfrey might also be taken, she noted, "Death is something I can think of calmly, but *not* torture for my husband or friends ... We feel as though all our security has gone—and are afraid to let our husbands out of our sight."[29] Everyone was feeling "about 100 years old," Gale noted in her diary.[30] Although her feeling of alarm would subside within a few days, her fear of, and anger towards, the Japanese was covered by only a thin veneer.

In addition to the threat of her potential separation from Godfrey—at Bridge House jail, for example, or an internment camp for men—Betty Gale worried about Margie's protection from illness and injury. Throughout her diary and in letters home during her internment, Betty would make note of Margie's health: pale ... listless ... rosy-cheeked ... eating well. Margie's well-being was a gauge of sorts to how Betty was coping with internment. With the exception of dysentery during the early days of the Columbia Country Club, Margie seemed remarkably healthy. However, on 12 January 1943 Margie had an accident from which she would carry scars on her hands into adulthood.

As an active toddler, Margie had been crawling around a lot under tables and chairs in the CCC lounge and then pulling herself up on whatever she could lay her hands on. At one point she grabbed at two metal pipes and heaved herself upright. Suddenly she let out a howl of pain; the pipes were carrying scalding water. The palms and fingers of both hands erupted immediately into a mass of blisters. After receiving a sedative and dressings from her father, Margie eventually settled. Her parents, however, felt horrified, believing they should have foreseen the accident and taken means to prevent it. The accident would be yet another reminder of their vulnerability.

In February 1943 the internees at the CCC received word that they were all to be moved to internment camps outside of Shanghai. All enemy aliens living in Shanghai were about to be "concentrated" and the CCC was about to become an official internment camp for Shanghai residents.[31] "We understand that we are going quite a distance," Betty Gale wrote her parents, "to the place where the CIM [China Inland Mission] had their training school, about 1896 or thereabouts—know the place, Dad?"[32] Betty's main concern was whether the food would be right for Margaret. She had good reason to worry: she herself would lose thirty pounds in the internment camps due to the scarcity of food; Godfrey would lose forty.[33]

Documents from the Canadian Department of Defence illustrate the difference between what the Japanese were communicating to the English-speaking public via radio broadcasts, and what confidential reports were describing. Radio broadcasts from Japan in April 1943, for example, reported that the internment camps in Shanghai were located in quiet suburban districts, that the houses were well built and that "many internees are even glad to be in the camps."[34] These broadcasts insisted that internment camps were being carefully planned, with special attention to accommodations required for group living, religious differences among internees, needs of married couples, and sanitary requirements. In contrast, a broadcast from Chongqing, Sichuan, reported that within a one-week period in March 1943, fifty-three Anglo-Americans in Shanghai who had been placed in "concentration camps" had been murdered or had committed suicide. Tokyo denied the story in their English broadcast to "the Americans" on 19 March 1943. The following month a Vatican broadcast reported that three Jesuit priests interned in Fuzhou had been killed."[35]

On 8 March 1943, two days before the Gales were scheduled to be transferred to Yangzhou Camp B, Betty went into a "J" (Japanese) shop to buy two warm nightgowns for Margie. Realizing when she returned to the ccc that she required larger clothes to account for Margie's growth during internment, she hurried back to the shop. When the Japanese shopkeeper refused to exchange them—even after Betty pled with him because of their impending internment—she got mad, tearfully shouting at him before storming out of his shop. On the sidewalk outside Betty leaned on her bicycle and began to "howl like a child with rage and frustration."[36] But she also immediately felt ashamed.

After a sleepless night of self-reflection, Betty Gale decided that she had made a moral error: "there is so much hatred in the world and I have added to it."[37] Returning to the shop the next morning, Gale surprised the shopkeeper by offering an apology for her rudeness. Although she did not receive a bigger nightgown, she felt rewarded by his smile and their mutual handshake over piles of children's underwear. As the shopkeeper graciously bowed as she left the store, Gale felt elated. For Gale, a clear conscience and peaceful relationships were more vital to her sense of well-being than obtaining necessary material goods. Through her years as a China mishkid and missionary nurse, she had been surrounded by people who earnestly believed that God would supply all their needs—be they physical, emotional, or spiritual. As she strove to understand the difference between her needs and her desires, she practised surrendering her concerns to God and was rewarded with a sense of serenity from which she drew strength.

On the night before the Gales were to be transferred to Yangzhou Camp, Betty stayed up late writing a last letter to her parents. Standing in the bathroom dressed in pyjamas and a fur coat (her dressing gown having already been packed and sent on ahead), Betty wrote, "I wish I could tell you of some of our recent experiences, but that would be [unwise] ... Here's hoping we'll be able to spin them off some night before a roaring grate fire when the lamps are dim and we can sit and munch fat rosy apples (without the absurd price of $2.50 being attached to one)."[38]

Last Vestige of Liberty

At the Columbia Country Club a committee was set up to work with the Japanese authorities on who would go to which internment camp. The internees would be dispersed to five camps—two set up in Shanghai in school and university buildings, and three in mission compounds upcountry, in the ancient city of Yangzhou. Each camp would hold three to four hundred people and would be assigned medical cover by interned physicians. In February 1943 the Gales received the news that they and the McAlls had been assigned to Yangzhou Camp B, a twenty-four-hour journey by boat from Shanghai. From what they understood, Godfrey Gale, Ken McAll, and Frances McAll—all physicians—would be responsible for the health of 350 internees at this camp. When Betty Gale heard rumours that they would be living in a Buddhist temple, she began to imagine a peaceful setting with the soft chime of temple bells. Meanwhile Dr. John and Georgina Lewis were assigned to Ash Camp in the centre of Shanghai; and a number of missionaries who had been under house arrest in Beijing and Tianjin were transferred to Weixian Camp: John and Mary Stanley, Rev. and Mrs. G.K. King, Bertha Hodge, Susie Kelsey, and Eric Liddell.[39]

The London Missionary Society had arranged for a small Red Cross parcel to be sent to the Gales every month; it contained milk powder, egg powder, and canned beef. They were allowed one trunk each plus as much hand luggage as they could carry. The McAlls, who had some money left over from Jinan, made the risky decision to spend the entire amount on a very comfortable upholstered settee that would unfold into a double bed at night. It was an "act of faith which paid off handsomely" in the coming years of internment.[40] The Gales and the McAlls set off to Yangzhou with the men carrying Margie and Eli in homemade slings while the women carried "all the clobber" to keep the children amused on the journey. On the night before they were to assemble at the Shanghai Cathedral courtyard with other Yangzhou Camp B internees, Betty Gale anticipated surrendering "our last vestige of liberty."[41]

Yangzhou Camp B

Standing on the grounds of the magnificent Shanghai Cathedral on a bitterly cold March morning with "hundreds of people—with stacks of luggage, all more or less unhappy, waiting for orders to march," Betty Gale felt strangely elated.[42] The six of them—three McAlls and three Gales—had received a warm send off by friends in Columbia Country Club after breakfast, and they were curious to know what life would be like in the ancient city of Yangzhou, where Marco Polo was once governor during the reign of

Kublai Khan (c. 1277). Their trip would involve a journey along the famous Grand Canal, built in 300 BC as a means to carry rice up to the Emperors Court in Beijing. Perhaps the thrill came from being free from the confines and uncertainty of the CCC. Perhaps it came from being reunited as a family for the first time in nine months. Or perhaps it was simply a sense of adventure: after the Japanese "barked out" the order to fill in and the group started making its way to the dock by foot through the streets of Shanghai, Betty Gale was astonished by the thousands of curious Chinese lining the streets to watch these new prisoners. With luggage in both hands and the toddlers on their fathers' backs, she felt encouraged by what she perceived as a sense of concern and compassion exuded from the crowds. As they wove their way along the Shanghai Bund, Gale felt that they were looked upon like heroes. Ken McAll, in contrast, felt humiliated.[43] At any rate, looking out across the Huangpu River towards Pudong, the dilapidated warehouse district where some foreign males had recently been interned, there was a sense of relief—at least they were not going *there*.

For all its uncertainty, the journey to Yangzhou was not unlike the journeys taken by Christian missionaries in China for the previous six decades. Heading to an uncertain future was the stuff of mission legend—as was travelling up the ancient Grand Canal. Still, when Godfrey Gale had gushed in a 1939 letter to Betty shortly after they met that "you must experience sailing along the Grand Canal sometime, if you have not done it already,"[44] travelling together to a prison camp is hardly what he had envisioned. While the notion of travelling by sampan, steamer, flat-bottomed junks, and rickshaws may have sounded exciting, in reality it was an exhausting ordeal. After being loaded onto a steamer, the women and children were separated from their husbands and locked into their cabins for several hours without food, drink, or toilet access. When they were allowed out to eat, they found only rice covered with a hot curry that burned their palates. While they attempted to scrape off the curry, the meal was simply not suitable for young children. They went to bed hungry.

Arriving the next morning in Zhejiang on the Yangtze River, the group of 382 internees was escorted up gangplanks lined by Japanese soldiers onto flat bottomed junks (barges) for the trip up the Grand Canal. Without a roof to protect them from the pouring rain, Betty Gale and Frances McAll crawled under a plank for some shelter, and settled down on the "hard dirty floor" with their daughters. Several hours later they arrived in Yangzhou, cold and wet through. After a forced march through the city streets the luggage-laden prisoners were relieved to arrive in the abandoned American Baptist Mission School for girls that would be their home for the next six months. In their relief they hardly noticed the "high brick walls and the large wooden gate which slammed shut behind us."[45] Nor did they notice that their steamer trunks had been rummaged through: most of the medical instruments Godfrey Gale had carefully procured from Qilu were gone, as were nearly all of Betty's winter clothes and many of Godfrey's and Margie's. Their belongings had been replaced by bricks. Betty and Godfrey Gale would share two pairs of trousers, while Betty Gale and Frances McAll would share pyjamas.

Mistrusting the Missionaries

For the Gales and the McAlls, heading off together to Yangzhou Camp B was reminiscent of their original call to China. Having been assigned to care for the medical needs of the 382 internees, they had a sense of mission not entirely unlike the one they had originally signed up for. One main difference was that they were not paid. They did not receive a salary during their four years of imprisonment, nor did they ever receive (or seek) restitution from the Japanese for their losses. Yangzhou would offer similarities in their working conditions in so far as they would be caring for people who were disenfranchised and living in poverty, and they would have limited resources. An advantage they would have was that of a common first language (English) and a shared (Western) understanding of medical care. Practising medicine and nursing in a prison camp, then, could be seen as an extension of conventional missionary work. Ken McAll came to terms with his internment by accepting the idea that God had called him to *China,* this did not necessarily mean to the *Chinese.*[46] Unfortunately, however, the internees did not wish to receive care provided by young, upcountry missionaries.

In some ways, the culture clash between the four Qilu missionaries and their prospective English patients was much greater than anything they had experienced with Chinese patients. While their relationship with the Chinese population at Jinan was rooted in decades of trust, forged within the bounds of the Qilu compound, the missionaries had little experience with the cosmopolitan expatriate world of Shanghai where most of the other Yangzhou internees were from. In fact, as a direct result of her recent experiences, Betty Gale was wary of the upper-class Shanghailanders: in her mind, not only had members of this community reportedly robbed them of their *Maru* berths, but four Shanghai expatriate women had had the nerve to visit the Columbia Country Club with the sole intention of satisfying their curiosity about the desperate living arrangements there. As it turned out, the four women who gawked at the internees at the ccc became internees themselves at Yangzhou Camp B.

Betty Gale was not impressed with the upper-crust English internees. When she stood, luggage in hand, on the grounds of Shanghai Chapel with the throng of newly arrested Shanghailanders, she wryly noted, "Some of those Shanghai ladies have not lifted anything heavier than a fan or a mirror for years."[47] To her surprise, the new internment camp would be comprised almost completely of members of the Shanghai business community—only nine others of the 382 were not. Living in close quarters with the Shanghailanders would prove more difficult than any of their confinements thus far. While Gale's China childhood and missionary years had prepared her to deal with adversity and scarce resources, her fellow-internee's virulent aversion to the idea of the young missionaries being placed in charge of their medical care would be completely unsettling.

Prior to this large-scale internment, the British Residents Association in Shanghai had arranged for several physicians and a dentist to be in each camp set up by the Japanese. When the McAlls and Gales, having volunteered their assistance while at the Columbia Country Club, were assigned to Yangzhou Camp B, they did not know to what extent the Japanese would support medical care. According to Article I, Clause 18, of the Regulations of the Civil Assembly Centre (a euphemism for internment camp), "members of a section shall take care of the sick in its section; when medical treatment is necessary, request shall be made for it to the Japanese officials in charge."[48] In reality, however, the Japanese made virtually no provision for medical care; they left the internees to care for each other under primitive conditions and with few resources. Ken McAll and Godfrey Gale took up the challenge before them by immediately organizing part of the camp into a space for medical care.

Yangzhou Camp B was on the site of an American Baptist school for Chinese girls called the Julia Mackenzie Memorial School.[49] The main school building was three stories high, constructed in grey brick ("Block A"). The first two floors, originally comprised of twenty-three rooms and four dormitories, were used to house 112 internees. The third floor—an attic—was used as a chapel and a school. Two smaller buildings on the grounds, originally used by school staff, became family residences: "Block B" contained eighteen rooms and "Block C" contained six. The Gales and McAlls were assigned a room in one of these. The church auditorium was used as a dining and recreation hall.

Washrooms, showers, and a laundry room were close by. Toilets were comprised of wooden tubs with covers, emptied once a day through a hole constructed in the encircling wall. On the other side of this wall Chinese peasants collected the excrement for fertilizing their gardens. Long cement troughs served as basins in which internees washed, using their own bucket. Once a week each internee was entitled to a bucketful of hot water to take the place of a hot bath. Small raised tanks were filled by hand pumps and used as showers. On the camp grounds there was an open area for growing vegetables, but no area big enough for "proper games."[50] A ten foot high wall surrounded the grounds, and the Japanese conducted twice-daily roll calls in the courtyard, rain or shine. The roll calls were unnecessary; no one even attempted to escape.

While the camp was under the jurisdiction of the Japanese Consulate of Nanjing, its internal administration was left entirely to the initiative of the internees. The camp representatives chosen from the beginning by the British Residents Association of Shanghai were in regular contact with the Japanese Commandant, Mr. M.S. Yamashita. There were seven subcommittees: a Sports Committee, Ladies Committee, Entertainment Committee, Gardening Committee, Canteen Committee, Billeting Committee, and Mothers Committee. A Chief of Police was appointed by the Camp Representative, and a Provisional Court acted as an arbitration body for grievances between internees. Although the internees were entitled to "comfort allowances" of CRB $700.00 each month to help fund some of their expenses (CRB was the Japanese-run Central Reserve Bank currency),[51] these were never received at Yangzhou.[52] Elsewhere, the allowances could only be used in the poorly stocked canteens.

Godfrey Gale and Ken McAll secured two larger rooms in Block B for a clinic and sickbay, and two smaller rooms for a dispensary and isolation unit. In order to gain a sense of the health needs of their new population, they started to make arrangements to conduct a physical examination of every person in the camp. The internees, however, refused. Betty Gale fumed: "They are all sure they will die if they get sick with such inexperienced medicals."[53] The internees, noted the McAlls, had been used to the "best of the pin-striped trouser medical attention for which they paid handsomely. Now they had to humble themselves to accept the only care available from the 'bloody young missionaries' as we found ourselves labelled. Missionaries had never ranked high in the business world's estimation. They found it hard to believe we could possibly know what we were doing and their security was seriously undermined."[54]

According to Godfrey Gale, the doctors decided to split up the work by specialty—Godfrey as an ears, nose, and throat specialist, Frances McAll as a cardiologist, and Ken McAll as a public health practitioner. In the role of public health officer, Ken McAll was able to use his medical knowledge to help the community adjust to unsanitary living conditions fraught with potential for widespread outbreaks of disease. And he used his considerable artistic ability to create illustrated instructions on how to prevent illness. His cartoons included basic advice about the use of mosquito nets, eating potato skins to get the maximum Vitamin B, and being careful to wash hands before eating and after using the toilets. Initially, however, the response to Ken's cartoons was "almost a riot."[55] The internees had no intention of listening to a young upstart telling them how to behave. They blankly refused to use nets over their beds, for example, "preferring, apparently, to risk malaria."[56]

The internees did not take well either to Frances McAll's recommendation that soya beans be added to the list of requests submitted to the Japanese authorities. She was concerned about the lack of a steady milk supply for Eli and Margie, but there were also older children in camp who required calcium for their proper development. When Frances was asked to be the "mother's representative" on a woman's committee that had been organized by some of the more vocal women in the camp, she was flattered, hoping it would be an opportunity to "propagate a few of my own ideas on child health."[57] One idea was that soya bean milk was an inexpensive and practical alternative to goat's milk for children. She brought the idea forward. However, "for some reason," Frances later wrote, the suggestion of soya milk "greatly enraged Mrs. M. who rallied her supporters and brought them to a meeting during which she accused me in eloquent terms of trying to poison them all and [of] being in league with the Japanese."[58] Rather than requesting soya beans from the Japanese, the committee voted to request a goat. The request was refused, leaving the internees with neither. Feeling that "the majority [of the committee] did not appreciate my great learning and experience," Frances resigned from the committee.[59] While she later came to believe that this odd behaviour was prompted by fear and loss, at the time she and Betty Gale found it incredibly frustrating ("a beautiful day, weatherwise, but hard to take *people*wise").[60]

As the internees tried to sort out how much authority the missionary doctors had, the doctors also became a target for complaints about poor camp conditions. The main problem in the camp was obtaining an adequate food and water supply. The Japanese carted in a daily supply of water from the canal in large containers used by the farmers for watering their crops. They provided seventy wheel barrow loads of water, amounting to approximately 4,500 litres each day, but the water was filthy; it had to be "settled with chemicals" before it could be used.[61] The internees had to rely mainly on hand-pumped water from a rainwater cistern conserved from the roof of the main building, or from water drawn by rope and bucket from a well. Outside the toilets, communal basins of water with a disinfectant added were set up. The toilet facilities consisted of a row of buckets with seats on top which the internees would take turns cleaning daily.

Food was also carted into camp daily in Chinese wheelbarrows. The meat was indigestible; it was comprised of lumps of pork fat with bristles still attached. On one occasion the internees who prepared the food for everyone did not, for some reason, wash or scrub the vegetables. The resultant stew, as Frances McAll remembered it, was "full of mud and swimming in grease, totally inedible."[62] The doctors were held to blame. "Utterly ridiculous," wrote Betty Gale, who was astonished by the response, "[it is the] British Representative [who] is to blame."[63] It was not, after all, up to the doctors to petition the Japanese for better food; their role was to care for the sick. But it would get worse. On 23 March 1943—Godfrey's thirtieth birthday—Betty wrote in her diary, "Twas a remarkable birthday! J.M Vitte died following an embolus. Mr. N. had a gastric haemorrhage and Mr. C. went crazy and threatened to kill Drs. and their families—because of the food! Awful!"[64] A member of the camp police had to guard Godfrey for the rest of the day.[65] The Gales and McAlls were baffled, but also worried.

In the midst of all this concern about food, internees started to complain that the doctors' children were getting preferential treatment. LMS missionary nurse Ethel Taylor had taken over the role of matron of the small camp "hospital" established by the Gales and McAlls. Because patients were allowed more nutritious rations than the general internee population, Ethel decided to pass some along for Eli and Margie. Upon seeing the little girls eating chicken with mashed potatoes and milk pudding, one internee commented: "Preferential treatment for the doctor's kids, eh?"[66] Betty Gale felt offended. "I am beginning to understand," she wrote, "why mothers of small children get belligerent, in areas where great poverty exists."[67] From Gale's perspective, if extra nourishment was available, the two toddlers *should* have priority: as the youngest prisoners in camp, they were also the most vulnerable. Perhaps she also felt a sense of entitlement: should there not be some benefit to being the ones responsible for looking after the camp's health needs?

The power struggles that characterized the early days of Yangzhou internment pitted the Shanghailanders against the missionaries. As Betty Gale and Frances McAll tried to make sense of the hostility towards them, they also sought reasons to empathize with the Shanghailanders. Empathy, after all, was an easier emotion to deal with than anger. Perhaps, they reasoned, the Shanghailanders' anger towards them was part of their process of coming to terms with imprisonment. Since it was not safe to openly resist the Japanese, maybe the Shanghailanders needed a safe target for their resentment. Or, perhaps the Shanghailanders had lost more—and lost it more quickly—than the missionaries had and were therefore in some sort of shock. The missionaries, after all, came to China with an expectation of living with less and adapting to difficult, wartime conditions whereas expatriates living in Shanghai were used to a luxurious lifestyle. Maybe some of the Shanghailanders were simply reluctant to give up what power or control they had left to members of a "lower" class—that is, the missionaries. Or maybe some of these internees were simply mean-spirited. Whatever the case, more than forty years after liberation both Ken McAll and Betty Gale would recall that it was the fifteen or so missionaries who did the majority of the manual labour at Yangzhou. According to Gale, "the missionaries did all the crummy jobs no one else wanted to do."[68]

Betty Gale had particular difficulty with "Mrs. M"—an attractive, clever woman who "delights in pulling to pieces anyone who does not 'kowtow' to her. Her special aversion seems to be doctors, especially woman doctors."[69] Although Betty never identified her by name, Frances McAll later confirmed her identity.[70] According to official camp records, this woman was a forty-six-year-old analytic chemist from New Zealand. It was Mrs. M. who, "in one of the vilest attacks I've ever heard," accused Frances of "being in league with the Japanese to poison us all," when Frances was rallying to have soya beans. To Betty, there were "a lot of foolish people in this Camp."[71] As Betty Gale and Frances McAll were processing their difficulties, an incident occurred that shifted the mistrustful atmosphere: the successful emergency surgery performed on a sixteen-year-old internee.

The acute appendicitis episode of a Russian teenager called Teddy Fleet galvanized the internees towards a common goal. Although the Japanese had planned to set up a hospital unit in Yangzhou Camp C, it was still not open in late March 1943 when the surgery was required. Between them, the Gales and the McAlls possessed one pair of surgical gloves, two pairs of artery forceps, one scalpel, and a very small bottle of chloroform. They set up a small room and performed the surgery, according to Betty's diary, on "a kitchen table."[72] When Teddy survived the crude surgery, everyone was surprised—not least of all Betty, who wrote:

> Within two hours of making the diagnosis, a table is made by Mr. T., a carpenter, while the doctors and nurses make an anaesthetic mask, wind sewing thread for sutures, boil up aprons, towels, swabs and their one pair of rubber gloves, and are well on their way, with the few instruments they can put together. [Ken and Godfrey] toss to see who actually operates—and G[odfrey] wins that, so he wears the gloves, and K[en] assists and F[rances] gives the anaesthetic. I stay upstairs with the babies and pray frantically ("why frantically?" asks Frances when I tell her afterwards).[73]

The incident brought the internees together on a common goal: even the formidable Mrs. M. joined in the cleaning of the room.[74] Betty Gale was relieved at the response of the upper-class British internees to the successful surgery: the missionary doctors were "not so bad after all, by Jove."[75]

Accommodation

Internment at Yangzhou Camp B required adaptation to a new, evolving set of social rules. First, there were the practical difficulties of sharing a room with the McAlls. Having each been brought up in "respectable homes in a respectable age,"[76] the problem of who should undress first was a real one. Arranging the children's homemade cots in the middle of the room provided a screen of sorts between the two couples, but "even so it took courage" to start undressing in the same room. It was something they would get used to over the next three years of confinement together; eventually they "never gave it a thought."[77] Still, the lack of privacy and modesty constraints undoubtedly hindered their marriage relationships: during four years of internment, neither woman bore a second child.

Second, the two women had to come to terms with differences in child-rearing styles. Because Betty Gale was most often in charge of watching the two toddlers, she depended on her own method of child care with both girls. Eli required extra attention because of some sort of digestive condition—certain types of foods would precipitate bouts of vomiting or diarrhoea. Although both girls ended up with health issues related to childhood deprivations—blackened lower teeth for Eli, vitamin-D-deficiency-related bone problems for Margie—Eli would be considered the sickly one. When later asked about how the camp got organized—how it was decided, for example, who was in charge of what—Betty Gale maintained that she had no time to pay attention to such things: watching out for two rambunctious toddlers in a setting ill suited to small children commanded her full attention.

In Betty Gale's accounts (diary, journal, letters, memoirs) there is no mention of any friction with Frances McAll. Frances, however, recalled "many times" in which she and Betty did not agree. Mostly their "rows" were related to their different approaches to child care. According to Frances, Betty had higher standards than she. Whereas Frances and Ken McAll were assertive and even feisty on occasion, Godfrey and Betty Gale tried to avoid conflict: "Godfrey had a marvellous way," Frances later recalled, "of escaping down to his little corner in the hospital and his books if there was a family row."[78] Frances found it "terribly hard to say sorry," and for a day or two there would be tension. But they always knew they had to "put it right; not just for [their] own sake, but for the sake of the camp."[79]

Modesty was a recurring concern in the internment camps. Although the McAlls and the Gales struggled through their own issues of privacy, they did have the privilege of sharing a closed room at Yangzhou. Others were not so fortunate, having to share large spaces with dozens of other internees. At Yangzhou Camp B, this meant sharing large dormitories. The experiences of Peggy Pemberton-Carter at Lunghua Camp give a sense of what it was like for those sharing a larger space. When first confronted with the hut that she would share with fifty-two other women, Pemberton-Carter chose to place her bedding near the communal toilet and shower room because that afforded her eighteen inches of extra wall space, and slightly more privacy from the other inhabitants: "There are many 'feelings' over re-measurement and re-allotment of hut space for each occupant and their baggage, so as to allow each person 9 feet by 4 feet, and a clear passage down the middle 4 feet wide. I rejoice, because it has been decreed that my bed cannot be shifted any nearer the wall, otherwise the door [to the washroom] will be obstructed …there are therefore compensations for slams and smells."[80]

In that small space Peggy Pemberton-Carter hung hooks for her clothes, a small shelf for books, and a curtain "made from my kimono" to cover her clothes. She had enough room for a small chair by a corner window, and filled the remaining space with a small trunk and three suitcases. Under the bed she stored a bucket, tinned food, and oddments of wire, wood, and glass "which one picks up because they may come in handy one day."[81] Against the head of her bed rested a folding table, washboard, and deckchair; above these, a shoe bag arrangement to hold toiletries. Other small shelves she made ("our pride over any bit of handiwork … is really pathetic") held thermos flasks, two saucepans, frying pan, coffee pot, teapot, plates, mug, kettle, and mirror. Finally, a top shelf held gumboots, a small medicine chest, dustpan, brush, tool basket, sunhat, and a cardboard box with food stores like tea, honey, sugar, and peanut butter. What is not clear is how Pemberton-Carter managed to hold onto her belongings at camp; in Betty Gale's camp experience, theft was rife and food scarce. Pemberton-Carter, in contrast, reported having "put on 9 lbs of weight in two months" at camp in 1943. Even so, "I am pronounced," she noted, "as quite badly anaemic."[82]

Describing the effort it took to stay clean at camp, Peggy Pemberton-Carter noted that being an internee meant standing in queues for meals, for washing water, for drinking water, and to register for taking showers—available on alternate days. To take a shower, internees were required to enter the bathhouse at the assigned time "with 47 other females of your batch, discard shoes, put on clogs, march to locker, undress, march to shower cubicle [at the sound of a whistle], water turned on for one minute to wet you, whistle, water turned off, soap yourself, whistle, water on so that you may rinse, whistle, march out and dress, march, change clogs for shoes" all to be completed in exactly twenty minutes.[83] "Oh Lord," Pemberton-Carter lamented, "how far removed from former hour-long wallowing in hot water with Gardenia bath salts."[84] Deciding that the showering process sounded "unspeakably exhausting," Pemberton-Carter decided to continue "in the bad old way with a bucket and kettle in the washroom trough, discreetly curtained from the public gaze by my counterpane thrown over a rope— *smells* from the temperamental cesspool notwithstanding."[85]

To Peggy Pemberton-Carter, camp life provided a study in human behaviour. Peering out from her corner of the crowded hut, she was intrigued by the ways in which her fellow internees, who would normally not be in contact with each other, responded to being placed in close quarters, dependent upon working as an organized unit for survival. These so-called Civil Assembly Centers were no respecters of class, status, or national hierarchies. Pemberton-Carter herself felt "ashamed to be seen by the Chinese who bring in the supplies when I am grovelling on the ash piles, scratching with a bit of stick for half-burned bits of coke and coal."[86] "No doubt I shall outgrow this relic of snobbery," she wrote.[87] From Pemberton-Carter's perspective the internment camps were little more than wartime labour camps—except that the labour benefited the internees themselves. Because the Japanese responsibility for the internees did not go beyond providing food and water, the internees were left to organize themselves. White collar office workers were "transformed into road builders, garbage collectors, stokers, stove builders, hot water firemen, cooks, butchers, and kitchen toilers"[88] Society women found themselves gardening, cooking, teaching, nursing, cleaning the dining rooms, cleaning vegetables, mending and "dol[ing] out the [boiled] drinking water for hours daily in all weathers— nearly scalded by the steam at their backs, whilst they freeze in front from the howling north-westerly winds."[89]

Camp life was the "merciless unveiler of every artifice" whether it be "dyed hair, alleged accomplishments or assumed qualities and virtues."[90] To Peggy Pemberton-Carter, "the essential personality emerges just as surely as the natural hair colour."[91] At Yangzhou Camp B, the Gales and McAlls noticed that, following the success of Teddy Fleet's appendectomy, other internees began to call on the Gales and McAlls to socialize in their room. "We are riding the crest of the wave," Betty Gale wrote. "We are aware that public sentiment can swing quickly from one extreme to the other— and know that at any moment another crisis may develop—and we'll be dropped like hot potatoes."[92] Some of the difficulties did persist. Life at Yangzhou Camp B was much different than the Columbia Country Club. There, the Gales were "just part of the crowd." But here, "the doctors are in a position of authority and power" and they were "finding out that when that happens one immediately becomes a target of criticism and abuse."[93] Furthermore, the missionaries had difficulty shaking the perception others had of them as bizarre creatures, eager to evangelize. "We must prove to them somehow," wrote Betty Gale, "that we are not the long-faced individuals depicted in cartoons, rushing around with an umbrella in one hand while delivering tracts 'to the heathen' with the other."[94]

The stark surroundings, strained relationships, and dirty conditions were exacerbated by the presence of "stink bugs" and centipedes. "I see a centipede today," wrote Betty Gale, "a terrible creature about 4 inches long—a shiny black body with two bright blue lines down its sides—and heaps of bright yellow legs and a shining red head. It runs out from under the box the kids use as a table—we try to catch it but it gets away. Ugh! They are almost impossible to kill—even if you can catch them. We always shake our shoes before putting them on."[95] The stink bugs were even worse. Flat, oval-shaped, winged creatures about one and a half inches long, they arrived in the "millions" over a three-day period in the summer, like a "great black cloud" settling on everything in sight.[96] If squashed they emitted a "loathsome stench"; the only way to get rid of them was to sweep them into "great heaps and set fire to them." During the few days of "the plague," Frances McAll described a feeling of "near kinship" with their Japanese guards who hated the bugs as much as they did.[97]

Betty Gale and Frances McAll sought refuge from the ugliness of camp life in the third-floor attic of the main building. They had discovered the space together one day. Noticing a piano there McAll, a gifted musician, began to play. Gale wrote:

> It is beautifully quiet up there—and through the windows I can see the street full of people, and I can also see into the neighbouring Chinese countryside [...]. It is a lovely evening—and I kneel on a chair, and gaze out, my elbows on the [window]sill with my chin resting in my hands. The sun sets in a blaze of glory—and gradually the sounds of children playing in the streets grow less—and soon fade away—everything is peaceful and dream like. I am far away, visiting family and friends in Canada when suddenly the music stops—and [Frances] says, "Come on Betty, it's time to go home…" I come to, with a start, and find myself once more in camp.[98]

Betty Gale sought ways to escape some of the more repulsive aspects of camp life, mostly by busying herself with the care and antics of Margie and Eli. One day she seized the opportunity to wash Margie's favourite—and rather filthy—green pillow while Margie was being taken for a walk by one of the teenagers. Seeing the sopping pillow "flapping in the breeze" on the wash line, Margie burst into tears, "my billow, Mummy, I want my billow!" Margie stood under the dripping pillow, its water mingling with her tears as she wept "copiously" until the pillow was dry. "I feel wretched," Betty wrote, "for as I hand it back to her she clasps it to her heart, looks at me over the top of it with wet eyes, and says accusingly, 'dad girl, Mummy!'"[99] On Margie's second birthday, 17 July 1943, a fellow internee arrived at the Gales' room with "an enormous cake, beautifully decorated, with pink and blue ribbons on it."[100] She had gone all over camp asking other internees for a spoonful of flour, or sugar, or milk powder until she got enough to bake the cake. On another occasion Margie threw a brick which hit Eli on her head, giving Eli a bleeding gash. "Eli howls, and her curls get all bloody. Margie is heart-broken—and she howls too, in sympathy. Fortunately it isn't a deep cut, and we put a big dressing on her head—and one on Margie, to cheer her up. And they go out to play with their arms around each other."[101]

In addition to watching the girls, Betty Gale took her turn in the camp kitchen, peeling vegetables and serving food to the queued internees, and cleaning the washrooms. She rediscovered her enjoyment of nursing by working in the clinic set up by her husband and the McAlls: "I am working in the clinic on Monday, Wednesday and Friday mornings—and also every evening, helping the doctors get through all the physicals [examinations of all the internees]. It's rather fun to be a nurse again—and infinitely better than being on 'lavatory duty.'"[102]

Betty Gale kept abreast of the health needs of internees through her husband's work. In August she reported on three patients—"Susan," who was "much better to-day," "Madeline," a seventeen-year-old with malaria, and "Olga," a Russian Shanghailander. Madeline was running a temperature of 107°F. Since there was no ice to cool her down, the teen-aged boys were recruited to work in shifts all day and all night, bringing in cool water from the deeper of the two wells. Betty and Ethel wrapped Madeline in cold wet sheets, changing them when they got warm. "It is an anxious night for everyone," wrote Betty, "but by morning she is much better."[103] Two days later Olga swallowed a number of sodium amytal tablets she had brought with her from Shanghai[104]—in an apparent suicide attempt.

Olga was one of several so-called "White Russians" in camp. The term generally referred to non-Communist Russians who were among those who escaped to China after the 1917 Russian Revolution. White Russian women, the internees believed, intentionally sought out wealthy Englishmen to marry for security and survival. Betty Gale considered the White Russian women in camp to be "rather wild."[105] Olga was a recently widowed mother of an eight-year-old "holy terror."[106] She had become attracted to a Roman Catholic priest interned in camp—an attraction that apparently was not mutual. According to Gale, "seeing no happy solution to her problem," Olga took the pills. After gaining consciousness the next day, she was "annoyed because she is still alive … she says she'll drink Lysol next time."[107] To Gale, Olga appeared "really desperate."[108] Caring for desperate others made Gale feel less desperate herself.

Resistance

Compared with their time of house arrest in Jinan, the Gales showed few signs of resistance against their Japanese captors in Yangzhou Camp B. Perhaps this was because there was scant opportunity to communicate with the outside world. Or perhaps they were simply preoccupied with the in-camp needs. No radios or newspapers were allowed into the camp, and the internees had no established relationships with Chinese nationals living in the area surrounding Yangzhou Camp.

For their part, the Japanese were eager to paint a positive portrait of life in the internment camps—partly through censoring camp mail, and partly through supplying propaganda to the media. For example, on 22 April 1943 the *Shanghai Times* reported that the internment of some 6,000 British, Americans, and Netherlanders who were living in Shanghai was almost complete. According to the report, the camps were located in "quiet suburban districts of Shanghai, and the houses are all well-built and in good condition."[109] As noted earlier, a very similar message was being broadcast by radio.[110] Furthermore, the internees included those who had lost their jobs with the outbreak of war and who had been "wandering aimlessly in the streets of Shanghai" before internment.[111] The internees were "peacefully settled" in the camps, "all satisfied and appreciative of the tolerant and considerate treatment" they were receiving. Inmates were "permitted to send and receive letters" as well as "read the latest papers and magazines and listen to the radios." Thus, the report concluded, "the internees are expressing their gratitude for the generous and just treatment accorded them by the Japanese Government Authorities, for they are now receiving more protection than ever before."[112]

The Japanese government had agreed to accept the terms of the Geneva Prisoner of War Convention, which included allowing civilian internees and prisoners of war to receive and send postcards administered through the International Red Cross.[113] Internees and POWs were also entitled to receive parcels of food and clothing. However, international humanitarian law, which seeks for humanitarian reasons to protect persons who are not or are no longer participating in the hostilities, is only as strong as those who must uphold it.[114] As Charles Roland has noted, the Japanese ignored or abandoned the Geneva Convention in many cases, claiming that they were not bound by it because it had never been officially ratified.[115] The Japanese did, however, agree that internees could start writing letters to next of kin in October 1942. Initially they required that the letters be written in Japanese or with a Japanese translation.[116] By 1943 the internees of all nationalities were instead required to write in English, or with an English translation, on a form supplied by the International Committee of the Red Cross.[117] On the front of the form the internees had six lines on which to write a twenty-five word message in block letters; on the back, family members could respond in twenty-five words. The message was to be "family news of a strictly personal character."[118] Twelve of Betty Gale's Red Cross letters from this period have survived, five from Yangzhou Camp B. However, these five did not actually arrive in Canada until after the Gales were transferred to Pudong Camp. By the time her parents' responses reached Betty Gale at Pudong, up to fifteen months had passed.

Because of the long turnaround times—not to mention Japanese censorship—the letters were hardly effective means of conveying reliable information. Still, they were invaluable to the recipients. For internees, letters were a lifeline to the outside world. For Betty Gale, correspondence with her mother had always been an important part of her existence. The Red Cross letters, in fact, were actually truncated versions of the correspondence mother and daughter had been writing for most of Betty's life. That is, while Betty's letters sought to reassure her mother of their health and safety, Margaret's letters were filled with family news. Betty found endless adjectives to describe Margie, now a toddler ("less pale," "getting fat," "flourishing," "walking," "thriving," "sturdy," "rosy," "mischievous"). In contrast, Margaret emphasized family births, marriages, and deaths ("Jean's, Gwen's babies due November," "Margery King widow," "Ruth's wedding September," "Sadie Loveless died"). In an April 1943 letter Betty wrote a congratulatory note to her father, stating, "You deserved it."[119] In subsequent letters she addressed her father as "Dr" Andrew Thomson. The congratulations were undoubtedly in response to the news that Thomson had been one of four recipients of an honorary Doctor of Divinity degree awarded by Victoria College in Toronto five months earlier.[120]

On one occasion, in August 1943, there was an unexpected opportunity for next of kin to get letters out to the internees at Yangzhou. The Thomson family wrote a one-page letter, each taking a different section. Margaret Thomson characteristically filled her section with family news, while Betty Gale's sister Muriel quipped, "This is confoozing—3 years' news to write in three lines. Guess I'd better talk about me and leave out the babies." Betty's brother Murray joked, "Hiya Betty, Worse half, etc., just a hail and hearty to you from the depths." The serious portion of the family letter came from Andrew Thomson, who chose to use the space allotted to him to encourage

Betty and Godfrey Gale in what he perceived as an extension of their missionary work: "You may not think so, but out there you are developing the finest kind of Christian living, just by being bright and cheerful, as you are making a contribution to the whole Church."[121]

Internalizing her father's advice, Betty Gale continued to write positively about her experiences at camp. By doing so, she was able to construct an image for herself, her husband, and the other missionaries as strong, physically, emotionally, and spiritually. Through her four years of internment she projected an image of someone determined not only to survive internment camp, but to find ways to thrive on it. By insisting both in her letters and her diaries that she and her family were fine—even flourishing—Gale came to believe it herself.

Smuggling and the Visit from the Swiss Consul

Faced with an opportunity to defy authorities more directly, Godfrey Gale and Ken McAll seized it. During the summer of 1943, the Gales received word that the Swiss Consul who had taken responsibility for Allied interests was coming to Yangzhou Camp B to check on camp conditions. He was to have an interview with M.S. Yamashita, the Japanese Commandant in charge of all three Yangzhou Camps, as well as with the doctors—albeit in the Commandant's presence. Godfrey Gale and Ken McAll had prepared a report which they "hoped to be able to smuggle somehow into the hands of the Consul."[122] They wanted to at least voice the dissatisfaction over the food, water, and medical supplies. Betty Gale noted in her diary: "The Swiss Consul arrived here all a.m. Reid [?] and Ken did their stuff—told them everything on the quiet and gave them all."[123] According to Frances McAll, the doctors discovered that the Consul, and perhaps even the Commandant, were prepared to collude:

> The group to meet [the Consul] sat around a table in the Commandant's office, the Consul asking and receiving non-committal replies. The Commandant, Mr. Y[amashita], was a pleasant kindly man who had himself experienced a short time of internment in Australia but he, like us, came ultimately under the authority of the military and so had to watch his step carefully. At one point, however, the telephone rang and the Commandant left the table to answer it and possibly deliberately, stood with his back to the others in the room. Ken felt a kick on his foot and caught the eye of the Consul as he nodded towards his open brief case which he held under the table. Letters and requests were bundled silently in and all was calm again when the Commandant returned to his seat.[124]

A copy of Swiss Consul M. Minutti's confidential report on the Yangzhou Camps, housed in the National Archives of Canada, paints a grim picture of internment there. Accompanied by the Chancellor of the Japanese Consulate at Nanjing and the Legal Counsellor for Chinese Affairs of the Swiss Consulate, the Swiss Consul's purpose in visiting the camps was to observe whether civilian internees were being treated in accordance with the Geneva Convention. These three met with the Japanese Commandant of each Camp (Mr. Yamashita for Camp B) with the understanding that, while Japan was not a signer of the Convention, they "undertook at the outbreak of hostilities to respect it and notably those clauses applicable to civilian internees."[125] Although Mr. Minutti found Mr. Yamashita "cold and stiff" at first, over lunch the atmosphere became "semi-cordial."[126] The visit to Camp B lasted from 9:00 a.m. until 1:40 p.m. and included interviews of the Camp Representatives and doctors in the Commandant's office. Mr. Minutti candidly wrote that Mr. Yamashita could barely hide his yawns during the interviews and left the room several times. The Consul "profited by his absence to speak freely to the Camp Representative or with the doctor. They even passed me notes, extracts of which follow."[127] He summarized his finding thus:

1 The two Japanese Commandants were doing the best they could.
2 The three Camp Representatives were filling their positions tactfully and conscientiously.
3 The general crowding and "promiscuousness which rises from it" was liable in the long run to make bad feeling.
4 The state of health was satisfactory. However, there was a danger of Vitamin D deficiency.
5 There was a poverty of medicines.
6 There was a lack of books, kitchen utensils, surgical instruments, ocular and dental equipment, small tools and accessories, and sports equipment.
7 The funds put at the disposition of the Camps were inadequate.
8 Food is monotonous and insufficient.
9 Stocks of cracked wheat were nearly gone.[128]

In an addendum to the report, Mr. Minutti reiterated the report that Godfrey Gale and Ken McAll had submitted secretly ("Confidential, handed over to M. Minutti without the knowledge of the Commandant"):[129]

We view with concern:
1 The primitive sanitary conditions of water supply and sewage disposal and the easy spread of diseases in this city.

2 The poor communications and possible interruptions of food and fuel supplies especially as regards the coming winter. In this matter of supplies we have already experienced delays.

3 There are 93 people over 50 years of age, many of whom could not stand primitive winter conditions. The doctors viewed "with concern" the primitive sanitary conditions.[130]

Furthermore, the doctors outlined the severe lack of adequate food, the urgent need for medicines, and their "grave concern" over the lack of facilities and equipment for general dental treatment.

In light of all the information gathered, Mr. Minutti concluded that "contrary to what we thought in the beginning, I have the definite impression that the internees of [Yangzhou], lost and forgotten in this inland city of limited resources, have a more unfortunate lot than those of Shanghai."[131] Whether or not Godfrey Gale and Ken McAll's reports had any impact on the decision, by September 1943 the Japanese authorities decided to close the three internment camps at Yangzhou and transfer the prisoners to other camps. Perhaps acknowledging the expectation of international humanitarian law that their provisions should meet a certain minimum standard of care, the Japanese were no longer able to meet even the basic requirements at Yangzhou.

In September Betty Gale was finding the food terrible: "Often we have no bread—or stew—just tea and cucumber or squash. We would be in a bad way if we didn't have those Red Cross parcels."[132] On 17 September the Gales and the McAlls heard that the Japanese were sending them back to Shanghai because of the difficulty of finding enough food. Even though they knew that they were only going to "exchange one concentration camp for another," the internees at Yangzhou were "wild with excitement."[133] According to Ken McAll, because the physicians had taken care of the Japanese Commandant's illness on occasion, he gave them the choice of which camp they could go to. Ironically, the reason they chose Pudong Camp was because it was an adults only camp; the abandoned building was considered particularly unsafe for children. The McAlls and Gales reasoned that a childless camp would, in fact, be safer for Eli and Margie because there would be much less incidence of communicable disease than with a camp filled with children.

On 30 September 1943 each of the internees was given twelve hard-boiled eggs and some bread. That would be their food until they reached their final internment site: the notorious Pudong Camp. Betty Gale looked forward to being reunited with some of the LMS missionaries who had remained in the Shanghai camps. She also confided ("I regret to say") that Mrs. M. was being transferred to Pudong Camp, too.[134]

Summary

The months from August 1942 to September 1943 were sadly ironic for Betty and Godfrey Gale. In the two years leading up to their internment at the Columbia Country Club and Yangzhou Camp B, the Gales lived in anticipation of being interned by the Japanese. When they found themselves stranded at Shanghai after expecting to be repatriated, they were caught completely off guard. Initially enraged and disappointed, Betty Gale soon chose to focus on all that was good or beautiful in her new setting. Her diary and letters from this period continue to be inordinately optimistic—a quality that was far more a reflection of her character and strategy for survival than of what might be expected given the conditions of the camps themselves. The gendered expectations of mishkid women who were simultaneously wives, mothers, nurses, and missionaries were put to the test in camp: Betty Gale would constantly struggle to find a balance of serenity, altruism, shrewdness, and tenacity. As her father wrote shortly before the Gales left Yangzhou Camp B, an internment camp was as much of a mission field as anywhere else: just by being "bright and cheerful" under the trying circumstances, Betty was fulfilling the expectations of a Christian, missionary, and woman. Whatever her private frustrations, keeping silent about them helped her to cope. So rare were Betty's public displays of anger—such as her outburst in the shop in Shanghai—they became highlights in the memoirs of her closest friends. Similarly, her refusal to identify Mrs. M. by her real name—even to her adult daughter Margaret forty years later—exemplifies the seriousness with which she held her standards of proper Christian behaviour.[135]

Just as Betty and Godfrey Gale's conditions at Qilu worsened almost imperceptibly over their eight months there, their internment conditions steadily worsened from Qilu to the ccc to Yangzhou. At Yangzhou Betty Gale's most difficult adjustment was to the poor food and, perhaps even more trying, the conflicts with Shanghailanders like Mrs. M. Whereas at the ccc most of the internees were missionaries, less than five percent of the Yangzhou Camp B population were missionaries.[136] Gale had little regard for the snobbish behaviour of the upper-crust residents of Yangzhou who treated the missionaries as lower class citizens who somehow owed them something. While this remedied itself over time, the transition to the new social atmosphere at Yangzhou was at least as difficult for Gale as the filthy and bare physical surroundings. Yet in this, too, she displayed remarkable resilience. Choosing to focus on the antics and needs of Eli and Margie, Gale managed to stay out of the centre of conflicts at Yangzhou. In fact, she developed her own islands of refuge to distract her from the reality of camp life—be it weekends at friends' homes in Shanghai, the attic of the main building at Yangzhou, or the fantasy world of two little girls wherever they were. Betty Gale's ability to mentally escape from the drudgery of camp life would serve her well for the final—and worst—two years of their internment, at Pudong Camp.

"The End of the World Has Come"
Pudong Camp (1943–1945)

They've jammed us like sardines in a go-down so derelict, so riddled with vermin, the British American Tobacco Company had to abandon it years ago as being unfit for storing tobacco.

—Desmond Power, *Little Foreign Devil*

Pudong Camp was a cluster of six abandoned *godowns* (warehouses) of the British-American Tobacco Company. It sat approximately half a mile from the bank of the Huangpu River, across from the famous Shanghai Bund—a group of nineteenth-century Western-style buildings along the embankment of the International Settlement that housed numerous foreign banks, consulates, and social clubs for expatriates. A symbol of foreign wealth and power in China, the Bund stood in sharp contrast to the prison camp that faced it across the river. The main building at Pudong Camp was a large three-story red brick structure consisting of sixteen large rooms with twenty-foot ceilings. Condemned since being bombed during the Japanese invasion of 1937, the warehouse had paper over most of its windows and gaps in the wooden boards between the floors. The second and third floors were used entirely for dormitories while the ground level contained dormitories, the dining hall, library, spare rooms, and two kitchens.[1] The ground floor was made of concrete, and this is where the Gales and the McAlls spent their first night at Pudong in October 1943—sleeping on blankets on the concrete floor.

Pudong Camp was never intended to house families. Its structure was considered too rough for women, let alone children. Six months earlier, in March 1943, the first internees went to Pudong. They were all men: 388 Americans, 658 Britons, 15 Netherlanders, and 1 who was "stateless."[2] Since then, 400 had been repatriated. Compared with the Shanghailanders at Yangzhou (Yangchow), this was a coarse crowd of civilian prisoners, comprised of labourers, crewmen, and even convicts. Pudong Camp had gained a reputation for being a tough place. According to Godfrey Gale, some of the residents had smuggled out letters to send to the Swiss Consul General

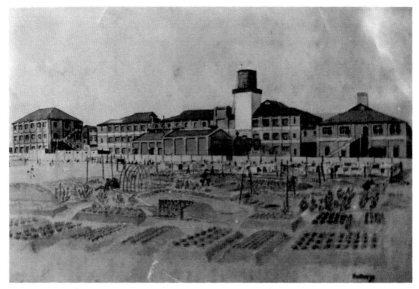

Fig. 7.1   Drawing of Pudong Camp

to complain about the conditions. Unfortunately the writers of the letters were identified and taken off to the notorious Bridge House jail in Shanghai for punishment. As they were being taken away "the whole camp turned out and demonstrated and the Japanese had to get out machine guns to restore order."[3] When the Swiss Consul made his first visit to the camp on 22 June 1943, he noted that a Mr. Mackenzie and a Mr. Forsyth—the former had been the British Representative in the camp—had been sent either to Haiphong Road Camp or to the Gendarmerie; "no definite information being obtainable on the spot" from the Japanese official concerned. "I had the firm impression that some trouble had occurred," reported the Swiss Consul, "for which they might have been made responsible. The representative of the protected nationals did not insist, but gave me by his attitude almost the assurance that there might have been some protest made by Mackenzie."[4]

On another occasion before the Gales arrived, a Chinese labourer was caught carrying a letter out of the camp. He was tied to a railing in full view of the prisoners and beaten "almost to death" as an example.[5] "No doubt," Godfrey Gale speculated, "the Japanese had decided that the addition of some women and children might improve the tone of the camp."[6] An additional 550 internees, including the Gales, were added to the camp in October 1943, bringing the total to 1,212.[7]

Betty Gale's first impression of Pudong Camp was of "dirty dilapidated old buildings—every window filled with wild bearded faces."[8] Stepping off one of the sampans that had taken her and 250 other internees across the Huangpu River, Betty was astonished to hear a band playing "Hail, Hail the Gang's All Here": a group of "old ccc friends" greeted them, took their baggage, and led them into a huge dining room for tea. "Terrible old buildings," Betty wrote in her diary upon arrival, "rats, bedbugs, barred windows; but a grand welcome."[9] Exhausted, she did not mind sleeping in a corner of the hospital at first, but after a while she was concerned that the toddlers, Eli and Margie, who were easily upset after their long trip, would disturb the patients. For the first week, Godfrey Gale and Ken McAll slept on blankets on the floor, Eli and Margie slept on pads, and Betty Gale and Frances McAll took turns sleeping on a hospital stretcher and dentist chair.

The rest of the 1,212 internees were being housed in sixteen large rooms which had been portioned off into six by four foot spaces—the minimum required by the International Committee of the Red Cross—identified by lines on the floor. On his first visit in June 1943, when the camp held 1,080, the Swiss Consul concluded that the overcrowding was insufferable. Now there were even more internees stuffed into the men's dormitories, women's dormitories, and dormitories for married couples. In the women's and married couples' dormitories (but not the men's), internees hung blankets or other forms of curtains to separate themselves from their neighbours. "The room is a mass of curtains," wrote Betty Gale, "and though sights are mercifully blotted out, sounds aren't ... the lack of privacy is going to be the biggest problem of all."[10] The only place where one could have a conversation without being overheard was in the hospital on the ground floor, or in the stairwell. At 10:00 p.m. the Japanese guards would turn out the lights in the large rooms, and everyone would be expected to be quiet and sleep ("the only good thing about camp," Betty Gale later quipped).[11]

A week after arriving, the Gales and the McAlls were shown their new lodgings: a 9 by 13 foot elevator shaft. The space in fact had two parts—a back portion, 9 by 7 feet, became the sleeping area for Ken and Frances McAll and the two girls. This opened up into a front portion, 9 by 6 feet, which was where Godfrey and Betty Gale slept. The front portion was the actual elevator shaft, fitted with a wooden platform. Oily elevator cables ran up two sides of the shaft to the elevator itself, which was suspended above. There was a large window at one end of the small room from which they could view the Huangpu River. A young boy lived in the elevator itself. "They promise the elevator won't fall down,"[12] Betty Gale wrote in her diary, later expanding in her journal, "I surely hope they are right ... we would look like waffles if it does, as the bottom of it has so many crossed beams. It's not a pleasant thought."[13] Still, theirs was the only space in Pudong Camp fitted with a door and, although part of the shaft was open to the large room housing seventy married couples, it was a relative luxury. Gale's aim was to keep the two children as quiet as possible at night since, with no soundproofing in the building, "about 600 people [would] be disturbed" if the girls cried.[14]

If the thought of a falling elevator or crying children did not keep Betty Gale awake at night, sleeping with "bed bugs by the million" and "huge fat rats that run around our heads in the beams" did.[15] The Gales and McAlls awoke once to a strange sound coming from Eli's bed ("Plop! Plop! Plop! Plop!"). Eli stood "transfixed with amazement—gazing at four baby rats, hairless and dreadful looking, lying knocked out cold in her bed."[16] They had fallen from the beams. Although Betty Gale and Frances McAll did their best to scrub the area clean, it was still "indescribably dirty." Not only could they not reach some of the higher, blackened areas of the walls, but also every movement in the elevator suspended above them would cause "cascades of dirt" to fall over them and their belongings.[17] They set up mosquito nets over the girls' beds, covered by an additional layer of heavy netting to protect them from the pieces of brick and other rubble that the rats would knock down into the room—and to protect them from the rats themselves. Of the seven internment camps around Shanghai—all in poor condition—only Pudong was reported to be infested with rats and bedbugs.

The Gales tried to make the space homey by installing shelves made from salvaged wood, hanging curtains made from an old bedspread, and putting up a frieze on the wall made of coloured labels from tins of fruit and vegetables. Although the space would remain cluttered and dirty throughout the internment, the preciousness of its semi-privacy was noted in a letter written to Betty and Godfrey Gale decades later by a fellow internee:

> May I thank you again, for the loan of your "lift room" in CAC [Civilian Assembly Centre, Pudong] 35 years ago, where we celebrated my 21st Birthday. It must have been one of the only "private" rooms in the whole of [Pudong]! Surely the most prized of all gifts in camp, was a few hours privacy. Such a kind thought on your part. Do you remember the party? Mrs. Habecost collected bits and bobs for weeks for the Birthday cake! And everyone collected and saved for the feast. It was a wonderful 21st Birthday Party, and I am sure no one has ever had such a unique one.[18]

Although the Gales recognized their relative privilege in gaining such a private space, it was still difficult to live in such close quarters. In a letter penned within two weeks of liberation and published in the *Missionary Monthly*, Godfrey Gale admitted that the last two years of internment had been the most difficult, particularly because of the confined space. "The main difficulty," he wrote, "was the lack of privacy between ourselves and all the other seventy married couples in the open dormitory, and the fact that we could never get away and be alone. It sometimes taxed our Christian forbearance to the limit."[19]

The Problem of the "Young Unmarrieds"

Pudong was considered too rough for women, let alone children. Margie and Eli were the youngest children until new babies were eventually born. The next oldest children were three eight-year-olds, plus a handful of teenagers. Eventually they were joined by a small group of school-aged children and teenagers who had been at the China Inland Mission boarding school at Zhifu. Initially these schoolchildren were sent to Weixian Camp, but they were later transferred to Pudong Camp when it was discovered that some of their parents were interned there. The relative lack of children can be seen in comparison to other camps. In September 1944 Pudong Camp reported only 27 children under 17 years of age—that is, 2.2 percent of the camp population. In comparison, Ash Camp reported 265 children under age 17, representing a full 60 percent of its population. At Pudong, children under three years old comprised 0.2 percent of the population; at Ash Camp, 40 percent was under three years old.[20]

Internment was especially difficult for teenagers. Some felt isolated and unsure of what to do with themselves. One solution was to encourage them to play sports. Next to the warehouse was an abandoned Chinese village that had been bombed in 1937.[21] A double barbed-wire fence surrounded the *godowns* and part of the bombed out village, which the first group of prisoners cleared of broken bricks and tiles to make a large playing field on one side and a space for small gardens on the other. There was no grass or trees at Pudong Camp, but the internees could grow vegetables and flowers with seeds from the Red Cross. By the time the Gales arrived, some of the gardens were surprisingly ornate, with terraces and rockeries. In one garden was a wooden signpost pointing to England with the poignant words, "8600 miles to Winchester and Helen."[22] Internees could use the space between 9:00 a.m. and 6:00 p.m. Initially there were many games played on the field; baseball in particular. Towards the end of the war, however, not even the teenagers had enough energy to play sports.[23]

The other main way to keep the young internees occupied was to have them attend a school of sorts. Two of the London Missionary Society missionaries, Anne Taylor and Ginger Anderson, were teachers. They divided the school-age children into groups and taught regular lessons, using textbooks that some of the parents brought with them. There were enough books at Pudong Camp, in fact, to organize a library of approximately a thousand books, including such authors as Dickens, Scott, and Shakespeare.[24] Some of these were brought by internees; others had been supplied through the International Committee of the Red Cross. A corner of the dining hall was used for the lessons, but the dining hall was also used for a number of other noisy activities. At any one time there might be the school in one corner, adult lectures in another, gymnastics in the centre, while all around people would be cobbling shoes, sewing, practising Russian or Italian or French, playing games of chess, bridge, mah-jong or solitaire, and practising music. It was cacophonic: "a wonder the students were able to concentrate at all."[25]

Still, a number of students took their studies seriously—perhaps as a way to feel that their time in internment had not been totally wasted. Anne Taylor and Ginger Anderson proudly recalled that, after liberation, their teaching was acknowledged through the distribution of certificates to the school children. In addition, a few of the teenagers who were of graduating age chose to take exams in mathematics. Two internees who were mathematicians created and set up an examination that the students wrote. These were later sent to Cambridge, and all but one of the students were granted matriculation.

There were classes for adults too. In fact, within the first week the internees had organized fifty different courses ranging from the study of eight different languages, commercial law, and naval architecture, to biochemistry and astronomy. There were so many professors, "brilliant businessmen," and scientists eager to teach that some of the adult internees started to view the camp as a place to gain knowledge that they would not otherwise have access to. Without some productive activity, noted Betty Gale, "we will tend to drift along aimlessly, waiting only to be released, and these months, or years, of our lives will be wasted."[26] Gale herself took lessons in conversational Chinese twice a week (her eleven classmates were businessmen) plus two weekly lectures on Chinese philosophy and religion with the distinguished F.A. Drake, who also taught the internees how to determine the age of broken pieces of ancient Chinese pottery they collected.

Not everyone was interested in studying, however. Almost immediately after the new internees arrived, the unattached girls were being "rushed off their feet" by the original Pudong internees, "and loving it."[27] The teenagers who had been "frowsy looking" at Yangzhou were all "sprucing up for conquest" within their first two days at Pudong Camp. There, dating meant walking round and round the abandoned buildings, along with hundreds of other people—a very public activity. Betty Gale started to worry, however, when after only three weeks one of the couples was engaged ("some of the other girls are also getting heavily involved; I hope not *too* heavily").[28] Most of the relationships that sprung up in camp did not end well. Of the three couples who married during the Gales' internment, only one was still on speaking terms by the end of the war. Camp was not an ideal place to start married life together. The first wedding involved a young girl who, four months into camp, was four months pregnant. The second wedding in camp was held two weeks later. "Maud" and "Jo," both widowed, were married by "Bishop W." in the front of the dining room.[29] Frances McAll played the wedding music and Betty Gale made confetti. "There will be no honeymoon, of course," wrote Betty, "just two camp-beds side by side in a big roomful of people."[30]

For those intent on finding them, there were *some* private spaces in the abandoned warehouses. Sexual encounters were not impossible; in fact, five babies were born to Pudong Camp internees in these two years. However, all were "out of wedlock."[31] Frances McAll had reason to believe that some of the teenage girls were being abused at camp.[32] The first pregnancy came early on; "Susie" was four months pregnant in February 1944, four months after the newcomers arrived. Betty Gale wrote, "a new baby will be about as welcome as an epidemic of the plague in the large dormitories."[33] Susie immediately married the baby's father, and the British Representative tried to find a small room where they could live when the baby was born—rooms currently being used by the carpenter, shoemaker, and "Public Works Department" as workshops.

Three of the later pregnancies were of young Eurasian girls (of mixed European and Asian descent) who had gotten involved with married men whose wives were in either England or the United States. Pregnancies, then, were not seen as signs of healthy relationships, but as a reflection of some of the more tragic aspects of camp life. Even so, the birth of a child was a celebrated event. Expectant mothers would be accompanied by sampan boat across the Huangpu River to the city of Shanghai to deliver the baby in a hospital there. One of the new mothers invited the Gales to her baby's baptism, again presided over by one of the interned ministers. Betty had been helping out by bathing the infant every day, and took Margie along to watch. Margie asked Betty if she could please go across the river to pick up a baby, too.

If camp was not a good place to start a healthy marriage, it was also not an easy place to keep one. After just a month at camp Betty Gale noticed, with some relief, that she had not seen the formidable "Mrs. M." very often.

And she never saw Mrs. M. with her husband in public; they had separated. Eventually Mrs. M. was being seen in the company of a "man we've never met before" with whom she would "sit together talking, for hours, under her green and white umbrella."[34]

For one young couple, tragedy struck in May 1944 when the husband, "Morris" (likely Maurice Weill), became suddenly ill with "tuberculosis meningitis" for which there was no cure. He had to be sent out to a hospital for infectious diseases in Shanghai. Dr. Keith Graham asked permission to accompany Morris's wife, Esther, across the Huangpu River to visit him, but the Japanese Commandant refused. When word came on 28 May that Morris was dying, Graham took Esther Weill to the Commandant to plead her case with him. She fell on her knees before him and with tears rolling down her cheeks, begged him to let her go just this once to see her husband. The Commandant reportedly "looked at her coldly and said, 'My wife and children are in Japan, and I want to see them too, but I cannot. Neither can you; we are at War.'"[35] The next day Morris Weill died.[36]

Perhaps the most tragic was the story of one young Russian woman whose husband died almost immediately after arriving at Yangzhou Camp. She was transferred to Pudong Camp where, towards the end of the war, she married one of the internees. Shortly afterward liberation the woman was taking a sampan across the Huangpu River to Shanghai. She accidentally slipped into the murky river—and simply disappeared. Betty Gale was horrified, and came face to face with some frightening new knowledge: that Godfrey Gale had been at greater risk than she had imagined every time he crossed the Huangpu River with patients who required surgery or specialized care at one of the still-functioning Shanghai hospitals.

Medical Care at Pudong

On their arrival at Pudong Camp, Betty Gale was happy to discover that there were three additional physicians there. Dr. Keith Graham was in charge, and he was assisted by Dr. Hodgkins and Ed Troop, a fourth-year medical student. Keith Graham was a surgeon from Tianjin. There had been four physicians at Pudong, but two American doctors had been repatriated before Godfrey Gale and Ken McAll arrived. Because Graham had been a senior physician, and because he was older than the others, he was put in charge of the medical work at Pudong. LMS nurses Ethel Taylor and Jean Gillison rounded out the team, with Betty Gale assisting when she could. However, there were even fewer medical resources at Pudong than at Yangzhou. Whatever Godfrey Gale had left from Qilu after the trunks were looted in Yangzhou, had been stolen en route to Pudong Camp. Even so, the doctors fashioned one section of the main floor of the warehouse into what was variously called a "hospital" or "sick bay"—an open ward with eight beds. There was also a small consulting room, a room for dental work, and a "little cubbyhole" where they could "boil things up" and store items.[37]

The physicians held daily clinics, seeing and treating patients as best they could with the supplies and information at hand. They also conducted regular rounds on the patients who required round-the-clock observation, rest, and care. Ethel Taylor organized women with nursing skills to assist her in looking after the patients who were hospitalized at Pudong. For example, when Frances McAll became ill with mononucleosis, she spent three weeks in the small hospital. Patients who required more specialized care were transferred by sampan boat across the Huangpu River to one of the hospitals in Shanghai; they would be accompanied by one of the physician-internees.

Relational conflict was one of the difficulties of living in internment camps. Although disagreements undoubtedly arose between the Gales and the McAlls, in their written accounts both couples glossed over any interpersonal conflicts. This is not surprising; to record disagreements could go against a missionary value system that emphasized patience, forgiveness, and respect. Moreover, an honest rendering of a disagreement would also require reflection on one's own role in the conflict. Keeping silent allowed everyone to avoid public embarrassment. Whatever the reason, the available written evidence (published and unpublished) does not reveal much about the extent or nature of inevitable disagreements between the Gales and the McAlls. However, oral interviews conducted decades later by Margaret Gale do give a glimpse into some potential sources of irritation between the couples. In these interviews, Betty, Frances, and Ken were more candid—undoubtedly due to their familiarity with Margaret and to the diminishing social importance of skirmishes with the passage of time. For example, the oral interviews suggest that Betty did not respect Ken's medical manners, something Ken seemed oblivious to. By his own account, Ken McAll did not get along with Keith Graham or Ethel Taylor. As he recalled it, the pair conspired to get him out of the clinic. The medical meetings had become rife with arguments and, in a fit of anger, Ken McAll insulted Keith Graham by calling him the "offspring of Australian convicts" ("which he probably was," he later insisted).[38] According to McAll, Keith Graham relegated him to the role of Public Health Officer because of the enmity between them. Betty Gale's recollection of the tensions between Ken and Keith, however, was slightly different. In her estimation, Ken McAll did not make a very good general practitioner; he "did not have a good way" with patients.[39] Godfrey Gale, Betty maintained, was the most popular doctor;

he held four to five clinics every day whereas Ken held only one. It irritated Betty that her husband would be working long hours in the clinic taking care of a long line of patients while Ken sat in an office close by "doing nothing."[40]

The three dentists who had originally been interned at Pudong Camp were also repatriated before the Gales' arrival. For the first two months that the Gales were at Pudong, a Japanese dentist visited once a week. Rev. Ken Parsons, a young Methodist minister, assisted the dentist and, when the internees were told that the Japanese dentist would no longer be coming, Ken Parsons took over the dental work. He also trained two assistants and together they became adept at filling cavities and repairing dental bridges and plates. Pudong Camp was the only internment camp without interned dentists.[41] The need was great—"hundreds" of internees were suffering from toothaches; there were usually 200–300 on the waiting list for care. If the cavities were too large, or the pain too great, Godfrey Gale would be called to pull the tooth: by the end of November 1943 he had already pulled more than 60, and by July 1945 he had pulled 604. Meanwhile Parsons had completed several thousand fillings. The significance of such care cannot be overstated. Four decades later one ex-internee wrote Gale thanking him for his care:

> [John Jackson] had a ghastly abscess on a molar tooth—there was no dentist. For 2 hours 2 doctors and an ex-medical student attempted to extract the tooth (without anaesthetic). Eventually Godfrey Gale was sent for. The patient by that time was almost frantic with pain, and he heard Godfrey say quietly, "I'm going to get hold of that tooth and not let go till it's out"— which he did! The feat was not merely an example of Godfrey's professional skill, but also of his great compassion.[42]

By July 1944 the hospital was getting dangerously low on certain drugs. The doctors decided to improvise. When they ran out of Kaolin, which was used for cases of diarrhoea, they collected clay from the garden, baked it, ground it into powder, and gave it to their patients—"with good results."[43] A pinch of tobacco, swallowed, was found to be a good substitute for "santonin"—a drug "for women" (possibly to relieve dysmenorrhea—menstrual cramps—or amenorrhea—to restore menstruation).[44] Beri beri was treated with boiled plantain seeds, which were considered to be rich in Vitamin B. Seeds containing castor oil grew wild in the garden so, when the doctors had their medical meetings, they would work on a little pile of seeds as they discussed problems—opening the seeds with their nails and extracting the oils. Frances McAll's thumb became infected at one point as a result; she had gotten a piece of seed under her nail without realizing it. Her thumb started to swell and she developed an acute asthma attack. This was followed by vomiting and diarrhoea, after which she broke out in a rash from head to foot. It took her several days to overcome the violent reaction. When several other people working on the seeds developed unspecified trouble, "Project Castor-Oil" was abandoned.

By the late summer of 1944 there had already been an inordinate number of tuberculosis patients—more than any of the other internment camps around Shanghai. The visiting Swiss Consul reported, "Special mention, however, must be made of the regrettable fact that in [Pudong], owing to the lack of isolated accommodation, ten T.B. patients, of which some [are] of infectious nature, are quartered in big dormitories with other healthy inmates."[45] In addition, Pudong was the only camp reporting (two) cases of rat-borne typhus. During the Swiss Consul's site visit there were five patients in the Pudong sick bay, and forty-one admitted to Shanghai hospitals, with an additional seven on the waiting list to be hospitalized in Shanghai.

In August 1944 Betty Gale came into their cubicle to find her husband and Ken McAll talking grimly. One of the nine-year-old boys—the son of China Inland Mission missionaries—had suddenly taken very ill with pneumococcal meningitis. "That dread word sends fear into the hearts of parents and doctors alike," Betty Gale wrote about standing there listening, holding Margie tightly in her arms.[46] Godfrey Gale, who was in charge of the boy's care, decided with the nurses to "roll up their sleeves," determined to "save that boy at all costs."[47] Discussing the case with the other physicians, they decide to try a new drug called "suephedrozine" (likely a type of sulpha drug), which had come in the American parcels. None of the doctors had heard of it before, but it was supposed to be for infectious illness, and the boy was so seriously ill they determined to treat him with it.

At the same time the doctors were treating this boy, a "Mrs. H." decided to give the doctors "a terrible blasting" for taking her two daughters off the extra rations list.[48] The doctors were responsible for keeping a list of internees who required extra rations due to illness. These daughters had been receiving extra food, but now that they were feeling better, their names had been removed. The mother accused the doctors of removing the names because "we don't belong to your mission." One of the daughters contended that her name was removed "because I'm not a prostitute,"[49] a reference to the fact that the five pregnant girls in camp were getting extra rations, none of whom was married.[50] Although the family continued to treat the Gales and McAlls with coldness, at first Godfrey and Betty Gale were too preoccupied with the critically ill boy to worry about their complaints. After six days passed, however, Betty decided it was "time to talk with Mrs. H."

Writing a note asking Mrs. H. to meet her in the garden, the pair talked for two hours about their mutual concerns. Mrs. H., a widow, eventually accepted Betty's explanation that there was no favouritism being shown; the other patients simply needed the extra rations more.

Two weeks after the nine-year-old took ill with meningitis, he started to recover. All were relieved and happy, but the high rate of illness among other internees tempered their excitement. One man, for example, developed renal colic and died on the way to a Shanghai hospital. The doctors were loath to send patients into the Shanghai hospitals unless absolutely necessary since the conditions in Shanghai were deplorable. There was no running water at the hospitals, so no toilets could be used between 9:00 a.m. and 4:00 p.m. Instead, patients used pots beside their beds, which were not emptied until 4:00 p.m. Recovering patients looked after the new post-operative patients, as there were few nurses in Shanghai. Chinese labourers would bring in the meals, dump them on the bedside tables, and leave. Each bed received one clean sheet on alternate weeks only, regardless of the condition of the sheets and how many patients had previously slept on them. At night there were no lights at all in the Shanghai hospitals. Thus, the Pudong doctors only sent camp patients to Shanghai as a last resort—or if they required surgery.

Patients requiring surgery could not stay at Pudong Camp. With no anaesthetics, few trained staff, and only eight sick beds, it was virtually impossible to cope with surgeries and post-operative care. On these occasions the doctors would seek permission from the Japanese Commandant to take patients to Shanghai. He could refuse—as he did when Ken McAll requested to take a patient who had a large abscess requiring surgery across the river. The Commandant argued, "If you are afraid to open [the abscess] yourself, I'll do it for you—with my sword!"[51]

In November 1944 there were three teenage girls expecting "illegitimate" babies by three married men in camp. There was a lot of criticism of the girls and, when Betty Gale and Frances McAll made plans to set up a newborn nursery in the carpenter's room, they were told that they were "encouraging vice."[52] The plan was for Gale to be in charge of the nursery under the supervision of British nurse Ethel Taylor, while Frances McAll would be the doctor in charge. The mothers would take turns sleeping in the nursery, along with one of approximately twenty volunteers, including Gale. "None of us would have wished for them to be born here in [Pudong], but since they are, we are going to give them the best start in life that we possibly can.[53] A carpenter crafted four small cots, the Red Cross in Shanghai sent material for their layettes, and several women started sewing and knitting blankets, mattresses, sheets, diapers, and clothing. Eli and Margie's outgrown clothing was cut down for the new babies. "Now if the mothers are able to nurse them," Betty Gale wrote, "they should be alright."[54]

By the time the first two babies arrived, the weather had turned cold—it was −10°C indoors. The internees wore "practically everything" they owned, the layers of sweaters making it difficult to bend their arms. It was so cold that one man who put his false teeth in a cup of water at night could not retrieve them in the morning because they were frozen in solidly. Betty Gale hung curtains in the nursery to try to mediate the cold, then smuggled a hot plate in to raise the temperature. The Japanese never discovered the hot plate.

Throughout her internment at Pudong, Betty Gale looked for opportunities to care for other internees. While much of her caregiving was directed towards Margie and Eli, it is clear from her diary entries that she also participated in the care of the sick. She gave vaccinations, helped to feed, wash, and otherwise provide comfort for patients, assisted with the care of newborns, and kept track of developing pregnancies. At one point she noted how she wished she had brought her nursing uniform with her to camp—presumably because uniforms were more utilitarian (and easier to clean) than street clothes. As someone close to three of the camp doctors, Gale seems to have been able to get as involved with caregiving as she desired. Her calling to minister to the needs of others, then, expressed itself as care to those who were sick or discouraged, including the doctors themselves.

Gangs in the Kitchen

Although the Pudong Camp was officially comprised of only British, American, or Dutch prisoners, in practice this stipulation meant only that one's father or husband had to be one of these nationalities. In fact, there were over thirty-eight nationalities represented in the camp. Equally diverse were the occupations of the internees. There were heads of banks and large corporations, university professors and chorus girls, engineers, doctors, nurses and lawyers, debutants, teachers, scientists and students, tinkers, tailors, old soldiers, and sailors. In addition the camp held the entire crew of the American liner *The President Harrison* as well as former inmates of Sing Sing prison.[55] Betty Gale found one man especially intriguing. Dr. Erban was a Russian doctor with long, curly, golden hair hanging down his back, and an equally golden, enormous beard. He wore scanty clothing, only khaki-coloured shorts and "wooden clops."[56] This man would lie on the matting roof set up over the outdoor stove, hour after hour, enjoying the warmth under him. Although it at first bothered Betty Gale when she would go out to do some cooking, "to see that great hairy body lying above us," she became so used to it that "we just look[ed] on him as part of the roof."[57]

What is not clear is whether this was the same man noted in the Swiss Consul's Confidential Report of an inspection made of Pudong Camp on 22 June 1943. According to that report, "the American Representative used the opportunity of my presence in the Commandant's office to ask very strongly for the removal of Mr. Erbon, a non-American who has been put into the camp under the belief that he was a United States national. This man, he said, is a very dubious character with communistic tendencies and is sure to cause trouble among the community, in which, otherwise, a [illegible] atmosphere would prevail."[58] In any case "Dr. Erban" would win the regard of the internees the following summer when, still perched on the roof most of the time, he would rummage through the garbage can for something edible. Coming across a stash of uncensored letters discarded by the Japanese, he hid them in his enormous beard before distributing them to exuberant internees.

The Japanese guards did not involve themselves with the day-to-day running of the camp. As long as the internees obeyed the rules the Japanese set out for them, they were mostly left to their own devices. When the Gales first arrived, a self-appointed "police force" was already in place, and seemed to be in charge of the internal running of everything in camp. Theft and bribery were rife, and Frances McAll noted that "people kept to themselves, sitting tight on their precious belongings in their corners."[59] Because laundry would be stolen while it was drying on the line, Betty Gale would park herself by her wet clothes for hours waiting for them to dry. However, it became apparent early on that the police force itself was corrupt. It was rumoured that the head of the police ran his group "by bribery and a leather whip."[60] Those who ran the kitchen and Public Works Department demanded "extra rations of food or clothing every time they lifted a finger to do a job of work, big or small."[61] A shady gang of men, then, were in charge of the most precious resources in Pudong Camp: the food. When it was discovered that the kitchen staff were themselves eating ten percent of all the food for camp, the Gales and McAlls decided to intervene the best way they knew how: by praying.

Ken McAll and Godfrey Gale, together with first one, then a number of ex-patients, began secretly meeting together each morning in a storeroom under the stairs to pray. The Japanese strictly prohibited meetings, except in very public places like the dining hall. Neither Betty Gale nor Frances McAll joined the group; it was considered too dangerous. The prayer group would first discuss the problem, and then be quiet to "allow God to put His thoughts into their minds."[62] One day the thought came to organize a "secret" police force. Without telling even Betty or Frances, the group set out to hand select "educated" men who were considered honest and upright citizens to comprise a new police force that would overthrow the corrupt one. Thirty-nine men were selected, and on the appointed day the internees who came onto the playing field for their daily roll call were surprised to see "a stalwart male at every vantage point round the building and by the laundry troughs, his hands behind his back, legs apart and a red armband with 'Police' sewn on loudly in black."[63]

The new police force had been prepared for open conflict, but nothing happened. The gang members "vanished like rats into a hole."[64] According to Frances McAll, there was a sudden release of tension in the camp, and with it an almost immediate sense of community. They felt a strong sense of accomplishment and affirmed faith.

At Pudong and, indeed, throughout her internment, Betty Gale made regular reference to spiritual disciplines that helped her to find meaning and strength during these years. In addition to attending and participating in weekly church services and Sunday School, she set aside time for a regular "Quiet Time" (QT) of prayer and scripture reading. In Pudong Camp she would go to the "canteen" between 6:30 a.m. and 7:30 a.m. for her "QT." In her notebook written during her last year of internment, Gale expands more on her inner spiritual life than in either her five year diary or journal. In August 1944, for example, she wrote about her reflections on a sermon: "Topping sermon for young and old yesterday by Tom Allan. 'What you are and what you can become.' Using story of Jesus and Peter—'Now you are called Simon, but you shall become Peter—a rock.' Jesus was a young man talking to a young man. How P[eter] had to be changed in all his ideas of things—what Christianity really is, how simple, etc. Not just church."[65]

Betty Gale took seriously the faith and ideals instilled in her through her missionary childhood. She looked toward Scripture and its interpretation by fellow Christians to make sense of her new world and her place in it. In recording this particular sermon, it seems possible that she identified with Peter in the sense that his relationship with Jesus and his experiences as being a follower of Christ in difficult circumstances changed his view of what Christianity meant. When Gale later reflected on her internment experiences—particularly Pudong—she noted how valuable a simple life, stripped away of all but the very basics, was. Having experienced severe poverty and hunger—and more quarrels and selfish behaviour than ever before—Gale started seeing a correlation between poverty and strife. Like fellow internee William Sewell, whose post-war book *Strange Harmony* she cited, Gale came to believe that "the poor of other lands … have so many characteristics which are *NOT National*, but that which poverty has given them. And if we want [those in developing countries] to be good citizens … [they must have] at least a measure of security."[66] If Gale grew up in China taking a view of the Chinese Other as somehow inferior in terms of the civil and refined English behaviour she and her family so valued, having experienced hunger and poverty herself (and having witnessed the "uncivil" behaviour of members of so-called civilized nations) she found herself re-thinking what it meant to be poor, and how poverty alone might influence behaviour. As someone who came to China to care for the poor, it was not until she experienced extreme and prolonged poverty herself that Gale came to really understand whom she was ministering to—and to relate to "strangers" as fellow sojourners. Through her own suffering, Betty Gale's view of Christianity, like Peter's, was transformed.

Ex-internees frequently commented on how camp disrupted existing social class barriers. Although like-minded internees naturally grouped together for socializing, work was a different matter. One morning Betty Gale was amused to watch the "Lavatory Squad" at work: the three men on duty together were a Bishop of the Church of England, a former manager of a large Shanghai bank, and a well-known street beggar from Shanghai. "They seem to work very well as a team," Betty Gale noted, "and in their old clothes, with messy overalls, you can't tell 't'other from which.'"[67] Wealth and position did not give a person status in camp; rather, "the only thing that counts is the contribution we make day by day to the general good."[68]

Resistance

Compared with Yangzhou Camp B the internees at Pudong Camp were more rebellious; they were more likely to find means to resist their Japanese captors. Perhaps this was because of the nature of the internees themselves; there were more men, 900 versus 250 women, and some of these men were, as Betty Gale called them, a lower sort of class—one that included convicts. The tallest man in camp was the Shanghai executioner, Mr. Roper. According to one LMS missionary, he had "no expression at all; no one talked to him."[69] At least one man in camp was a murderer: "He was a very nice man, actually. He came to our sick bay with malaria or something and kept very quiet. It was funny to be sitting beside him at night [in the hospital]. But he wasn't at all dangerous. After he left the sick bay, a mother with a little girl said he came in and played with the baby and was very nice. Someone later told the mom that he was a murderer […] He said that the person he killed needed to be killed."[70] There were rumours that in the first six months of Pudong Camp, when it only housed men, there were breakouts of violence, and even attempted murders.[71] Unlike the predominantly missionary population of the ccc and the predominantly affluent population of Yangzhou Camp B, the population of Pudong Camp was rough—and bold. They were, it seems, more ready to take risks to undermine the Japanese.

They were also closer to a major city. Although surrounded by barbed wire and guard towers with armed Japanese guards, there were ways to get into Shanghai across the river. One of the more legitimate ways to accompany those patients who required surgery or hospitalization in Shanghai. In addition to Japanese escorts, a physician and stretcher bearers were required. Once when it was Dr. Ken McAll's turn, eight American internees volunteered to go along as stretcher bearers. The Japanese guard became incensed, insisting that only four were needed. The guard grabbed McAll's arm and twisted it behind his back until he demanded that four of the men withdraw.[72] On another occasion Dr. Keith Graham was in the hospital with the patient, not realizing that the stretcher bearers were treating the Japanese escort guards to enough alcohol to make them drunk, and then ditching them in Shanghai, returning to camp with only Keith Graham. With a little imagination, then, these hospital trips could be used as a way to acquire alcohol or other contraband items to bring back to camp.

Those who were especially daring could sneak out of the camp at night and return before daybreak. For example, one side of the *godown*—a side that Japanese guards could not see from their watch tower—was right against the bank of the Huangpu River. For a while a group of five teenagers regularly escaped out of their window after dark, taking boats across to Shanghai where they would purchase tobacco. This carried dire consequences, however. One night at 10:15 p.m., when the internees were settling down to sleep, there was a sudden clanging of bells and a "tremendous uproar broke out in the Commandant's office."[73] Soon the whole area was "swarming with J[apanese] all armed to the teeth." Betty Gale and Frances McAll grabbed their dressing gowns, wrapped their children in blankets and obeyed the shouted command to line up immediately for roll call. They stood for almost three hours, trying to keep Eli and Margie in hand. Finally they were allowed back to bed. Five teenagers had escaped; they had been caught by the guards and were brought back to the camp in chains.

At first there was talk of shooting the boys then and there. Instead, they were taken to the guardhouse where they were each given a thorough beating. One boy fought back, and had his jaw broken. "The poor kids had to stand all night, and when they fell from exhaustion—were beaten again."[74] Women in the dormitory next door could hear the violence through the walls. Some, including the "mothers and sweethearts of these boys" became hysterical. The doctors gave them all sedatives, "but no one in Camp sleeps for the rest of the night."[75]

The next day the boys were paraded up and down before the rest of the internees, in their bare feet, fastened together with chains—a "harrowing site" for the entire camp. The boys were sent to jail in Shanghai for three months of solitary confinement. According to camp records, a total of four men were arrested at Pudong: it is unclear whether these were the "teenagers" from this incident; those arrested were ages seventeen, nineteen, twenty, and twenty-one at the time.[76] The rest of the internees were punished by being barred from the "garden" (playing field) for one week (those living in the same room as the boys were barred for two weeks); by having planned activities cancelled; by having outdoor roll call twice a day; and by having an extra roll call in the middle of the night for three weeks.

Betty Gale and the others felt sympathetic towards the boys; life in camp was so "intensely dull" for young people, that this must have seemed an exciting diversion and a "challenge of wits."[77] Years later one claimed that he had been "over the wall" twenty times to buy tobacco in Shanghai to sell to the internees.[78] Tobacco was in high demand too: by February 1944 smokers were becoming so desperate for cigarettes that they were exchanging coats and gold Swiss watches for them. To Betty Gale, the "former chain smokers look terrible, so haggard and thin; they can't sleep, but prowl around like restless animals all night long."[79] Cigarette butts were saved from ashtrays, the floor, or the ashcan, and rewrapped for future use. The most desperate wrapped tea leaves in toilet paper as a substitute for the tobacco they craved. The boys who were caught escaping to Shanghai in May 1944 would buy all the cigarettes they could find and then bring them back to Mr. "Z" who would sell them to the internees at a "terrific profit."[80] The internees were incensed at Mr. Z., whom they considered the "real villain" in this incident.[81]

Betty Gale described Mr. Z. as a "strange looking man, very short and flabby, with a huge bald egg-shaped head."[82] The day that the boys went to jail, Mr. Z. was called into visit the Japanese Commandant. "Feeling is running high against him," wrote Gale, "and if the J[apanese] don't beat him up, some of the internees may."[83] Hundreds of internees watched as Mr. Z. climbed the steps to the Commandant's office, looking pale and frightened. After a few minutes he came out—smiling. "We wonder how much money passed across the table in those five minutes," Betty Gale wryly questioned. The rest of the internees "cold-shouldered" Mr. Z., but to Gale's relief, no one struck him.

Although it was clearly possible to do so, none of the Pudong Camp internees escaped during the two years that the Gales were there. Out of the approximately 13,544 prisoners in the civilian internment camps in China, thirteen reportedly escaped successfully, while eight others tried but failed.

It is not clear what happened to those who failed.[84] According to Betty Gale, there was a small group that escaped to West China when Pudong was just a men's camp, but the details of this are unknown. When later asked why those who left the camp—to buy tobacco, for instance—did not "just keep running," Ken McAll surmised that it was because they knew that, even if they were free, their escape would mean severe punishment for those left behind. According to McAll, while still at Qilu, he and Frances had been offered an opportunity by some of their students to escape to Free China (Chongqing), but they were afraid of what punishment might befall those left behind, so they turned it down.[85]

On 5 November 1943, three American men were caught with a radio they had made themselves. They were taken to the guardhouse for questioning. Although, as Betty Gale wrote in her diary, "everyone feeling rather scared, to say the least," nothing happened and they returned unharmed to their rooms that evening.[86] However, five days later the entire camp was punished by having their hot-plates confiscated, their visits to the dentist and "oculist" cancelled, and their Saturday night dances temporarily banned. ("What a howl there will be from the teenagers over this," Gale wrote.)[87] More unfortunately, the three men were sent to solitary confinement in a Shanghai jail for three months ("how *grim* for them," worried Gale).

Apparently this punishment did not deter them. For the duration of the war, there was at least one radio at Pudong Camp, hidden in the belly of a stuffed toy. Furtive arrangements had been made to have radio parts smuggled into camp in tins of food. Godfrey Gale and Ken McAll were among those privy to the reports from the radio broadcasts. In fact, they were among the first to know about the atomic bombing of Hiroshima and Nagasaki in August 1945 and the subsequent surrender of the Japanese. They told their wives but could not share the news with others in camp until it came out through more official means.

One unusual source of information was a Russian man who lived down the road from Pudong Camp and worked for the Japanese. He was in charge of a fire hall and every time there was good news to share about the war, he would ring the fire-bell and a friend in camp would run outside onto a little front porch. The Russian would ride by on his bicycle and, looking straight ahead, would call out the latest news, in Russian. Although what he was saying could not always be clearly understood, Betty took heart to know that at least the news was good.

Acts of resistance sometimes also emerged unexpectedly. A year after their arrival in Pudong Camp, the Gales were enjoying an evening concert performed by the camp orchestra. The director had worked out a medley of well-known songs for the last number, into which he wove a section of notes from the British anthem "God save the King." The song was so skil-fully blended into the others that the Japanese guards, sitting in the front row, did not recognize it. "*We* all do," wrote Betty Gale, "and we had a hard time not jumping to our feet and *singing* the words."[88]

On more than one occasion Betty Gale was glad to be interned under the Japanese Consular Police rather than the Japanese Military. Once when the Japanese Military was inspecting the camp, a "rough burly" military man stalked into one of the bathrooms where a large group of women were in various stages of undress. "He strides across the room," Betty Gale wrote, "scattering us before him as though we were so many cattle." He "relieves himself" against the wall and then stalks out again, staring contemptuously at us as he goes and slams the door behind him. The hate smouldering in his eyes sends chills up and down our spines."[89]

Camp Conflict

Nothing seemed to gall Betty Gale more than signs of selfishness in other internees. Five months after they arrived in Pudong Camp, "huge" Ameri-can Red Cross parcels arrived, filled with food and medicine and clothing. There was great "jubilation" in camp … until it became clear that some of the American internees perceived themselves as the only ones entitled to the contents. Betty Gale fumed:

> It is hard to believe this, but a group of the Americans say, "these parcels are from the U.S.A., therefore they are for Americans only, and not one goes to a ruddy Britisher." We are at first incredulous, and then furiously angry. The Red Cross is an international organization, and all parcels are for all allied prisoners, irrespective of the Country that sends them, U.S.A. this month—hopefully Britain next month […] We overhear one Britisher say, "But this is ridiculous, of course we should have our share! Well—hang it all—it was England that started the war!!"[90]

After two days of negotiation between the British Representative and the American internees, the food in the parcels was divided up, "fair and square." The Gales revelled in real butter, tinned ham, egg powder, milk, and chocolates. However, the "Britishers" were told that they were not allowed to have any of the clothing. This struck Betty Gale as ludicrous, consider-ing that there was only one American woman in camp. This woman got her pick of the clothes, and other clothes were parcelled out to women who were dating some of the American male internees. The rest were "smuggled into [Shanghai] to girlfriends, or sold on the black market."[91] Forty years later Gale would still feel vexed by this display of extreme selfishness, and for good reason: most of her own clothing had been stolen. "It's a real disgrace," she penned, "for there are so many internees who have lost nearly all their clothing through looting on our journey here, and need things so badly."[92]

Letters were becoming scarce. Although the rules changed at times, generally the internees were allowed to post one letter a month to family overseas, and one local letter. They were to receive an unlimited number of letters. During their three on-site visits to Pudong Camp, the Swiss Consuls invariably found internees complaining about the lack of mail. Internees requested having the number of outgoing letters increased to three per month, but the Japanese objected. As it was, they were finding it difficult to keep up with the censoring involved. According to the Swiss Consul: "The staff engaged in this task [of censoring internee letters] find it difficult to cope already with the present volume of correspondence as a result of which transmission is usually considerably delayed."[93] While incoming messages were supposed to be freely accepted and delivered, the International Committee of the Red Cross discouraged the local population in Shanghai from writing too many letters lest the Japanese "enforce restrictions."[94] Still, Betty Gale did not receive letters from her family for over a year. She did, however, receive one from Mary Stanley, in September 1944: the letter arrived on Betty and Godfrey's fourth anniversary. Although Gale did not comment on the contents of Stanley's letter, it does confirm that each knew where the other was.[95]

Despite Japanese assurances that a canteen would be provided for the purchase of extra food items, soap, and other toiletries, in reality none of the Shanghai internment camps had properly functioning canteens.[96] Most were without any stock. Orders placed with the Japanese canteen contractor took weeks to fill even partially. Furthermore, the "comfort funds" provided through the Swiss Consulate and ICRC were rarely made available to the internees. Initially allotted CRB $200 to $300 per month, the amount was increased to CRB $3,000 to $4,000 by 1944 because of inflation, but even then it could not buy much. Friends of the internees who had been supplying food parcels were less inclined to do so by 1944 with prices of an average parcel exceeding CRB $6,000 in the inflated Shanghai war economy.

According to Frances McAll, violence erupted regularly in Pudong Camp. A tough group already, it sometimes did not take much for heated arguments to get physical. One day the men who worked on the outside grill asked the "Committee on Baths" if they could be allotted an extra shower on the days they worked the fires. Having been refused the men retaliated by removing all the fire from the grill—meaning that those who had bread in the oven had their precious food ruined. "A terrific row follows," Betty Gale wrote, "everyone is furious, one man brandishes a knife and threatens to kill another chap."[97] Eventually the Committee on Baths compromises by allowing the men an extra bucket each, and they started the fire going again. On another occasion two women got into a fight. Gale described it thus:

> Molly is a large, beautifully formed young woman with the mental age of about 12 years. For some strange reason she is attracted to Mr. B.—a horrible little man, dirty, slovenly, and twice her age. He was a beggar on the streets of Shanghai before the J. brought him into Camp. Mrs. B. is a little Eurasian woman, usually very quiet, but today she becomes angry and shouts at Molly, and the latter, who is as strong as an ox, hits her, and shakes off the combined efforts of six young girls who try to hold her. Fortunately some men arrive who can control her, while Mrs. B. makes her escape. Molly is being moved to another room, at the far side of the Camp.[98]

The string of fights continued when some men who had formed a camp band obtained some liquor from the Japanese guards. At a party in the dormitory, one boy got in a fight and fell down a high flight of iron stairs, sustaining a concussion, broken arm, and severe internal injuries.[99] Godfrey Gale and Ken McAll were up "nearly all night" with him, and accompanied the boy to Shanghai at daybreak, in very serious condition.

Keith Graham was attacked one afternoon by a man who had gone berserk. "He might have been killed if Ken McAll hadn't arrived in the nick of time," Betty Gale wrote. The man was a patient of Graham's who had tried to get extra rations for himself but had been refused. He had been brooding about this for weeks and on that day was out for revenge. He came to the clinic with a piece of old piping hidden inside his coat. When Keith Graham sat down to write out a prescription, the man took a swing at his head. Just at that moment McAll came in, saw what was happening, grabbed the man's arm, and then wrestled him to the ground. Rumours about the incident somehow made it as far as Chapei internment camp, where it was said that, after being hit over the head, Graham "went crazy and stabbed 2 men at night!"[100] The man who attacked Keith Graham was sent to a Shanghai hospital for psychiatric treatment.

Keeping Fed and Warm

As winter approached in 1944, the rooms in Pudong Camp became bitterly cold. On a day that the inside temperature dropped to 6°C, Godfrey Gale and Ken McAll pasted up every crack they could find to keep out the wind, "but it doesn't make any difference."[101] Margie and Eli's faces were "blue with cold" and their hands "icy." Betty Gale wrapped them up in blankets and read to them by turn. The older folks in camp had such difficulty with the cold, many would simply stay in bed under their blankets for days on end. The cost of coal was rumoured to be CRB $22,000 per ton in Shanghai; at that price, the Japanese didn't even try to heat the warehouse where the internees were living. They did, however, have heat themselves, via stoves in the guardhouse and gatehouse.

By wintertime the food was also getting worse. "Our rice these days is horrible," Betty Gale wrote, "full of mud, husks, and rat droppings."[102] Gale counted fifty-nine weevils in Margie's porridge one morning; she fished them out while Margie watched, fascinated. According to some sources, internees were forbidden to remove the weevils from their cracked wheat, since these creatures would add some much needed protein to their diet.[103] Perhaps this is, in part, why Margie and Eli were fed in their room rather than in the dining hall. Feeding the girls in their room gave some much desired privacy; it also allowed the parents to feed them the more nutritious hospital food on occasion without prying eyes—and criticism—from other internees. Eli in particular had constant trouble with the food and, as a result, often looked thin and pale. Once, when two-and-a-half-year-old Eli became violently ill with vomiting and diarrhoea in the middle of the night, her parents lit a small candle to help them to see as they assisted her and tried to clean up. The Japanese guards, who took their 10:00 p.m. lights-out rule very seriously, shouted at them to put out the candle, leaving the McAlls to attend to Eli in total darkness.

The summer of 1944 brought the problem of intense heat—and less food. The cost of food had skyrocketed in Shanghai, and the internees were being allowed only 1,300 calories a day. The fare was meagre: breakfast consisted of tea and sour bread, lunch of rice with marrow soup, supper of rice with "watery (beef?) stew"—what the internees referred to as "S.O.S.": Same Old Stew.[104] The bread, comprised of soy bean flour, soured very quickly in hot weather. The meat was of very poor quality, mostly buffalo meat containing a "comparatively large percentage of bone and offal."[105] The food was barely enough to live on, and not enough to supply the internees with enough energy for their work—never mind playing games or putting on concerts. The Swiss Consul who visited determined that the food was deficient in proteins, fats, vitamins, and minerals; the situation was critical for children.[106]

Every month the Shanghai Red Cross sent the Gales parcels that had been arranged by the LMS before they left the Columbia Country Club, but the British Red Cross and International Red Cross parcels were not coming—in part because of the difficulty in sending overseas shipments. All of the internment camps around Shanghai were receiving fewer Red Cross parcels than expected. In September 1944 the Swiss Consul reported that on average only thirty-eight percent of the six thousand internees in the seven Shanghai camps were receiving parcels; more than one-third of the camp populations did not receive any regular parcels at all.[107] By the end of the summer, the old people were lying on their bed most of the time, conserving their energy. Many were experiencing bleeding gums, extremely slow healing of wounds, and scratches that turned septic—all indicative of inadequate nutrition.

Fewer internees felt up to playing outside sports games. This may have been because everyone was feeling weaker. It might also have been because of a fear of what too much expended energy might do to their weakened bodies. At the end of August 1944 a group of teenage girls challenged some older men to a game of baseball. They had a lot of fun but it ended in tragedy as one of the men had a stroke and became paralyzed on his right side as a result.

By the winter of 1945, the food situation was even more dire. In Shanghai rice was reportedly CRB $52,000 per sack, flour was $150 per pound, and jam was $600 for a small tin. One small, flat biscuit was $15.[108] When the internees' second International Red Cross parcel arrived on 30 January 1945, they were "wild" with "rejoicing."[109] By strange coincidence their first British Red Cross parcels arrived on the same day. Two days earlier their monthly parcels from Shanghai had arrived. "We are buried in them," Betty Gale wrote, "but how marvellous it is. We haven't seen so much food all at once since before the war began."[110] Margie was so impressed that she changed her evening prayer to fit the occasion: the line "quickly, quickly passes each happy day" became "quickly, quickly *parcels* each happy day." There was no problem dividing up the American food parcels this time, but the men were fighting over the clothes again. One of two men who fought over a particular jacket got his front teeth knocked out. By the spring of 1945 Godfrey Gale had lost forty pounds, while Betty Gale had lost thirty—she weighed in at ninety-seven pounds.

Making Pudong "A Happy Place"

"Perhaps it is better that we cannot see ahead," Betty Gale wrote at the end of 1943, "but just live as fully, and as happily as we can, *one day at a time.*"[111] Gale felt it was very important for their morale to try to accept Pudong Camp as their permanent home, to do what they could to make "our small corner" a happy place, "especially for the children, for this will be the first home they will remember."[112] At one point she observed that the two girls were "loving it" at Pudong. "They have so many kind 'uncles' and 'aunties' waiting to spoil them with love and overindulgence."[113] As the only pre-schoolers at Pudong Camp, Eli and Margie were the centre of attention for many of the internees. The teenagers loved to babysit and take the little girls for walks.

Even the most rough of the male internees would delight in the little girls. On Sundays Betty Gale was in charge of arranging flowers for the weekly church service, presided over by one of the many interned ministers and held in the dining room. To prepare, on Saturdays Betty would take Margie out to one of the gardens where flowers were growing to request if they could have a small bouquet for the church service. The men would invariably agree, and Margie would carefully carry the flowers home, where she would help Betty arrange them in their only glass tumbler. After the Sunday service, Betty and Margie would bring the flowers to the little hospital.

A few days before Easter in 1944, Betty Gale and others asked if the Japanese guards might provide them with some branches of fruit trees that were in blossom about half a kilometre down the road. She could see the trees from her window. To her delight, the guards brought them the next day. Gale kept the blossoms in two large buckets of water in the dining room. "How glorious to see and touch and smell their delicate beauty," she raved. "I bury my face in them, and am right back in my uncle's orchard in Ontario, green grass under my feet, the sun warm on my back, and the drowsy hum of bees in my ears."[114] (Margie buried her face in the blossoms, too, but remarked, "I can't hear any bees, I guess my blossoms don't have any on them.")[115]

On Good Friday 1944, the Pudong choir sang Stainer's *Crucifixion*. On Easter Sunday some of the internees got up early to decorate the dining room by hanging blue curtains across the front, with a white sheet in the centre, in front of which they placed a "pulpit" table. A wooden cross was placed on the table. Four stools were covered with blue cloth and topped with pots of white paper lilies attached to branches of oleanders. Side tables were banked with willow branches, weeds, and blossoms. The 11:00 a.m. service was "packed"; "those who can't get in look through the doors and windows [...] For some, it was their first Easter Service, and we all find it a very moving experience."[116]

The sheets used to decorate the dining hall were sent by the Shanghai Red Cross for theatricals. "There is an incredible amount of talent locked up here," Betty Gale wrote. There were regular concerts and plays, from Hamlet to cancan dancing. Some internees had brought instruments and costumes with them to camp. Whatever else was needed was crafted, improvised, or imagined. The creation of beauty—be it visual, oral, or auditory—seemed an important preoccupation. In her experience as a missionary nurse outside of the internment camps, Betty Gale was used to a sort of ebb and flow between the difficulties of work and the pleasures of "off" times. As predominantly educated, middle-class women, who enjoyed the relatively inexpensive indulgences available in China of cooks, amahs, and labourers, mishkid nurses worked in a world where they had the luxury of stepping out of the poverty and sickness they faced by coming home at night to lovely homes and gardens, and spending holidays at seaside resorts. Evenings and weekends were filled with socializing and creating concerts and other events. In the internment camps, there was no longer the opportunity to separate oneself from one's work—or from those one cared for as a nurse or physician. By creating and attending social events, missionaries and other internees replicated a social scene familiar to them while also providing a distraction from boredom and anxiety.

To many of the internees, Eli and Margie were an important source of entertainment. Their playful innocence was refreshing, and while younger internees vied for chances to babysit or take the girls for a walk, older internees found reasons to give gifts and affection, spoiling them with attention. On their third birthdays, the girls were showered with homemade gifts. A paragraph in the day's camp "Bulletin" called the girls "the Centre's Cinderellas" and went on to describe the sentiments of the internees: "When, last year, on a wet day, the wee lassies arrived at [Yangzhou], the compassionate hearts of the Camp were touched. Since that time they have been regarded as miniature mascots, and have found a warm niche in the hearts of all of [Pudong]."[117]

Through the miserable summer months of 1944 the girls also kept their parents entertained. For example, when Betty Gale was napping one afternoon, the McAlls surreptitiously watched as Margie began to undress herself in her crib. Ken McAll later wrote a poem describing the "Pootung Incident":

> During rest time little fat one
> In her cot then meant for sleeping
> While her mother gently snoring
> Turned her back on what was happening,
> Quietly pulled her bed to pieces,
> First the pillow then the blankets
> Flung regardless o'er the cot side
> Followed quickly by her clothing

Tugged from off her little body
Pants and vest and lastly nappy
Joined the pile beside her mother.
Then, while mother still unseeing
Little streamlet gently trickled
Through the furrow made to guide it,
Dripped down plip plop to the sick bay
Where the Red Head sat absorbing
Knowledge from the books around him
Bald one and his long-nosed woman
Split their sides with silent laughter.[118]

Even the Japanese guards took notice of the girls at times; some even took photos of them. Once a guard surprised the Gales and McAlls by bringing two pears and two cookies to their cubicle. He laughed and talked with the girls (in Japanese), patting them on the head. When the parents motioned to him to sit down, he did, bringing out a stash of photographs of his family, including two children aged four and six. "He looks so young," wrote Betty Gale, "and so homesick; how incredibly *beastly* is this war."[119]

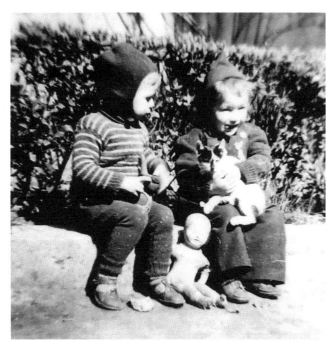

Fig. 7.2   Eli and Margie at Pudong Camp (photo taken by Japanese guard)

One April day, two-and-a-half-year-old Eli was standing on a chair looking out the window. It was a cold, miserable day with a strong wind blowing. She watched a group of small Chinese children holding their coats tightly as they struggled against the wind. Sorrowfully Eli said, "Poor little Chinese children, they haven't got a nice home like I have."[120] Betty Gale and Frances McAll looked at each other, and around the messy elevator shaft cubicle, "with its grimy walls, broken windows, rotting floors, and the rubber sheets hanging over the beds keeping off the rain," and felt a surge of awe and gratitude. "Thank God," Gale wrote, with an air of amazement, "that she feels she has a 'lovely home.'"[121]

For their second Christmas at Pudong Camp, in 1944, the internees pulled out all the stops. Carpenters fashioned a realistic mantelpiece to cover a very real-looking fireplace created by an electrician. On the wall above it, Ken McAll painted a clock, candlesticks, a picture in a frame, and a bunch of holly and mistletoe. "The fire looks so real," Betty Gale wrote, "that people stand in front of it all day trying to warm themselves."[122] McAll also painted four huge murals on the walls using lime, soot, and red brick dust mixed with scrapings from the rice cauldron. The internees worked together to put on a Christmas tableau on Christmas Eve, complete with "Mary" looking "absolutely beautiful in Frances's rose wool dress, with a deep blue curtain falling from her shoulders like a cloak, and a white veil over her hair."[123] It was a huge success.

After the Christmas service on Christmas Day, Betty and Godfrey Gale invited twenty-six people over for tea. As was always done for a party, Betty and her friend Ginger Anderson collected ingredients in advance from the guests who were coming, and then made as much as they could with what they collected. It was a "hilarious do" since the cubicle really could not accommodate so many people, but they had all enjoyed the sandwiches, two cakes, and a few plain cookies. The guests brought gifts for the girls. The prize gift was a dollhouse made out of two cardboard boxes. It was filled with painted furniture made of papier mâché. In addition to a completed kitchen, bedrooms, and living room with fireplace, it included a bathroom with a tub, sink, toilet, and even towel racks with tiny towels and an infinitesimal roll of toilet paper. The girls spent hours playing with the dollhouse, but did not know what to make of the furniture and pictures ("a bath-tub? What's *that* for?").[124] As her present to the girls, Betty Gale made nurses' aprons and caps. When she later took the girls to the hospital to deliver some presents, they wore their new uniforms, much to everyone's delight.

To keep Margie entertained one day when she was recovering from bronchitis, Betty Gale decided to tell her about things she has never seen— like ice cream, bananas, candies, and other fresh fruit. "But how do you tell a child who has never eaten it, what ice cream tastes like?" she wondered.[125] For Gale, the presence of the two children provided important ballast in her altered life. With everything else so completely changed and even unrecognizable, the children acted like, well, children. That is to say, they brought a sense of normalcy and familiarity to the squalid surroundings, and gave Gale a focus and mission that were more important, and more enduring, than her nursing practice.

Bombing Shanghai

From their window overlooking the Huangpu River, Betty Gale and the others could watch the movements of the ships in the harbour there. They could tell which were Japanese military ships, for example, and tried to look for clues as to the status of the war based on the activity on the river. Being so close to the harbour, the Pudong Camp internees recognized that, were warfare to break out, Pudong would likely be a target—intentionally or not—of bombing. As with most things in camp, a committee was struck to help the internees to prepare for such an event. In January 1944 Godfrey Gale was appointed the Chief Medical of the Air Raid Precaution Organization. The task of the committee was to prepare for two very serious contingencies—"either a direct hit and a collapse of our rickety buildings from blast" or "being caught between the fire of an American expeditionary force advancing on Shanghai from the south, and the fire of the J. defending the city."[126] Their concerns would prove to be well founded, although the air raids would not occur for another five months. "I think it is somewhat like facing the birth of a first baby," Betty Gale wrote. "We want the baby to come, we can hardly wait for it, but a thread of fear runs along the back of our minds, when we think of the actual delivery—a fear of the unknown, and of pain."[127]

Godfrey Gale began to teach courses in first aid, while another internee, who was a member of St. John Ambulance, was training men and women for rescue work. One day in April 1944 the internees awoke to the sound of machine-gun fire. "We don't know what is happening," Betty Gale wrote. "We pack an emergency bag to be grabbed in case of need."[128] By the end of May, forty people had completed the first aid training and received certificates created by LMS missionary Ginger Anderson. Eleven days later, on 11 June 1944, the internees experienced their first air raid. Hearing the siren the Gales and the McAlls leaped out of bed, threw on their clothes, and dressed the children. Godfrey Gale and Ken McAll went to their posts: Godfrey to set up an emergency hospital in the library area; Ken to evacuate the eight-bed hospital ward downstairs. Betty and Frances took their daughters to join the other internees in the playing field. Standing under the nearly full moon, the girls were excited to see the sky filled with stars ("Oh Mummy, see all the baby suns," Margie exclaimed.")[129] Off in the distance they could hear the crash of bombs and anti-aircraft guns, while tracer bullets shot across the sky "like golden rain." Eventually the all-clear sounded and everyone went back to bed.

The bombing would continue for the next ten days. Preferring to stay inside, Betty Gale and Frances McAll would take the girls into bed with them, and pile pillows around them to protect them from flying glass. "They usually go back to sleep quickly," Betty wrote, adding, "We do not."[130] By June 1944 it was becoming clear that Shanghai was becoming a battlefield again, and that Pudong Camp internees were in a most vulnerable spot. Pudong Camp was less than a kilometre from the Huangpu River, where there were "dozens of war ships of every kind."[131] There was an ammunition factory about three hundred metres north of the camp and an oil and gasoline dump ten metres from the Gales' window. The Japanese naval headquarters were less than a kilometre down the road, and anti-aircraft guns stood on three corners of Pudong Camp. On 23 June the internees watched as the Japanese lay mines in the road in front of the camp. There were "pill boxes" every 200 metres, communication trenches, and tank traps. Although the internees presumed the American military knew about their existence, they also realized that it would want to destroy the Japanese ammunition supply.

Betty Gale felt the same sort of anxiety she had felt in the fall of 1941 when war was imminent in Qilu. As the bombing increased over Shanghai, she started to wonder, "Will we be caught in the line of fire? Will we be transported to Manchuria or Japan to face all kinds of new danger? Will we be lined up and shot? Or will a 'miracle' happen, with a Japanese surrender and the disappearance of our guards overnight?"[132] Internees made plans for the evacuation of their buildings should there be a direct hit or a fire. There were no air raid shelters, since being on the banks of a river meant that water was only a metre below the ground. "When bombing gets too heavy," Betty Gale wrote, "we are told to congregate in the center of the rooms on the first floor, and to stay as far from the windows as possible."[133] As a mishkid, danger was a familiar concept. But this was the most perilous situation Gale had ever experienced.

Although young Margie Gale would have few memories of the bombings, as an adult she had recurring nightmares involving the sounds and smells of bombing and darkness, accompanied by an overwhelming sense of anxiety.[134] Frances McAll would remember looking out of their window as bombs fell, and then looking down at young Eli beside her. Eli, she noticed, was not looking out of the window at the falling bombs; she was looking intently up at her mother's face. Frances realized that Eli's own response to the air raids would be shaped by the emotion she found there: Eli would be afraid only if she saw fear reflected in her own face.[135] The air raids would continue for the next fourteen months, until the end of the war.

On 14 July 1944 one of the internees who acted as an interpreter heard over the Japanese "wireless" that Hitler had been assassinated. "Wild excitement in camp the last two days," Betty Gale wrote in her notebook. "Rumours?"[136]

The bombing intensified. On 8 August 1944 an American plane dropped a bomb right into the middle of the *Conte Verde*, a ship anchored in the Huangpu River harbour. The noise was "deafening" and vibrations shook the whole camp. "Everyone shrieked with joy," Betty Gale noted, "and all ran to the windows to see what was happening. The J. Guards were scared stiff."[137] Seeing the much-battered ship lying on her side in the mud at daybreak, Gale wrote, "How the Chinese will be laughing over this!"[138]

The bombing did not always frighten the internees. In November 1944 Betty Gale wrote that they had had "a most exciting day," because there were several huge American "Flying Fortresses" bombing Shanghai.[139] The planes were above Shanghai for three hours as the Gales and McAlls watched from their ringside seat: "One J. plane goes up to attack, but as soon as the pilot sees what he is up against, he returns even quicker than he went up. A second J. plane goes up, and is promptly shot down by J. anti-aircraft guns. This war is getting more ridiculous every day."[140]

By January 1945 Pudong Camp was having daily air raids. Occasionally news would seep out from the four men who still possessed the radio stuffed in a child's toy. A broadcaster from West China told his audience to "prepare for big developments any day now."[141] Betty Gale started having recurring "frightful dreams" where she, Godfrey, and Margie were back in Toronto, standing across the road from her family home at 33 Rose Park Drive. The door would open and out would rush her parents and siblings and all their families laughing and calling out. "Suddenly a metal fence slides out of the road," wrote Gale, "barring the way. It rapidly grows higher and higher until we can no longer see the roof of the house. We call and call, and they answer, but their voices are muffled and gradually fade away. We stand there desolate, weeping … and I awake to find my pillow wet with tears."[142]

The internees watched a second Japanese plane being shot down by Japanese anti-aircraft guns. One guard explained this to the interpreter (Charlie) by saying that the Americans had tried to camouflage the plane with a fake Japanese emblem, but that the Japanese saw through the plan and shot it down. The sergeant was "more honest" saying, "You were all gentlemen not to cheer when we shot down one of our own planes."[143] Whoever the plane belonged to, Betty Gale found it "horrible sickening" that a young man crashed to the ground in flames in front of them. The next day the Japanese Commandant issued a warning that "any internee seen at a window, on a balcony or on a roof during one of the 'alert' periods will be shot and killed."[144]

On 5 February 1945 Betty Gale counted sixty-eight Japanese warships in the river, all visible from the third floor window. One of the guards told a Japanese interpreter, "Japan will never be beaten, because we will ask for peace terms before we are offered them, so that we need never say 'we were beaten.'"[145]

By 16 April 1945 bombing by the American military had begun in earnest. One bomb dropped only 150 metres away and the blast threw several people out of their beds. Windows were smashed and numerous people had small cuts from the shards of glass. The Japanese authorities said, "Americans machine-gunned us because lights were seen in the Camp."[146] Realizing that her husband would often have to be outside during the air raids, Betty Gale made him a helmet out of their one and only tin wash basin.

As the air raids wore on, Betty Gale buoyed herself with the idea that the war was coming to an end. One can imagine that she was starting to picture herself again in peaceful times, reuniting with friends and family. The reality of what they had risked (and gained) by staying must have hit home again on 17 April 1945, when Betty Gale received word that Eric Liddell had died in Weixian Camp two months earlier, on 21 February. "Oh how frightful for Flo to get that news in Toronto, so far away from him, with their three little girls. I cannot bear thinking about it," Betty reflected. "He was so universally beloved and admired—and he and Flo had such a wonderful marriage."[147] The missionaries at Pudong camp were stunned. In her notebook Gale wrote, "Terribly shocked by the news of Eric's death—on Feb. 21—due to brain tumour and sudden haemorrhage. Find it hard to believe it [*sic*]. Florence constantly in our thoughts and prayers. It just seems too awful for her. Had a memorial service here on Good Friday, for him."[148] Florence Liddell would not receive word of her husband's death until after the Pudong memorial. It was not until 2 May 1945 that Rev. G.K. King and Rev. A.E. Armstrong of the United Church mission board would deliver the news to her in person, in Toronto.[149]

Towards the end of April rumours abounded. On the same day the internees heard that Germany had collapsed, the Japanese guards got very drunk, suggesting that perhaps the rumours were true. On 29 April one of the large American planes was struck with tracer bullets directly over Pudong Camp. Pushed two hundred yards beyond the camp, it caught on fire, lighting up the whole area before it crashed, the bomb it was carrying detonating as the plane hit the ground. "We are all terribly saddened and sick at heart," wrote Betty Gale, "as we think of all those young men on board dying in such a way."[150] The next day's paper announced that the Japanese were offering a CRB $1,000,000 award for any American airman found in or around Shanghai.

By May rumours about Hitler's death resumed in earnest, followed by rumours of the death of his Nazi leaders, and of Mussolini. With the European war seemingly over, the waiting and the tension at Pudong Camp seemed even worse—"almost unbearable at times."[151] At one point the internees were told they were going to be moved again, but it was not true.

After months of unrelenting bombing, Betty Gale was feeling the strain of internment. Just one month after receiving the news of Eric Liddell's death, she was watching her husband climb the stairs when she realized that he was seriously ill. "Today I see G. coming up the stairs slowly and painfully, on his way to visit a patient, pulling himself up by the banister," she wrote. Later, in a reflection likely penned after the war had ended, Gale wrote:

He is looking so pale and thin and tired, I cannot bear it, and want to do something violent. But what? And to whom? I find it so easy to understand now why there is so much fighting where there is poverty—for poverty breeds violence. Any wife will revert to the tactics of the cave-woman when she sees her husband hungry and over-burdened—and any mother will fight to protect her child if her well-being is threatened. We are finding out, in Camp, that the veneer of culture of our civilization is pretty thin.[152]

Undoubtedly Betty Gale's sensitivity to the possibility of Godfrey's injury or death in camp was heightened following Liddell's death. Still, given her later interest in the writings by internee William Sewell, it seems likely that her analysis of the situation as written in her journal was layered on afterwards. Her reflection suggests that seeing her husband ill triggered some powerful, unfamiliar, and uncomfortable emotions—ones that she would, as a Christian and a missionary, expect herself to control and not give into. Gale was, by this time, fiercely in love with her husband. In the intervening years since the couple had first met during her summer of light-heartedness and fun in 1939, they had experienced extraordinary hardship, but also great joy. In her notebook in May 1944, Betty Gale reflected on their relationship at Pudong:

Godfrey and I have had an exceptionally nice time together lately. He gets grander all the time. I can't remember or imagine what life was like before he came along. And the fact that he asked me to marry him must forever remain the 8th Wonder of the World. But praise be he did! And praise be I didn't go home in 1941 when I had the chance. We've gotten closer together these last two years than 10 other ones in normal life. This internment has been marvellous for me in some ways, and I am very very sure that God intended Margaret and me to stay here with Godf[rey].[153]

Undoubtedly the death of Eric Liddell and imagining what life was like for Florence now triggered Betty Gale's reflections on her own decision to stay in China. It would remain the defining moment of her life—a sign of her dedication to her husband, of her desire to have her daughter's father close by, and of her faith in the God of her missionary ancestors.

On 3 June 1945 there was a "terrific amount of noise and excitement" at Pudong, which was "literally crawling with [Japanese] troops, for horses, men and ammunition are pouring in." The men were busy digging trenches around the camp, which filled up almost immediately with water because of the high water table there. The Japanese, it seemed, were expecting an attack. Margie and Eli piled all the furniture into one room of their dollhouse because "today it's bomb-day."[154]

Air Raids: "The End of the World Has Come"

The end of the war was drawing near. Everyone could sense it. On 15 June 1945 the medical team at Pudong Camp received word that the two general hospitals in Shanghai were closing to the public so that they could be used by military troops. The tension was mounting around camp, and Betty Gale hoped that there would not be too many internees requiring hospital care. Godfrey Gale had graduated 120 men and women from the St. John Ambulance First Aid course, and "Sarge" had trained seven sets of stretcher squads, four rescue squads, and two demolition squads. The doctors had set up a blood donor service with sixty volunteers, first aid casualty stations, an emergency operating theatre, and casualty wards. The interpreters had told the Gales of accounts in the paper of the direct bomb hits on Stanley Camp in Hong Kong, and of American prisoners killed in camps during a raid on Japan, "so we are aware of the possibility of accidents."[155]

The 22nd of July brought "the heaviest air raid yet" and Betty Gale counted at least sixty planes over them at one time (the ban of watching through the windows having apparently been lifted).[156] Large numbers of bombs were dropped; the noise was "indescribable." Betty Gale and the others on her floor evacuated to the main floor and stayed in the centre, away from the windows. "F.S. Drake [who gave four lectures a week over a two-and-a-half-year period] is sitting studying at his small table with piles of books around him," Betty Gale wrote, "so completely absorbed that I honestly think he doesn't know there is an air raid going on."[157] Margie, too, was unperturbed, and sat drawing rabbits. Betty and Godfrey had made up a bag of Margie's special toys and kept it beside their emergency bag to grab when the air raid sirens went off.

Three days later Betty Gale again reported the worst raid yet. It was "absolutely terrifying," she wrote," a bomb explodes one hundred yards north of us, and all the glass in all the windows on that side of our building falls in—while shrapnel flies around like hail."[158] Amazingly no one was hit: Keith Graham stepped away from his chair a second before a large piece of shrapnel came through the window, went through the back of his chair, and smashed into the wall behind. While Godfrey Gale and Ken, Frances, and Eli McAll headed to the emergency stations, Betty Gale gathered Margie and sat together with her on a box in the hall. "Bomb after bomb crashes down," Betty wrote:

> The plaster falls and we are soon covered with layers of dust and plaster. Boxes and thermoses can be heard falling on the floor in the cubicles to the accompaniment of breaking glass. It really feels as though the end of the world has come, for us, at any rate. Everyone is quiet, white and tense, but no one cries. During all the turmoil Margie is sitting on my knee drawing pictures, and does not seem the least bit alarmed. Suddenly there is a crash to end all crashes, and we are again littered with debris from head to foot. Then there is a deep, deep silence, no one seems to be even breathing, and into this silence Margie's voice rings out unnaturally loud and clear, "Mummy, shall I colour this grass green, or blue?" Some of the ladies begin to cry, then.[159]

That raid left gaping holes in the walls of two rooms, made by machine-gun bullets from the planes diving on the anti-aircraft guns, and fragments from the shells came through the roof. Several people were cut, but none seriously; again this seemed miraculous to Betty Gale. At Stanley Camp in Hong Kong, the prisoners were not as fortunate: fifteen died in air raids there.

The next evening a group of internees sat together in the garden for a while. They reviewed the events of the past few years and how they had been affected by them. After talking for a long while the group came to the consensus that "we do not regret these years, or consider them wasted."[160] According to Betty Gale's journal, she asked her husband to sum up the discussion for her that evening, and he wrote the following:

> Life in [Pudong] has been a true democracy. We have mixed with all sorts and conditions of men, and have all been on an equal footing, lining up in the same queues, doing the same "fatigues" and so on. We have learned a tremendous lot about human nature, and not all of it was pleasant. We have learned that many of the trimmings of civilization are not essential for happiness, and so have got a new and truer sense of values, learning how to improvise to supply our needs, and how to enjoy the simpler things of life.
>
> We have learned the hard lesson of living at very close quarters with those not necessarily our chosen friends. In circumstances not always congenial, and where there has been no privacy, and no escape from each other. And in the give and take of this rabbit warren-type of existence, we have learned lessons of cooperation and patience and mutual appreciation which will help us all to build more soundly in the reconstruction years ahead.[161]

Although it is difficult to say for certain whether Godfrey Gale penned this reflection at the time or later, its message is consistent with the notes that Betty Gale later slipped into her camp notebook, written approximately ten years post-liberation, likely for a speech. Their greatest fear, Gale noted, was what would happen after the war ended. Would they be caught between the line of fire as the Allies advanced to take Shanghai? Would they be transported to Japan to face all kinds of unknown dangers? "Or," wrote Gale, "would we be lined up and shot to get us out of the way?"[162] Like her husband she concluded that she did not regret those years of internment because of the opportunity it provided to test one's character and perseverance, deepen self-understanding, and develop life-long friendships.[163] Interment was a difficult but invaluable opportunity to understand and live out the mission that God had placed in their lives—one that was as much (if not more) about personal transformation as it was about the transformation of others.

On 27 July 1945 the Japanese Commandant finally agreed to let the internees paint large white crosses on the roofs of the Pudong Camp building. The arms of the cross were eight feet wide. Another gigantic white cross was created on the playing field, using sheets nailed down with wooden pegs. Less than two weeks later, the American military dropped atomic bombs on the cities of Hiroshima and Nagasaki, triggering the surrender of the Japanese and the end of the war.

Liberation

On 6 August 1945 the Gales and McAlls heard, via hidden radio, that "an enormous bomb has been dropped by the Americans on the city of Hiroshima. It is called an 'atomic bomb' and they say it has wiped out the whole city, men, women and little children. My mind boggles at such an immensity of horror and wickedness," Betty Gale wrote.[164] On 9 August the internees heard that Russia had declared war on Japan. "Coming on top of word about the fiendish atomic bomb makes us feel that the Js must surely soon give in," Betty noted.[165] At 8:00 a.m. on 10 August 1945, a Russian walked by the camp and shouted out over and over as he went: "Peace has been declared! *Peace has been declared!!*"[166] The internees became wild with excitement, wondering if it really was true. All morning long Chinese streamed past the camp, talking and laughing and shouting over the fence, "The war is over!" Three young Chinese men gazed up at the Gales as they watched from their window. Grinning ear to ear they "point to the Japanese sentry at the gate and slowly, and with great relish, draw their hands across their throats."[167]

The next day a new rumour came via the hidden radio—that the American Navy would be in Shanghai within twenty-four hours. "We wonder what will happen when Japan capitulates," wrote Betty, "and under what circumstances we will walk through the gates to freedom. We hope there will not be a fight between our men and the guards, for some of them have openly boasted that they will break the neck of every J. they find when the war is over."[168] The Russian who had earlier rung his fire-bell to tell of good news, also told his friend in camp that when the war news was *extra* good, he would hang a towel out of his window as a sign. On 12 August "he hangs out not just a towel, but a huge white sheet!"[169]

The rumours continued, playing the internees emotions like a roller coaster. On 13 August they were told "there is no truth at all in any of the rumours" of Allied victory.[170] The internees were stunned into silence. Betty Gale found the quiet frightening after all the shouting and noise and confusion. Most of the internees laid on their beds, faces to the wall, too exhausted to do anything else. Godfrey Gale, however, took his wife aside and told her, in the strictest confidence, that news from the hidden radio confirmed that "IT IS TRUE; THE WAR *IS* OVER" and that the American fleet would arrive in a few days.[171] The McAlls knew too, but they could not breathe a word of it until it came out publicly.

Setting down Eli and Margie to play with their doll house, Betty Gale laid on her bed. She turned her face to the wall, covered it with a pillow, and cried, and cried, and cried. Suddenly the room was quiet and Betty looked to see Margie and Eli standing beside her "with the greatest concern and anxiety written on each little face."[172] Reassuring them that she was not sick, but happy, Betty took both girls downstairs to the nursery to give the babies their morning bath.

The tensions were mounting. On 14 August Betty wrote, "The J. military seem very [keen] on keeping the Chinese away from us. This a.m. the Chinese men came to take away the garbage as usual and a Jap[anese] plain-clothes man walked in with them—carrying a paper parcel. He opened the parcel, took out a revolver and kept it pointing at the head of the head Chinese [labourer] all the time he was working."[173] The Japanese did not want the Chinese to bring any news to the internees; there was fear that the internees might rush the gate.

Finally, on 15 August 1945, the British, American, and Dutch Representatives were called to the Swiss Consul in Shanghai to receive an important message, "as a crisis was imminent."[174] The internees were, as Betty Gale put it, "all agog!" Rumours began to circulate during their three-hour absence: "(1) J's in S'hai were not giving in; (2) We were to be handed over to the military; (3) Civil war in Japan; (4) The war is still on; (5) The Empire was kicked out, etc., etc."[175] The three men returned at 2:00 p.m. with the news: the war was over. The unbelievable had happened; Japan had surrendered.

Immediately the internees began singing the British, American, and Dutch anthems, and as each was sung the corresponding flag was unfurled. "It is an emotion-packed hour," wrote Betty Gale, "as everyone weeps un-ashamedly and goes altogether 'crazy.'"[176] They awoke the next morning to find that all of the Japanese guards had gone. The internees organized an impromptu "Thanksgiving Service" and sang "with all our hearts that grand old hymn, *Praise God from whom all blessings flow.*"[177] Godfrey and Betty took Margaret to the empty Japanese sentry box to play. It was "terribly exciting," wrote Betty. But also, oddly, sad. Betty was "heartsick" when she saw the Japanese soldiers after receiving the news. Ever compassionate, she wrote: "they look so sad, pale and *small.*"[178]

For the next three days thousands of people came over from Shanghai to see the "inmates of Pudong." An American plane circled several times around the camp on 19 August, while internees rushed from window to window to watch, many screaming hysterically. Pamphlets came floating down and on them the internees read the words: "Japan signed the Peace Terms today."[179] Seven American aviators came into the camp to bring medicine, food, and encouragement. They had not been given permission to land, so did so at great personal risk. Friends of the Gales in Shanghai also came to visit. "It is wonderful to see them, absolutely wonderful," Betty Gale wrote, "but we are so tired."[180]

For years we have longed for the war to end, and thought how we would celebrate, and how carefree and happy and young we would be. And now it has ended, but almost every joyful emotion we had expected to feel is swallowed up by this terrible state of exhaustion. We are happy, yes, but not carefree, and definitely not young. I feel very, very old. We have only one wish in the world, at this moment, and that is to escape from all noise, and crowds of people, even those whom we love, and find a quiet corner where we can sleep, and sleep, and sleep.[181]

Godfrey Gale, who was on the verge of collapse, was hospitalized with amoebic dysentery.

On 30 August British and American ships came into Shanghai and the streets were white with sailors. Two days later, after tearful farewells, Betty, Godfrey, and Margie Gale left Pudong Camp with Ken, Frances, and Eli McAll. The children were excited and ran ahead of their parents down the steps towards the wide open gates. "We expect them to run right through," Betty Gale wrote, "but force of habit is too strong, and they stop dead in their tracks right on the threshold."[182] The girls looked at each other, then back at their parents who reassured them, "it's alright darlings; you can go out now." Hand in hand, and with a shout of joy, Eli and Margie ran through the gate.

For the next six weeks the Gales and the McAlls stayed in Shanghai reorientating themselves and making plans to leave. At first Godfrey wanted to return to Qilu—at his own expense if necessary. But uncertain conditions made it impossible to consider that possibility yet. The McAlls were invited to stay in an American mission compound run by an ex-internee. The Gale family, on the other hand, moved into a room in a former brothel in Shanghai. The rooms had been converted to Japanese-style. "Marvellous to be able to shut the door," wrote Betty.[183] Godfrey and the male internees continued to work at Pudong Camp. Although it is not clear what they were doing, it allowed them to "claim parcels from Parachutes and other things like milk and eggs."[184] On Thursday 28 September the Gales received the news that they were booked to leave the following morning on the *HMS Glenearn* to return to England. Betty Gale's last entry in her China Notebook was from aboard the *Glenearn* on 2 November 1945. "Busy since sailing trying to get our winter clothes ready for wearing when we leave Gibralter," she noted.

The Gales and the McAlls arrived in London together, on 9 November 1945. While the McAlls settled in to await the arrival of their second child, Godfrey Gale began studying for his Fellowship of the Royal College of Surgeons qualifications at the University of Edinburgh. Britain was recovering from war and, although Godfrey had family in England, their means and accommodation were limited. Betty Gale, now pregnant with their son Kendall, decided to return to Canada in April 1946 to stay with her family in Toronto until Godfrey could join them five months later. In July, on the morning of the day Godfrey was writing his final exam, he was diagnosed with tuberculosis and admitted to hospital. When he did finally sail for Canada in the spring of 1947, he went directly to the Toronto Sanitorium to continue his treatments. He was not well enough to go back to work until after their third child, Patricia, was born in 1950—and then only part time. Eventually Godfrey Gale took a full time position at the same hospital where he had been a patient in Toronto, now called the West Park Healthcare Centre. By then the door to China had closed. Gale remained at West Park throughout his career, retiring as the Chief of Medical Staff.[185] Their marriage lasted forty-six years. Godfrey Gale died of cancer on 3 April 1986 at the age of 73. Betty Gale died on 17 June 1995 of congestive heart failure just days shy of her eighty-fourth birthday.

Summary

Pudong Camp was by far the most difficult of the four sites in which the Gales were interned between 8 December 1941 and 1 September 1945. Not only were the facilities more sparse, filthy, and cold, the internee population was more crude, aggressive, and at times violent. Glimpses of interpersonal tension between the McAlls and the Gales is undoubtedly reflective of relational conflicts around camp: chronic fear, hunger, and boredom, coupled with living in close quarters, and compounded by the increasing frequency of air raids would have placed extraordinary stress on interpersonal relationships. The risks were greater, too. The Huangpu River that separated the camp from Shanghai had a strong current; the trips that Godfrey Gale took when accompanying patients to Shanghai hospitals by sampan would have meant certain death were he to have fallen overboard. In addition to the usual concerns about food and shelter, the Gales and the McAlls—and Ken McAll in particular—had to find ways to deal with a corrupt internee police unit that ran the Camp with bribes and threats. Most significantly, Pudong Camp was close to Japanese military instalments and was therefore vulnerable to the incessant and increasingly vicious air raids through the last year of the war.

Unlike the earlier chapters in this book, this chapter draws almost exclusively from first person sources—particularly Betty Gale's journal, diary, and notebook, Ken and Frances McAlls' published memoirs, and interviews with Pudong ex-internees Betty Gale, Frances and Ken McAll, and three LMS missionaries—Annie Taylor, Ginger Anderson, and Jean Gillison—in

1991. There is good reason for this: prior to Pudong, there were multiple forms of communication that shed light on different aspects of Betty Gale's life and the period in which she was living. Not so in Pudong: the prisoners were quite effectively shut off from the rest of the world. What is striking about Betty Gale's diary from Pudong Camp is that she ceased to write as "I" any more, using instead the pronoun "we." It is not always clear who that "we" is—Betty and Godfrey? Betty and Frances? The Gales and the McAlls? The missionaries? It is significant, though, because it indicates Betty Gale's complete absorption into communal life. She rarely separated out her own thoughts and experiences from those of the other internees. Pudong Camp had no privacy. There was barely private space for a married couple, let alone one person needing some solitude. Perhaps F.A. Drake managed to tune out the rest of the camp as he absorbed himself so much into his studies that he did not even hear the bombing. But he was surely the exception.

But there is something else that is striking due to its contrast with Betty Gale's earlier writing and, in particular, the letters she wrote prior to internment at Pudong Camp: the absence of Godfrey. The demands of his job as camp physician kept Godfrey Gale incessantly occupied—holding four to five clinics each day, doing his share of rounds on the eight-bed hospital/sick bay on the main floor of the building, taking turns accompanying ill patients across the Huangpu River to Shanghai, training 120 internees in first aid, and being involved in medical meetings. He also donated blood. When Betty saw Godfrey, pale and weak, struggling up the staircase to visit a patient less than a month after she received the news of Eric Liddell's death at Weixian Camp, it is little wonder she felt a surge of anger—at the Japanese, at the injustice of the situation, at those who demanded Godfrey's time, and even Godfrey himself: after all they had endured, Godfrey Gale was being worked to death.

Today Margaret Gale's overriding memory of her camp childhood sixty years ago is of her parents' love. Margaret felt—and feels—that hers was a *privileged* childhood. She received the unconditional love and undivided attention of her parents—not to mention an entire camp that adored her and Eli enough to consider them the camp mascots, the Centre Cinderellas. To her mother, Margie was a source of innocent happiness that brought inestimable joy and a semblance of normalcy to the "rabbit-warren" life in Pudong Camp. Betty Gale later credited Margaret with their very survival in camp: she was their "thread of gold" who kept them grounded, distracted, and determined to face their indeterminate days as internees with a sense of purpose, to craft a strong childhood experience out of the misery they were living in.

Perhaps most telling are the dozens of letters Margaret Gale (now Wightman) collected for the occasion of her parents' fortieth wedding anniversary in 1980. Most were written by fellow internees, each of whom had been asked to recall a memorable anecdote about Betty and Godfrey Gale. They remembered with humour the long days of internment, the rats, the rain, the lack of privacy, and the roll calls. One remembered with pride the first aid certificate he had earned under Godfrey's tutelage.[186] Only a few wrote about the more horrific times—the bombings, for example—although some remembered their own moments of private agony that Godfrey or Betty managed to soothe. Florence (Liddell) Hall's letter is particularly moving. With a shaky hand she wrote: "Then a few brief months in the Spring of '39 when the clouds of war and possible separation from our husbands hung heavy on our hearts. Then after you finally came home in 1946—Godfrey was in hospital and Eric had died."[187] Although these women had chosen very different paths—Florence by returning to Canada, Betty by staying in China—each had suffered much.

After the war Betty Gale and Florence Liddell, each aged thirty-five, drew on the strength of their China childhood to come to terms with the trauma of their China adulthood. Betty no longer kept a diary; perhaps she no longer needed to. "Our friendship," Florence professed forty years later, "was a sustaining force."[188] Their friendship helped them make sense of the defining moment of their lives—when one chose to stay and one to quit China—and its aftermath. It also helped Betty Gale to reset her compass for a future in which only one thing was certain: once she was safely back on Canadian soil, neither she nor the other mishkid nurses could return to the land of their birth; the era of mishkid nursing had ended.

Internment and the Reshaping of a Canadian Missionary Community

At the beginning we had thought that internment was going to be good for us all. We should learn through suffering and living together a better way of life. Now we saw that while some of the best among us had been made better, many were not refined but degraded, the thin cover of culture having fallen away. Internment had gone on too long.

—William Sewell, Stanley Camp internee, in Austin, *Saving China*

There were 300,000 Allied nationals in Japanese hands during the war.[1] Japan held 13,544 civilian men, women, and children as captives in China and Hong Kong, including 311 Canadians, ten of whom were missionaries.[2] Of the 189 Canadians who remained in internment after the 1943 repatriation, only six were missionaries—all of them women. Five had been North China missionaries; four were nurses; three were missionary kids—Betty Thomson Gale, Mary Boyd Stanley, and Georgina Menzies Lewis.[3] Hamish Ion has argued that, although the numbers are relatively small, the significance of the Canadian experience in Japanese camps lies not in its scale, but in what can be garnered from it about broader issues.[4] As a social history, the internment of mishkid nurses was not a discrete event, but rather an extension of the history of the United Church of Canada North China missionary community. Wartime reshaped this community from a fairly remote and insular group in the 1910s to a diaspora of relocated missionaries by the 1930s. While the dispersed missionaries kept in contact with each other through letters and visits, internment served to drive a wedge between them, cutting them off from the larger Canadian missionary community. Internment forced internees to mix with disparate communities of imprisoned strangers. However valiantly the missionaries adjusted to their changing circumstances in the early twentieth century, they did not—they could not—keep pace with concurrent political changes in China. By the time Betty Gale and the others emerged from internment, China and the missionaries had disengaged from each other.

Japanese internment was the final chapter in the history of mishkid nursing in China. Less a story of the unravelling of the global missionary movement than of the resilience of individuals within it, the history of mishkid nurses before and during Japanese internment reveals something of the sustaining nature of missionary communities. It was their missionary childhood that set the stage for mishkid nurses' later, unreasonable faith in God, his mission, and their place in it. Here I use the term "unreasonable" not with disapproval, but with thoughtful observation—for within the context of deteriorating wartime conditions and diminishing financial and moral support from the church at home, the decisions of missionaries to go to, and remain in, Japanese-occupied China were not reasonable by most Canadian standards. However, within the social context of a missionary community that viewed China as a place of intersecting humanitarian and spiritual transformation, such faith in God and such decisions *were* a reasonable response, despite the uncertainty and danger that accompanied them.

Road to Internment

The Canadian missionary community in China was well-established by the time China-born missionary kids returned to assist with the medical side of the missionary enterprise. Their parents were committed to China: on average, mishkids' fathers and mothers worked with the North China Mission for forty years.[5] The first mishkid (Jean Menzies) was born in China in 1896. Her return to China in 1923 after studying nursing in Toronto coincided with a shift in mission emphasis from spiritual to physical ministrations. Whereas preaching the gospel and nurturing the spiritual development of Chinese Christians had been a priority for the North China Mission in its first thirty-five years, now Canadians were turning their attention to care of the sick as an expression of the Christian gospel. Like many other mission organizations across China, they were taking up the challenge to develop modern hospitals and medical and nurses training schools that were rooted in a Christian ethos of care. After a generation of laying the groundwork by building relationships and infrastructure, the Canadian missionary community was poised to impact their corner of China's health care landscape. In the meantime, however, public opinion of missions had taken a downward turn as Canadians started to question the value (and expense) of the missionary enterprise.

In the 1930s China missions were under critical scrutiny at home. The Depression made it difficult for donors in Canada to justify the cost of building new hospitals and paying for the related equipment and supplies. Furthermore, leading mission organizations in the United States and Canada were calling for missions to reinvent themselves if they were to be "adequate to the demands of the hour."[6] A 1932 *Time* magazine report of the release of *Re-Thinking Missions*, the contentious multi-denominational appraisal of Protestant work in Eastern Asia, emphasized that church members at home were concerned that missions were becoming obsolete. Initiated by John D. Rockefeller and a group of Baptist businessmen, the appraisal committee "knew that gifts to missions had fallen off alarmingly," reported *Time*; "People no longer thought missionizing the best way, as they thought 30 years ago to spend their charity-money. Most people did not know or care much about conditions in foreign mission fields."[7] *Re-Thinking Missions* recommended that missions become less concerned with evangelism and preaching, and more concerned with working cooperatively with other denominations, agencies, and religions to make an impact in Eastern Asia.

The United Church of Canada responded to critiques in *Re-Thinking Missions* by re-emphasizing the value of evangelism, even while pointing out its own efforts to align more closely to what was going on elsewhere in China, namely, an increased emphasis on preventive health, education, and medical service. Under increasing pressure from the broader missionary community to modernize their health care services in Henan, the United Church was also dealing with a lack of denominational support for doing so. Key to their success was the recruitment of missionary nurses to train a new generation of Chinese nurses. As it turned out, the outbreak of war in China in 1937 interrupted the shaky vision to modernize health services in Henan. It also introduced a new recruitment message for prospective missionaries: China at war was desperate for nurses. Yet mishkids were the only ones to respond.

It cannot be overstated that being the children of missionaries influenced mishkid nurses' most salient life decisions, including becoming missionary nurses, wives, and mothers. Over time their missionary identities became more established: they were Christian women in China for a God-ordained purpose. Over the course of her years as a missionary nurse in wartime China, Betty Gale made sense of her experiences through the view that even pain or struggle could ultimately serve a higher good. Thus, while her 1941 decision to stay in China brought new trauma into her life, Gale chose to view internment as ultimately beneficial; it allowed her (and Godfrey) to provide practical support to family, friends, and patients, and it contributed to her personal spiritual formation and character development. Gale constructed a view of internment as a place where she could best enact the missionary impulse that brought her to China in the first place.

The Incongruence of Camp as a "Happy Place"

Betty Gale, Georgina Lewis, and Mary Stanley spent most of their internment years in separate camps. Most of what we can glean about missionary internees' social lives comes to us through the writings of Betty Gale. There are some surprises. For example, there are unexpected vestiges of privilege, at least in the early years. Life at Qilu, even under house arrest, included personal cooks, amahs, and gardeners, and the Columbia Country Club had a swimming pool and bowling alley, however defunct. Gale's early descriptions of games, sports, music, and drama are not very different than what she described as part of her missionary experience before imprisonment. Perhaps most surprising is Margaret Gale's early assumption that her childhood in a "camp" meant she had lived at an idyllic "summer camp" rather than a prison camp. Her recollection of a content childhood contrasts sharply with versions of Japanese prison camps described in popular books like Ballard's *Empire of the Sun*, Power's *Little Foreign Devil*, and Boulle's *The Bridge over the River Kwai*—that is, as cruel settings filled with sadness and sadism.[8] Tens of thousands died in POW and internment camps throughout the Japanese Empire and occupied territories.[9] Why, then, this incongruence between what one might expect to read about internment, and Betty Gale's narrative?

One explanation relates to the different purposes of wartime camps. Japanese and German prison camps were roughly differentiated into "concentration camps" for criminals and dissidents, "prisoner of war camps" for captured enemy soldiers, and "civilian internment camps" for foreigners living in a country that was at war with their homeland. In addition, Germany had "extermination camps" to support their policy of genocide. Medical historian Charles Roland has noted that prisoners in civilian internment camps in Hong Kong and Japan were no less incarcerated than in other camps but that in general the Japanese treated internees "somewhat less badly" than they did the POWs.[10] Still, Hamish Ion has argued that wartime bureaucracy contributed to the deaths of thousands of prisoners.[11] This might explain why the "mere" neglect of the Gales' earlier years in Qilu and the CCC devolved into lethal negligence by the time they reached Yangzhou, and especially Pudong Camp.

The second explanation for Betty Gale's unexpectedly optimistic renderings of her experiences in China is that she used a redemptive narrative framework to interpret her life. Gale's acceptance of the biblical story supported her belief in a grand narrative of history in which everything, even the most disastrous catastrophes, would ultimately make sense—if not now, then at some point of illumination in the future.[12] Whether she was writing letters or diary entries during the war years or answering questions in a recorded interview almost fifty years later, Gale was consistent in her message: she did not regret her time spent at camp. According to all those interviewed, she never wavered from her assertion that internment was ultimately a valuable experience. It served a higher purpose: living in such close proximity as a family was good for her marriage and for Margie's social development; internees required sound medical care and Godfrey was uniquely qualified to provide it; Margie's innocent playfulness acted as ballast for her parents; Margie was the object of affection for childless parents, aunts, and uncles.

The moral messages underpinning Betty Gale's internment narrative are consistent with the Christian message she was taught: having surrendered her life in service to God, her life became an instrument for God. Her life was for God to use for his purposes, his grand design. Her story, however it unfolded, was part of a larger biblical narrative within which God was bringing his children ever closer to himself over the course of history. Suffering was an avenue through which one could grow closer to others and, ultimately, to God. Gale described her internment experience as transforming her perspective on the world—particularly her place in it as a privileged person. No longer viewing poverty, for example, as something belonging to others (the less privileged, the foreign, the sick), Betty Gale, through internment, came to see herself as more aligned with—and having more in common with—those outside of her missionary community. That is, while Canadian missionaries had made it their mandate to care for those who were poor, ill, hungry, and displaced, prior to internment their privileged position as Westerners meant that they could retreat from the disadvantaged communities they came to serve. Caring for the sick during the day, missionaries could withdraw to a socially rich expatriate community in the evenings and on weekends and holidays. In the internment camps, however, there was no longer a clear class, racial, or cultural distinction between caregivers and care receivers. Regardless of background, internees were, for the most part, equally impoverished, hungry, and at risk with regard to illness and injury. Evacuation, retreat, or even respite from the suffering masses was not an option.

In 1943 Betty Gale wrote of her determination to accept Pudong Camp as if it were their permanent home, to do what they could to make it a "happy place" for the children. This set into motion a socially constructed version of her life in which camp-as-prison was replaced by camp-as-home. In February 1945 Gale started to write a letter to her mother from Pudong Camp (never sent) in which she reflected once more on the question of whether she had made the right decision by staying in China. She wondered if her mother had been "a bit hurt" that she had seemed so keen to stay behind when she "had a ticket and an open way to No. 33 four years ago."[13] Yet now that it was clear that Godfrey would have faced long years of imprisonment alone, Betty believed she would have regretted leaving. She wrote: "Godfrey and I are closer to each other now than we could have been at the end of 10 years of ordinary living in peace times."[14] While Gale missed her family in Toronto, she was "as sure as I ever was of anything that God intended me to have these years here, learning how to live with other people (some most amazingly uncongenial—awful!!) and to learn to depend on Him for strength to meet the demands of others, criticisms, lack of privacy etc. of each new day."[15] With regard to Margie's role in Pudong Camp, Gale wrote, "I can hardly keep from weeping when I see the looks on the faces of a lot of these men, whose babies are far away. You know they aren't really seeing our kids at all, but trying to picture what their own must be like, after all these years."[16] Internment, however difficult, had some redeeming qualities.

A Redemptive Narrative

A helpful framework for understanding the expressed experience of internees is one known as a "redemptive narrative." In their respective studies of Japanese Canadians who were interned in camps in Canada between 1941 and 1945, Mona Oikawa and Pamela Sugiman found that their subjects used redemptive narratives to make sense of their experiences. These *Nisei* (second-generation) Japanese Canadians often referred to their internment experience as a "blessing in disguise," suggesting that they actually benefitted from their exclusion and incarceration during the 1940s.[17] In her interviews with seventy-five *Nisei* women and men, Pamela Sugiman heard moving descriptions of suffering and injustice; vivid memories of forced relocation, restricted mobility, registration, and curfews; the loss of privacy, ticks, bedbugs, and separation of family[18]—descriptions that sound hauntingly familiar to the story told by Betty Gale. Moments later in the same interviews, Sugiman noted that these same people recounted happy stories and even suggested that internment offered Japanese Canadians acceptance into the dominant society, the promise of upward economic mobility, movement from one part of the country to another, and a better life for subsequent generations. Stories of triumph were shared alongside recollections of suffering. In spite of the hardship and injustices of the internment camps in Canada, the message delivered by these internees was: life is sweet.

While the details of Betty Gale's internment story differ in many respects from the *Nisei*, the moral message is similar: internment was a blessing in disguise. Betty and Godfrey Gale agreed on this point. Godfrey reflected: "We gained something that could not have come otherwise. We learned how many things we can get along without." Furthermore, "we learned to what heights of achievement humble people can rise, and we learned to know and understand what it means to be poor."[19] Or, as Betty put it: "We were shown by the lives of ordinary men and women the possibility of triumph over adverse circumstances."[20]

Sugiman questioned the blessing-in-disguise metaphor used by her interviewees. She argued that it was less a reflection of forgiving and forgetting than an attempt to bridge the past with the present in a way that conveys recovery and survival rather than victimization and defeat.[21] Using the notion of composure introduced by Alistair Thomson, Sugiman suggested that the internee narrators "composed" or constructed their memories using the public language and meanings of their culture.[22] They also composed memories which helped them to feel comfortable with their lives, giving them a feeling of self-control—or "composure." Memories of experiences "which are still painful or 'unsafe' because they do not easily accord with our present identity or because their inherent traumas or tensions have never been resolved" are remade or repressed.[23]

Betty Gale's narration of her life through her letters, diary, and recollections certainly resists victimization and defeat. So do the recollections of other missionaries and mishkids described here. Gale came to terms with the injustice of having their berths stolen on the repatriation ship *"Wangle" Maru* in the summer of 1942 by considering the advantages to other prisoners of having the services of a physician and nurse. She came to terms with the injustice perpetrated by a Japanese shopkeeper who refused to allow her to exchange clothes for Margie by telling herself that there was too much fighting in the world already without adding her anger to it. She explained the rude and discriminatory actions of the Shanghailanders as a natural outcome of their sudden fall from wealth and privilege. And she felt compassion for the departing sad, pale, and small Japanese guards from Pudong Camp after Japan's defeat was announced. Empathy, then, became a strategy for survival, as well as an extension of the Christian ethos. By the time she arrived at Pudong, Gale had learned to consciously look for ways to relate to, and ideally to feel sorry for, those whom she feared—including Japanese guards, whom she decided were lonely and missing their families, just like her.

One important difference between the study of Betty Gale and those of the *Nisei* is the timing of the reflections. Whereas the recollections of the *Nisei* were attempts to come to terms with the past, the chronicles of Betty Gale were attempts to come to terms with both the present and an uncertain future. In this sense Gale's redemptive narrative was both retrospective (journal, recollections) *and* prospective (letters, diary, notebook). From the time Gale made her initial decision to return to China at the behest of Bob McClure in 1938, she composed and then lived out a narrative that anticipated both suffering and survival. If her life before Pearl Harbor was spent preparing for unknown disasters, her life afterwards was spent coming to terms with the meaning of those disasters.

A redemptive narrative served Betty Gale well. Her construction of camp as a place to find meaning fits with psychiatrist Viktor Frankl's theory that the search for meaning is a primary motivation in life.[24] Frankl came to this theory—and a related revolutionary approach to psychotherapy—during and through his experiences as a prisoner in a Nazi extermination camp. "There is nothing in the world," Frankl ventured, "that would so effectively help one to survive even the worst conditions as the knowledge that there is a meaning in one's life."[25] Finding meaning, to Frankl, is not a retrospective or even an introspective exercise, but rather a future-oriented one. In his view prisoners of war who were able to focus on the meanings to be fulfilled by them in the future were more likely to survive. The search for meaning in one's life, Frankl asserted, is built on the belief that the meaning itself is "unique and specific" in that it must and can be fulfilled only by the person searching for it. Mental health, in his view, requires a certain degree of tension—between what one has already achieved and what one still ought to accomplish, or the gap between what one has already achieved and what one ought to achieve. Survival does not require the removal of all tensions but the call of a potential meaning waiting to be fulfilled.

In China, each of the interned missionaries had to come to terms with their internment in their own way. While Betty Gale and some of the others found meaning in and through her experiences, American missionary Dr. Hattie Love Rankin did not. A 1911 graduate of Woman's Medical College of Pennsylvania, Dr. Rankin joined the Methodist Church's missionary program in 1913. She served in Suzhou and "Changchos" (Changzhou?) and supervised the Margaret Williamson Hospital in Shanghai. After her marriage to a medical missionary with the Fundamentalist Mission, she established a clinic in "Chenju" (Chengdu?) and later, a hospital in Shanghai.[26] Dr. Rankin described her difficulties in learning the Chinese language and customs and combatting "ignorance and malpractice" in Shanghai. In her memoirs, entitled *I Saw It Happen to China, 1913–1949*, Rankin detailed her "harrowing stay" as an internee in Chapei Camp.[27] After the war she remained in China until the Communist victory in 1949. By then she was completely dispirited. Shortly before fleeing China, she wrote: "Today I am sixty-five years old, just a plain, old, good-for-nothing, kau-feh-zu (unreliable), worn out missionary."[28] Dr. Rankin had lost her sense of purpose; it is not difficult to imagine that there were other ex-internees who felt the same way—even if they were not so candid.

In her study of interned Japanese Canadians, Pamela Sugiman noted that some of the women and men who shared their stories moved from descriptions of misfortunes to "blessings" in an attempt to bring coherence to their life stories, to help the past meet the present, and to tell their audience that they are more than their wartime experiences—"however profound the past has been and however strong it may live in memory."[29] Like the *Nisei* internees, Betty Gale worked at bringing the empirical content of her narrative in line with the moral message that defined her life story. She and Mary and Dorothy Boyd—if not the others—returned to China in 1939 believing they had a purpose to fulfill. Surviving trying experiences with their faith and sense of integrity intact was a way for them to fulfill the legacy started by their families a generation earlier. While their parents' presence and privilege in China was made possible through the politics of the imperial power of Britain, their incarceration was a consequence of the politics of the imperial power of Japan. Their calling, however, was the same: if their life in China was to be an expression of their faith in God and the biblical narrative, they would have to find ways to exemplify the most salient of Christian values—that is, to love their (Chinese) neighbours as themselves. In internment, however, their neighbours were no longer Chinese.

Within a redemptive narrative, the mishkid nurses responded to the unfolding events around them in four ways: (1) by gazing through mishkid eyes, (2) by resisting separation, (3) by acting appropriately, and (4) by continuing the legacy. While these themes emerge most clearly during the internment years as described by Betty Gale, they are rooted in the mishkid nurses' early China lives. They provide clues about how mishkid nurses came to terms with internment. Although Betty Gale, Mary Stanley, and Georgina Lewis survived camp, even emerging as "better" persons, they did not return to missionary work after liberation. They would thereafter be *former* missionaries. They had fulfilled their mission.

Gazing through Mishkid Eyes

While the mishkid nurses' view of China carried some of the characteristics of Said's Orientalist gaze or point of view,[30] being China-born tempered their representations of the Chinese as the cultural "other." On the one hand, their China childhood reinforced a sense that, as Canadian subjects allied with Britain, they could expect a certain level of privilege and security. Their relative wealth and education granted them a lifestyle unattainable by their Chinese nursing students and staff, never mind their amahs, cooks, and house servants. On the other hand, living and working alongside Chinese colleagues—most of them female, Christian nurses—instilled a sense of solidarity that minimized cultural differences. Ethnic difference was trumped by a degree of religious and professional similarity. That the Canadian missionary community in North China perceived itself as allied with the Chinese against the Japanese occupiers also gave them more common ground. Being acculturated in China shaped the mishkid nurses' view of the Chinese—at least Chinese Christians—as belonging to the same social community and sharing a common purpose, even if this view was not reciprocated by the Chinese. Indeed, in the case of Betty Gale's work as a missionary nurse, her greatest crises and resolutions with cultural "others" were not with the Chinese at all, but with the Westerners she was later interned with. These included the Shanghailanders, labourers, and petty criminals with whom she had little in common, and whom she did not trust. Thus, even more striking than an Orientalist gaze that positioned the Chinese as "other" was Gale's deep struggle with the "otherness" of fellow Westerners, particularly those who viewed missionaries with both suspicion and contempt.

Seen through a mishkid gaze, China could be a threatening place. Foreigners who lived there simply had to come to terms with the danger. Mishkids learned how to carve out a space of security, a place of calm in the centre of various storms within which they carried on the normal activities of life. During their upbringing this sometimes meant being evacuated out of Henan to safer regions of China. At other times it meant simply being expected to adjust to threats, such as when young Ruth Lochead was required to eat a sandwich while she and her father crouched in relative safety in an open grave as warlords opened fire nearby in the 1920s. By the time Betty Gale, Dorothy Boyd, and Mary Boyd returned to China they had learned to feel comfortable and enjoy life within safe regions (Beijing, Beidaihe, Jinan) while Henan was under military attack. Before Pearl Harbor, Betty Gale seemed to readily accept the incongruence between her desire to help the poor and disenfranchised, even under the imminent threat of war, and the privileges afforded Westerners living in China. The university campus at Qilu was an island of refuge from the realities of life experienced by most Chinese in the region. After she was placed under house arrest, Gale sought opportunities to continue social events, the scarcity of supplies adding to the challenge and reward of events like birthdays and Christmas. As internment progressed it became increasingly difficult, and important, to find opportunities to share laughter and fun; these activities kept fears at bay.

It was during the air raids at Pudong—the worst moments of internment—that Betty Gale's mishkid childhood came full circle. Margie's innocent voice ringing through the post-raid silence asking Betty what colour she should make the grass exemplified the need for (and ability to create) normalcy. Just as North China mishkids had done a generation earlier, Margie and Eli found their own fun. That is not to say that the children did not feel threatened, but rather that their parents were successful in creating a sense of security, and saw it as their responsibility to do so. Eli's careful gaze at Frances McAll's face during a Pudong air raid was to gauge the seriousness of the attacks in 1945. Eli and Margie's gazing at Betty Gale's tearstained face after the news of Allied victory was to gauge whether they should be frightened or happy. The mishkid gaze, then, involved discerning threats on the countenance of those in authority.

In her study of civilian internment, Bernice Archer has noted that children of internees frequently abdicated their anxiety onto their parents.[31] In fact, those who were used to a "pampered, pearl egg-spoon" existence in colonial ports enjoyed a new-found freedom and independence at camp. While their parents ran the camps and worried about their children's health and safety, the children felt a strong sense of security. Kids let their parents do the worrying for them. "The grown-ups," one Stanley Camp internee recalled, "were quite removed, they were sort of busy trying to survive. They had a lot of problems," she continued, "We didn't."[32] Margie Gale's childhood ability to entrust her anxieties to the adults in her life reflected Betty Gale's and other mishkids' own upbringing in China. As Margie searched her mother's face for signs of fear or threat, Betty responded as her parents had done a generation earlier: she rearranged her expression to convey a level of serenity she did not feel.

Resisting Separation

Although her mishkid upbringing was the impetus for her return to China in 1939, Betty Gale resisted some of the unquestioned practices of missionary life, particularly that of familial separation. Her singular refusal to be separated from her husband led to her crucial decision to stay in China against consular advice in 1941. Betty came to terms with the possibility of internment by determining that she would rather face imprisonment with Godfrey than isolation without him. It was a risky decision with far-reaching implications. For the next four and a half years, Betty drew on the values instilled during her missionary upbringing and nurse's training to adapt to an increasingly deprived existence in a series of internment camps.

As Betty Gale moved from house arrest at Qilu to displacement at the Columbia Country Club to imprisonment at Yangzhou Camp B and Pudong Camp, there were fewer physical resources, but also fewer social ones: for the first time in her life Gale was living as a cultural outsider, removed from the familiarity of the China missionary community within which she had always lived, whether in China or Canada. Housed together with hundreds of other expatriates representing diverse nationalities, ethnicities, religious beliefs, occupations, levels of wealth, education, and social status, Gale had to learn to adapt to ever-changing demands and resources. She emerged, emaciated and depleted, from the most demanding of the camps in September 1945. Her daughter had rickets and related scoliosis; her husband, advanced tuberculosis. And yet thereafter Betty Gale would insist that it was worth it. Compared to the fate of her friend Florence Liddell, it probably was. But it took a toll.

It is unlikely that we will ever know the extent to which Betty Gale and Florence Liddell discussed the painful outcomes of their 1941 decisions about staying in China. Florence chose separation and security. She and her children were spared the neglect and suffering of the camps, but they lost four years of being with Eric while he still lived. Betty and her family survived, but they paid an emotional, physical, and economic price for their decision. Both women, it seemed, found solidarity in their suffering, however, and perceived suffering as a necessary part of spiritual and personal growth. This view of suffering reinforced—and was reinforced by—the views of the missionary community in which they were reared.

Acting Appropriately

Betty Gale's response to the Japanese occupation of China was shaped by expectations surrounding perceptions of gender roles, religion, ethnicity, and class. The dignified behaviour that characterized her China life was more than a personality trait; it was a means for survival. Bernice Archer argues that, beyond the obvious needs for food, shelter, and health care in civilian internment camps, the most important Western social and cultural traditions that assisted survival were the maintenance of "civilized" and "dignified" patterns of behaviour.[33]

Both before and during internment, Betty Gale's kind and gentle demeanour belied an underlying tenacity and shrewdness. For example, when considering ways to help two Chinese students resolve their differences, Gale invited them into her home for tea. She intentionally laid out Christian literature on the table to draw them into a conversation about the need for Christian unity. With Japanese guards at Qilu, she strategized about the best way to win their favour and thus increase her independence while shopping. And, by placing flowers in the entrance to her Qilu home to welcome the Japanese soldier's wife she imagined would be living there, Gale demonstrated one of her deepest convictions: even enemies could be won over by kindness and generosity.

Although Betty Gale had been working as a nurse after Margie was born at Qilu, after internment she did not seek many formal opportunities to provide nursing care. While one may argue that missionaries held conservative or traditional views on married women working, or that the absence of childcare in internment made working impossible, this was not the case with her friend Dr. Frances McAll. In Yangzhou and Pudong, Betty Gale moved quite readily into a position of support not only for Godfrey, but also for Frances. Certainly part of this could be explained by the degree to which nurses were acculturated to privilege the work of physicians, but such inequality was also often informed by gender roles—physicians as males, nurses as females. Yet the inequality between Betty Gale and Frances McAll is striking; even though Betty worked as a nurse on occasion, she was more involved with Eli's care than Frances was with Margie's. While Gale may have determined that hospitality and childcare were more appropriate ways to spend her energies than on nursing, she may also have simply preferred to avoid conflict. Frances and Ken McAll had more assertive personalities, and they readily admitted that there was conflict at times between the McAlls and the Gales. In fact, of the four, Betty was the only one to exclude disagreements with the McAlls from her memoirs.

Betty Gale worked hard to avoid interpersonal conflict. Her measured reactions to disappointment and conflict belied an underlying anxiety and desire for approval. There were several times that she wrote privately about her frustrations with others, and yet she rarely confronted these people with her concerns. Some exceptions stand out—such as when she approached her colleague at Qilu Hospital to inquire why she had not offered her much assistance in her new role. The conflict was easily resolved through an honest dialogue, and it contributed to Gale's peace of mind. Or again, in Shanghai Betty Gale did confront a Japanese clerk who refused to allow her to exchange a purchase of too-small pyjamas for Margie. Yet her outburst bothered her so much that she returned to apologize; she was embarrassed that she had not behaved in a more dignified way. That Gale did not expect or demand justice in this situation exemplified her approach to internment as a whole: she determined that behaving honourably in an unjust situation was its own reward; she accepted the Japanese clerk's opinion that he owed her nothing.

Continuing the Legacy

One way to evaluate the legacy of China missions is to gauge the impact of mission policies and practice in China by simply counting the number of new converts, hospitals, nurses, or patients listed in missionary records.[34] Another way is to consider the longevity of programs initiated by missionaries in China.[35] Still another way is to examine what legacy missionary children themselves sought to continue in China; what was the legacy passed from missionaries to their children?

Mishkids were aware that their parents had come to China on the wave of the Student Volunteer Movement of the late 1880s, a movement whose goal was the "evangelization of the world in this generation."[36] Yet the mishkids did not tend to describe their work in China in terms of saving souls or seeing others converted to Christianity. Mishkid nurses seemed prepared to carry on the work of hospital-based nursing and the training of Chinese nurses, but they did not seem especially committed to gaining new converts or expanding existing work. While it is true that the evacuation of the North China Mission in 1939 made it difficult for them to invest in the future of the institutions their parents had established, mishkids did not emphasize the development of hospitals, schools, or churches in their letters and memoirs. Rather, they focused on their personal growth, plus their relationships with others.

Betty Gale's writings emphasize a personal striving to discern and follow the will of God and the example of Jesus Christ. Selflessness, humility, forgiveness, kindness, empathy, and peace—these formed the legacy she understood as the essence of missionary work. Shaped by her upbringing, tested by her China challenges, and constructed in her writings as a moral message to her daughter, the legacy that Gale strove to pass on had more to do with how one acted in relationship to others than in the continuance of Christian institutions. Program development did not resonate; character development did.

By the end of her internment, Betty Gale no longer wrote in the first person; nor did she and Godfrey separate their individual voices in their post-internment recollections. Pamela Sugiman has noted that, in a shared group memory, narrators adopt recounted events as their own, even though they themselves may not have personally experienced the events.[37] While it is not clear how often or readily Betty Gale shared her China experiences publicly after returning to Canada, she was certainly known and respected among her peers as someone who practised Christian altruism. In her post-China recollections, including the draft of a speech written approximately ten years after liberation, Gale's key moral message was this: Suffering is abundant and should not be ignored. Nor should it be abandoned. Choosing to enter into another's suffering provides opportunity to change lives—not least of all our own.

China Interrupted

It is difficult to speculate on how Canadian missions might have evolved had Japan not invaded China, but it seems unlikely that they would have continued indefinitely. Even before Japan's occupation of China, the future of China missions seemed uncertain. As the 1932 *Re-Thinking Missions* report made clear, Christian missionaries had always been uninvited guests among people of other cultures and faiths. Their work was dependent on continuous financial donations. Yet by the 1930s church members who had previously supported missions were starting to ask whether missionaries had outlived their usefulness; whether there was a decline in the value of missions to the Far East.[38] Although the Laymen's Appraisal Commission recommended that China missions continue, they made it clear that much needed to change in the field. Medical missions, in particular, would need to be consolidated, standardized, and improved through increased collaboration between missions, government, and private (philanthropic) organizations. Nurses training, they believed, would need to be a priority for mission hospitals that were properly resourced to do so. More attention would need to be paid to health education, preventive medicine, and public health nursing, all in cooperation with the state. In other words, to remain relevant, missionaries would need to be committed to a very different vision of the future—one that was less autonomous, less insular, and frankly less attractive to long-serving missionaries who had already invested considerable effort in the establishment of churches, hospitals, and nursing schools.

By the 1930s the Canadian missionary enterprise had grown in China into a richly interwoven, familial community. For mishkids, China was a place where committed Christians went to live out their faith in tangible ways. If mishkid nurses were aware of the debates over the future viability of China missions, they did not publicly engage in them. Their approach to missions was very personal; they were committed to continue the work (and lifestyles) of their parents. Whether they agreed with the broader vision of nursing as increasingly collaborative, state-run, and preventative did not seem to matter; in the end, none of the mishkid nurses occupied positions of authority in the North China Mission. Indeed, only Jean Menzies and Georgina Menzies actually worked on-site as nurses at the mission in Henan. Even if the 1930s and '40s had been peaceful, it seems unlikely that mishkid nurses would have been the ones to lead the envisioned transition of nursing to a state-run, Chinese-administered one: by 1941 they had all married and were turning their attention from nursing to family concerns.

As I asserted at the beginning of Chapter 7, Japanese internment re-shaped the North China missionary community in part by driving a wedge between missionaries, separating them from each other and forcing internees to integrate with new, disparate communities. But what happened after the missionaries departed China? Although the lack of mission records makes it difficult to trace the missionary diaspora, we do know that by the 1960s missionaries were much less visible in Canada than they had been two decades earlier. Disappearing from view, they nevertheless stayed in close contact with each other, as the dozens of letters sent from other missionaries to Godfrey and Betty Gale on their fortieth wedding anniversary in 1980 attest. Some missionaries, like Bob McClure, went on to practise missionary medicine in places like Korea and Taiwan. Others, like Clara Preston and Susie Kelsey, practised missionary nursing in Aboriginal communities in Canada. It seems likely that still others joined postwar humanitarian agencies like the United Nations Rehabilitation and Relief Administration or the World Health Organization. We know that Don Faris, for example, worked on UN-sponsored projects in Korea, Thailand, and India after leaving China and played a crucial role in the founding of the Canadian University Service Overseas (CUSO).[39] Whatever missionaries did after China, we do know that missionary work was not as valued in postwar Canada as it had been in the past.

In an article describing the last days of the North China Mission during China's civil war, in 1947, I have argued that the closure of China missions triggered a silencing of missionary nursing that continues to this day.[40] That is, given the popularity of missionary nursing in early-twentieth-century Canada, it is surprising how little is known today about missionary nurses, even in nursing academia, and especially given the current interest in global health. There are three explanations for the silence: a postwar view of China missions as a shameful "failure," an expectation that returning missionary nurses were to keep silent in order to protect Christian Chinese colleagues living under Communist rule, and an academic critique of missions as an arm of colonialism. Alvyn Austin and Jamie Scott have similarly noted that missionaries disappeared from the radar of popular culture and academic history in Canada after the 1950s. China missions were re-cast as a tragic mistake. Worse yet, missionaries "had become a historical embarrassment."[41]

The notion of missions as a shameful history was affirmed when I visited China in 2006 with a group of Canadian mishkids who had been children in China during the 1930s and '40s. They explained that it was their experience that, in Canada, one did not readily admit to having a missionary past. Missionary parents were akin to skeletons in the family closet; "missionary" was an offensive word. After our Chinese hosts plied the mishkids for memories about their parents' work in China, one mishkid told me that this was the first time she could remember voicing the word "missionary" in public. The reshaping of the missionary community, then, did not end with internment, but continued well into the postwar period. Indeed, its most dramatic revision likely happened after the missionaries returned to Canada. But alas, that is another study for another time.

Alvyn Austin and Jamie Scott assert that Canadian missions have had a larger impact on Canadian identity than they did in, say, the United States because of the relatively large proportion of Canadians who worked as missionaries.[42] The relational reach of the China missionary community into influential circles is exemplified by a letter written in 1950 by Dr. Jesse Arnup of the United Church of Canada Board of Overseas Missions to West China (and quoted by Austin in *Saving China*):

> Did I tell you about my trip to Ottawa to urge upon the government of the new regime in China? I found a curious situation. The Minister, Lester Pearson, is the son of a well-known Methodist Minister; his deputy [Escott Reid] is the son of an Anglican minister; his Secretary is Jerry Riddell, whose father was Principal of Wesley College, Winnipeg; the specialist on the Far East is [North China mishkid] Arthur Menzies, son of Jimmy [J.M.] Menzies of [Henan]; his Number One man in Japan is Herbert Norman, Dan Norman's son; and his leading representative in China is Ronning, who is the son of a missionary. I felt quite at home among them all.[43]

Even if it was no longer clear by the 1950s to the Canadian public what missionaries had bequeathed the newly-communist China, it *is* clear that China had given a lot to missionaries. China had been a testing ground for nineteenth-century missionaries eager to see the outcome of a concerted worldwide evangelistic effort. In the early twentieth century it became a testing ground for mishkids keen to contribute in a tangible way to the place of their youth. In the 1940s internment camps became social laboratories for testing Christian principles of kindness, long-suffering, and service under the most trying circumstances. For many, China had been a good place to develop strong family ties. And for mishkids, it had been a place of belonging.

Betty and Godfrey Gale spent the rest of their lives describing a China that had done much to enrich their spiritual lives—that is, their relationships with one another, with others, and with God. Like most China missionaries, they never lived to see how, or whether, their efforts in China impacted those they came to serve there. Settling in Canada while Godfrey continued his long recovery from tuberculosis, the Gales had two more children by 1950.[44] For the most part their post-China lives were unremarkable. Godfrey Gale eventually took up full time medical practice in Toronto where he was recognized for his expertise in the care of tuberculosis. The Gales lived quiet lives absorbed in church life and in a strong family, with Betty's parents and siblings close by. They both died—Godfrey in 1986 and Betty in 1995—without ever having the opportunity to re-establish contact with China.

There is an important postscript to the social history of mishkid nurses in China that begs to be told. That is, the internment of civilians in Japanese camps remains a largely overlooked aspect of the Second World War. Even though Betty Gale chose to emphasize internment as an opportunity for personal and spiritual transformation, we cannot—and should not—overlook the point that internment was an act of political and social injustice. In 1988 the Canadian government offered a formal apology and compensation package to those Canadians of Japanese heritage who were interned in Canada during the war. While the of internment of Canadians by their own government is not the same thing as internment of Canadians by enemy occupiers in a foreign country, it is worth noting that the silence that shrouds Canadian missionary history in China also shrouds the history of civilian internment there. More recently, on 8 December 2011, Canada accepted the Japanese government's apology for the horrendous treatment of approximately 1,000 Canadian prisoners of war held for five years after the Battle of Hong Kong.[45] To date, however, there has been no apology offered to the 13,544 civilians imprisoned in China. Betty Gale seemed to recognize that there was something inherently important about her role as a witness to, and participant in, the internment of missionaries and other civilians in China. She found many ways to capture the story—through letters, diary, notebooks, a journal, and at least one recorded interview. If, as Pamela Sugiman has noted, "the personal act of remembering, woven into an analysis of culture and society is, after all, a political project,"[46] then we would be remiss not to also attend to the political message underlying Gale's narratives.

Kindness, self-sacrifice, and empathy formed part of the moral message Betty Gale passed along through her journal in particular. However, one senses a deeper, more controversial political message skirting around the edges of her writing: the issue of internment as politically unjust. By focusing on the question of personal agency ("Should I have stayed?"), Gale avoided directly answering a more dangerous question: Are we being victimized by the Japanese? There were good reasons not to commit these questions to paper while she was a prisoner. Yet, while Gale's acceptance of suffering as having redemptive value served her well in coming to terms with her internment, it also kept her—and likely others—silent in any political sense. Self-censorship during the war and afterwards served to protect Canadian internees from future harm; it also helped keep the tragedy of internment from Canadian public attention.

Hamish Ion has recently pointed out that the Canadian government has "long since forgiven the Japanese for any wrongdoing against Canadian POWs and CIS [civilian internees]."[47] A political decision was made back in 1952 that it was "more important to win the goodwill of the Japanese government than to stand on principle and demand justice for Canadian servicemen and civilians."[48] Despite the small numbers, it seems doubtful that Japanese internment was inconsequential for Canada. Yet to date civilian internment of Canadians has received little attention. In contrast, the extent to which civilian internment influenced survivors' mental and physical health has been a question of great interest in the Netherlands, for example, and Dutch internees who immigrated to Canada after the war have recently started raising similar questions in this country.[49] Does the postwar policy of not demanding justice for Canadian prisoners reflect a Canadian acceptance of civilian internment as an inevitable consequence of living in Japanese-occupied areas? How might a deeper understanding of the health effects of wartime internment influence current Canadian health care policy and practice, as surviving internees become part of Canada's aging population? These are questions as yet unexplored in Canada. What we do know is that the era of mishkid nurses in China ended when the prison camps were liberated. By the time the North China Mission was evacuated for the last time—under gunfire in 1947—mishkid nurses had already disappeared from the China landscape. While mishkid nurses continued the legacy of their missionary parents, it was not in a way anyone expected. Internment became the devastating pinnacle of their missionary careers. Yet through it, Canadian mishkid nurses developed private legacies of their own.

Appendix A

Canadian Missionary Nurses in China, April 1941

	Name	Birthplace	NCM Missionary Parents	Nurse's Training School	Graduation Date
1	Margaret Gay	Toronto 1886	–	VGH	1926
2	Clara Preston	Boissevain, MB 1891	–	RVH; McGill (Education); UWO (Hosp admin); UWO (Pub Health)	1922; 1928; 1931; 1938
3	Susie Kelsey	?	–	WGH	1923?
4	Anna Marion (Fisher) Faris	?	–	UBC	1923
5	Jean (Menzies) Stockley	Anyang 1898	James R. & Davina Menzies	TGH	1922
6	Georgina (Menzies) Lewis	Huaiqing 1906	James R. & Davina Menzies	TGH	1929
7	Elizabeth (Thomson) Gale	Anyang 1911	Andrew & Margaret Thomson	TGH; U Toronto (admin)	1935; 1938
8	Florence (Mackenzie) Liddell (later Hall)	Tianjin? 1911	Hugh & Agnes MacKenzie	TGH	1933?
9	Dorothy Boyd	Huaiqing 1916	Herbert A. & Jessie Boyd	TGH	1938
10	Mary (Boyd) Stanley	Huaiqing 1913	Herbert A.& Jessie Boyd	TGH; U Toronto (public health)	1938?
11	Hilda McIllroy	Toronto?	Mr. S. & Mrs. Henrietta McIllroy	St. Johns Hospital School of Nursing (Toronto?)	1939?

Dates in China as Missionary	Married to China Missionary	Mission	Years Interned	Camp
1910–1941	–	NCM	–	–
1922–1947	–	NCM	–	–
1924–1949	–	Anglican Church of Canada	1941–1943	Weixian
1923–1941	Rev. D.K. (Don) Faris	NCM	(Don 1941–1942)	(House arrest at Qilu)
1927–1940/41	Dr. Handley Stockley, 1927	NCM; English Baptist Mission	–	–
1931–1945	Dr. John Llewellyn Lewis, 1939	NCM; Baptist Missionary Society	1941–1945	Ash
1939–1945	Dr. Godfrey Gale, 1940	NCM; LMS	1941–1945	Yangzhou B; Pudong
1934–1941	Eric Liddell, 1934	NCM; LMS	(Eric 1941–1945)	(Weixian, d. 21.02.45)
1939–1941	(m. non-missionary Mr. Johnson, 1941)	NCM	–	–
1939–1945	Charles Johnson Stanley, 1940	NCM; (College of Chinese Studies)	1941–1945	Weixian
1939–1945	–	Church Missionary Society or Canadian Missionary Society?	1941–1945	Yangzhou A & B; Pudong

Appendix B

All Canadian Nurses Interned in China

Surname	Given Names	Age in 1943	Husband	Children	Husband's Nationality
Missionary Nurses					
1 Gale	Elizabeth Durie	33	Godfrey Livingstone	Margaret Mackay	British
2 Stanley	Mary Boyd	31	Charles John	Charles A.	American
3 Lewis	Georgina Robb	38	John Llewellyn	John Menzies; Margaret Ann	British
4 Kelsey	Susie	?	–	–	–
5 McIllroy	Hilda Elizabeth	37	–	–	–
Non-Missionary Civilian Nurses					
1 Campbell	Amy Isabel	35	–	–	–
2 Robinson	Ethel Estey	60	–	–	–
3 Turner	Marie Yvonne	30	William George	William George; Carol Louise	Canadian
4 Burgess	Myrtle Lanndon	50	John Cecil?	–	Canadian
5 Williams	Nellie	44	–	–	–
6 Christie	Kathleen	34	–	–	–
7 Coleman	Helen Elsie Marsh	35	Archibald Bryan McDonald	–	Canadian
8 Fairburn	Mary Constance	45	–	–	–
9 Greaves	Alys	59	Aubrey Vernon	–	Canadian
10 Needham	Florence Pearl	42	G.K. Needham	?	?

Husband's Occupation	Organization	Camps	Out Date
Medical missionary	London Missionary Society	Yangzhou B; Pudong	Aug 45
Librarian	Yenching University	Weixian	Aug 45
Medical missionary	Baptist Missionary Society	Ash	Aug 45
–	Anglican Church of Canada	Weixian	Sept 43
–	Canadian Missionary Society	Yangzhou A; Yangzhou B; Pudong	Aug 45

–	SM Nursing Service	Ash	Sept 43
–	–	Chapei	Sept 43
Police Sergeant	SM Police	Chapei	Sept 43
Secretary Treasurer	Shanghai General Hospital	Lunghwa; husband at Haiphong	Sept 43
–	Country Hospital	Lunghwa	Sept 43
–	Canadian Army	Bowen Road; Stanley	Sept 43
Refrigeration Engineer	Dairy Farm Ice & Cold Storage Co.	Stanley	Sept 43
–	–	Stanley	Sept 43
Bacteriologist	Hong Kong Public Health Department	Stanley	Sept 43
Military? (Hong Kong POW)	Military?	Stanley	Sept 43

	Surname	Given Names	Age in 1943	Husband	Children	Husband's Nationality
Non-Missionary Civilian Nurses, cont'd						
11	Stokes	Winifred Anne	51	–	–	–
12	Waters	Anna Mary	42	–	–	–
13	Chan	May	43	Guy H.	Guy; Eugene J.	Canadian
Military Nurses						
1	Christie	Kathleen G.	–	–	–	–
2	Waters	Anna May	–	–	–	–

Husband's Occupation	Organization	Camps	Out Date
–	Matilda Hospital	Stanley	Sept 43
–	Military?	Bowen Road; Stanley	Sept 43
Physician	British American Tobacco Co.	Iltis Hydro; Weixian	Aug 45

–	Canadian military	Stanley	1943
–	Canadian military	Stanley	1943

Notes

Notes to Introduction

1 Betty Gale, "The Journal of Betty Gale: A Personal Account of Four Years of Civilian Internment in Occupied China" (Unpublished journal, July 1941–September 1945), Margaret Wightman Private Collection (hereafter MWPC), 15.

2 Ibid.

3 Born Elizabeth ("Betty") Durie Thomson, she is referred to in this book both as Betty Thomson (generally in reference to her childhood) and as Betty Gale. Mishkids Mary Boyd, Georgina and Jean Menzies, and Florence Mackenzie are similarly referred to by both their maiden and married names (Mary Stanley, Georgina Lewis, Jean Stockley, and Florence Liddell).

4 My gratitude goes to one anonymous reader of an earlier version of this manuscript, whose succinct description of the three main aspects of this story captured them so well that I have repeated them here much as they were presented to me in that reader's written report.

5 See, for example: Peggy Abkhazi, *A Curious Cage: Life in a Japanese Internment Camp, 1943–1945* (Victoria, BC: SonoNis Press, 2002); Bernice Archer, *A Patchwork of Internment: The Internment of Western Civilians under the Japanese, 1941–1945* (New York: RoutledgeCurzon, 2004); Pierre Boulle, *The Bridge over the River Kwai* (New York: Presidio Press, 2007); Bruce Elleman, *Japanese American Civilian Prisoner Exchanges and Detention Camps, 1941–45* (London: Routledge, 2006); Greg Leck, *Captives of Empire: The Japanese Internment of Allied Civilians in China, 1941–1945* (Bangor, PA: Shandy Press, 2006); Oliver Lyndsay and John R. Harris, *The Battle for Hong Kong, 1941–1945: Hostage to Fortune* (Hong Kong: Hong Kong University Press, 2005); Elizabeth Norman, *We Band of Angels: The Untold Story of American Nurses Trapped on Bataan by the Japanese* (New York: Random House, 1999).

6 The Japanese Consular Police were a private police force attached to Japan's consulate office in China. See Erik W. Esselstrom, *Crossing Empire's Edge: Foreign Ministry Police and Japanese Expansionism in Northeast Asia* (Honolulu: University of Hawai'i Press, 2009).

7 Janet C. Ross Kerr, "Nursing History at the Graduate Level: State of the Art," *Canadian Bulletin of Medical History* 11, no. 1 (1994): 230.

8 Sonya Grypma, "Withdrawal from Weihui: China Missions and the Silencing of Missionary Nursing, 1888–1947," *Nursing Inquiry* 14, no. 4 (2007): 306–19.

9 The broader issues identified and discussed by Ion were the influences of humanity on warfare, just penalties for war crimes, and differing perspectives of war across

cultural boundaries. See A. Hamish Ion, "'Much Ado about Too Few': Aspects of the Treatment of Canadian and Commonwealth POWs and Civilian Internees in Metropolitan Japan, 1941–1945," *Defence Studies* 6, no. 3 (2006): 292–317.

10 In the last decade more attention has been paid to the history of Canadian missions in China—both in Canada and in China. See Sonya Grypma, *Healing Henan: Canadian Nurses at the North China Mission, 1888–1947* (Vancouver: University of British Columbia Press, 2008).

11 Grypma, "Withdrawal from Weihui," 316.

12 Hilda Elizabeth McIllroy was with the Church Missionary Society. She was interned at Yangchow B, Yangchow C, and Pudong Camps. Leck, *Captives of Empire*, 688.

13 Leck, *Captives of Empire*, 679.

14 A *Globe and Mail* newspaper article in 1945 describes Hilda McIlfroy as the daughter of Mrs. Henrietta McIlroy, 139 Galley Ave, Toronto. It also identifies McIlroy as a member of the Canadian Missionary Society, and a graduate of "St. John's Hospital" in Toronto. She had gone to China as a missionary nurse six years before and was "stationed at a hospital in Hanchow when captured by the Japs [*sic*]." "Canadians Believed in Japanese Hands," *Globe and Mail*, 31 August 1945, Democracy at War: Canadian Newspapers and the Second World War, Canadian War Museum website, http://www.warmuseum.ca/cwm/exhibitions/newspapers/intro_e.shtml.

15 Grypma, Healing Henan.

16 See Norman, *We Band of Angels*.

17 See Betty Jeffrey, *White Coolies* (Sydney: Angus and Robertson, 1985).

18 Second World War poster featuring the Nurses on Corregidor. "Women Prisoners of War," Website of Captain Barbara A. Wilson, USAF, 1996, http://userpages.aug .com/captbarb/prisoners.html.

19 Norman, *We Band of Angels*, 129.

20 Norman, *We Band of Angels*; United States Department of Defense, *We All Came Home* (1985), documentary film.

21 Jeffrey, *White Coolies*; Australian Government Department of Veterans' Affairs, "Australia's War 1939–1945: Nurses Recovered," http://www.ww2australia.gov.au/ behindwire/found.html.

22 Leck, *Captives of Empire*, 620 and 652.

23 Utsumi Aiko, cited in Ion, "Much Ado," 294.

24 Ion, "Much Ado," 303; see also Charles Roland, *Long Night's Journey into Day: Prisoners of War in Hong Kong and Japan, 1941–1945* (Waterloo, ON: Wilfrid Laurier University Press, 2001), xv.

25 Grypma, *Healing Henan*, 106–7.

26 Elizabeth McKechnie and Harriet Sutherland respectively.

27 Alvyn Austin, *Saving China: Canadian Missionaries in the Middle Kingdom, 1888–1959* (Toronto: University of Toronto Press, 1987), 85.

28 Alyvn Austin and Jamie S. Scott, *Canadian Missionaries, Indigenous Peoples: Representing Religion at Home and Abroad* (Toronto: University of Toronto Press, 2005), 4.

29 Austin, *Saving China*, 85.

30 See Yuet-wah Cheung, *Missionary Medicine in China: A Study of Two Canadian Protestant Missions in China before 1937* (Lanhan, MD: University Press of America, 1988); Austin, *Saving China*; Grant Maxwell, "Partners in Mission: The Grey Sis-

ters," in *Assignment in Chekiang: Seventy-one Canadians in China, 1902–1954* (Scarborough, ON: Scarboro Foreign Mission Society, 1984). See also Sister Rita McGuire, "Grey Sisters in China 1929–1943; 1946–1952" (unpublished history), Grey Sisters of the Immaculate Conception, Pembroke Archives.

31 Austin, *Saving China*, 32–35. See also George Leslie MacKay, *From Far Formosa: The Island, Its People and Missions*, 4th ed. (New York: Fleming H. Revell, 1895).

32 The North China Mission hired twenty-one single nurses and the West China Mission hired twenty-four, compared with five Grey Sisters of the Immaculate Conception associated with the Scarboro Foreign Mission Society. Kenneth Beaton, *Serving with the Sons of Shuh: Fifty Fateful Years in West China, 1891–1941* (Toronto: United Church of Canada, 1941), 233–35. According to a list of West China missionaries between 1891 and 1939, there were 14 female physicians and 32 married RNs. Added to Beaton's count of 24 single RNs between 1894 and 1952, the ratio of RNs to MDs in West China was 56 to 14. See also, Janet Beaton, "Canadian Missionary Nurses in China: 1894–1951" (Paper presented at the 14th Annual Conference of the Canadian Association for the History of Nursing, University of Manitoba, Winnipeg, 9 June 2001). It appears that the Grey Sisters who went as nurses were Sisters St. Oswald, Mary Anthony, Mary Genevieve Anderchuk, St Angela Lynch, and Mary Daniel O'Connor. The record, however, is not clear regarding their training. One Grey Sister, Mary Catherine Doyle, was apparently trained as a pharmacist. Nine Grey Sisters went to China altogether between 1929 and 1952. McGuire, "Grey Sisters."

33 This estimate includes married nurses; the West China Mission, for example had 32 married nurses in addition to the 24 WMS nurses.

34 Sonya Grypma, "Missionary Nursing: Internationalizing Religious Ideals," in *Religion, Religious Ethics and Nursing*, ed. M. Fowler, B. Pesut, S. Reimer-Kirkham and R. Sawatzky (New York: Springer, 2011), 129–50.

35 Liu Chung-tung, "From San Gu Liu to 'Caring Scholar': The Chinese Nurse in Perspective," *International Journal of Nursing Studies* 28, no. 4 (1991): 315–24.

36 Ibid., 320.

37 Ibid., 322.

38 Sally Chan and Frances Wong, "Development of Basic Nursing Education in China and Hong Kong," *Journal of Advanced Nursing* 29, no. 6 (1999): 1300–07. The early period of Chinese nursing was chiefly under the leadership of missionary nurses from the West. The Chinese Nurses Association was developed in 1914; by 1915 examinations were offered to certify nurses.

39 Barbara L. Brush et al., *Nurses of All Nations: A History of the International Council of Nurses, 1899–1999* (Philadelphia: Lippincott, 1999), 65.

40 Grypma, *Healing Henan*, 136.

41 Patricia D'Antonio, "Revisiting and Rethinking the Rewriting of Nursing History," *Bulletin of the History of Medicine* 72 (1999): 268–90.

42 D'Antonio, "Revisiting"; Patricia D'Antonio, "Nurses—and Wives and Mothers: Women and the Latter-day Saints Training School's Class of 1919," *Journal of Women's History* 19, no. 3 (2007): 112–36.

43 M. Louise Fitzpatrick, "Historical Research: The Method," in *Nursing Research: A Qualitative Perspective*, 2nd ed., ed. Patricia Munhall and Carolyn Oiler Boyd (New York: National League for Nursing Press, 1993), 364–70.

44 Alice Wexler, "Emma Goldman and the Anxiety of Biography," in *The Challenge of Feminist Biography: Writing the Lives of Modern American Women*, ed. Sara Alpern et al. (Urbana, IL: University of Illinois Press, 1992), 34–50.

45 Geertje Boschma et al., "Oral History Research," in *Capturing Nursing History: A Guide to Historical Methods in Research*, ed. Sandra B. Lewenson and Eleanor Krohn Herrmann (New York: Springer, 2008), 79–98.

46 Jacquelyn Dowd Hall, "Second Thoughts: On Writing Feminist Biography," *Feminist Studies* 13, no. 1 (1987): 23.

47 For studies on first-generation missionary women, see Ruth Compton Brouwer, *New Women for God: Canadian Presbyterian Women and India Missions, 1876–1914* (Toronto: University of Toronto Press, 1990); Ruth Compton Brouwer, *Modern Women, Modernizing Men: The Changing Missions of Three Professional Women in Asia and Africa, 1902–69* (Vancouver, University of British Columbia Press, 2002); Rosemary Gagan, *A Sensitive Independence: Canadian Methodist Women Missionaries in Canada and the Orient, 1881–1925* (Montreal: McGill-Queen's University Press, 1992); Rhonda Anne Semple, *Missionary Women: Gender, Professionalism and the Victorian Idea of Christian Mission* (Rochester, NY: Boydell, 2003).

48 Christoffer Grundmann, *Sent to Heal! Emergence and Development of Medical Missions* (Landham, MD: University Press of America, 2005), 154.

49 Ross Kerr, "Nursing History," 230.

50 Grundmann, *Sent to Heal*, 154.

51 Sally Chandler, cited in Geertje Boschma, Sonya Grypma, and Florence Melchior, "Reflections on Researcher Subjectivity and Identity in Nursing History," in *Capturing Nursing History: A Guide to Historical Methods in Research*, ed. Sandra B. Lewenson and Eleanor Krohn Herrmann (New York: Springer, 2008), 99.

52 Ibid., 100.

53 Pamela Sugiman, "'Life is sweet': Vulnerability and Composure in the Wartime Narratives of Japanese Canadians," *Journal of Canadian Studies* 43, no. 1 (2009): 186–218.

54 Ibid., 191.

55 Godfrey Gale, "Pacific War" (unpublished memoir/diary, n.d.), MWPC. The first two typewritten pages serve as an introduction to the compiled diary entries. Hereafter the introduction is referred to as Godfrey Gale, "Pacific War," whereas diarized entries are dated (e.g., Godfrey Gale, "Pacific War," 8 December 1941).

Notes to Chapter 1

1 Marnie Copland, *Moon Cakes and Maple Sugar* (Burlington, ON: G.R. Welch, 1980), 9.

2 The Menzies arrived in 1895, the Thomsons in 1906, the Mackenzies in 1909, and the Boyds in 1912.

3 In Margaret Brown, "History of the Honan (North China) Mission of the United Church of Canada, Originally a Mission of the Presbyterian Church in Canada" (unpublished, n.d.), United Church of Canada Archives (hereafter UCCA), 46: 4.

4 Sonya Grypma, *Healing Henan: Canadian Nurses at the North China Mission, 1888–1947* (Vancouver: University of British Columbia Press, 2008), 58.

5 Brown, "History of the Honan Mission," 57: 12.

6 Ibid.

7 Grypma, *Healing Henan*, 66. See also Sonya Grypma, "James R. Menzies: Preaching and Healing in Early 20th-Century China," *Canadian Medical Association Journal* 170, no. 1 (2004): 84–85.

8 Brown, "History of the Honan Mission," 73: 15.

9 A wealth of scholarship exists for those interested in the political and cultural history of this period, particularly works by Jonathan Spence. See, for example, Jonathan D. Spence, *Search for Modern China* (New York: W.W. Norton, 1990).

10 Alvyn Austin, *Saving China: Canadian Missionaries in the Middle Kingdom, 1888–1959* (Toronto: University of Toronto Press, 1987), 208.

11 Grypma, *Healing Henan*, 103.

12 Louise Mackenzie McLean, interview with the author, April 2003.

13 Georgina Menzies, "Ward Rounds," 1936/37, UCCA 83.058C, box 58, file 26, series 3.

14 Ibid.

15 Ibid. (emphasis added).

16 Brown, "History of the Honan Mission," 96: 7.

17 Jeannette Radcliffe [*sic*], "War in Weihwei," *Canadian Nurse* 34, no. 7 (1938), 357.

18 Ibid.

19 The five left were Margaret Gay, Jeannette Ratcliffe, Janet Brydon, Clara Preston—and Coral Brodie, who had been seconded to Jinan since 1928. The three who resigned to marry were Allegra Smith (1935, returned to Canada), Isabel Leslie (1937, to NCM missionary John Flemming), and Georgina Menzies (1938, to Baptist missionary John Lewis).

20 "Georgina Menzies," UCCA Biographical Files (Bio Files).

21 Austin, *Saving China*, 228–29.

22 "Religion: Re-Thinking Missions," *Time*, 28 November 1932, http://www.time.com/time/magazine/article/0,9171,744802,00.html#ixzz1MxACE48d.

23 Commission of Appraisal, with William Ernest Hocking, Chair, *Re-Thinking Missions: A Laymen's Inquiry after One Hundred Years* (New York: Harper, 1932), 325–29.

24 Changed shortly before from its original name "Board of Foreign Missions."

25 Austin, *Saving China*, 230–31.

26 John H. MacVicar, foreword to *Life's Waking Part: Being the Autobiography of Reverend James Frazer Smith, Pioneer Medical Missionary to Honan, China, and Missionary to Central Asia*, by James Frazer Smith (Toronto: T. Nelson, 1937).

27 Bob McClure, "Memories of Betty Gale" (unpublished, written on the occasion of Betty and Godfrey Gale's fortieth wedding anniversary), MWPC.

28 Ibid.

29 Ibid.

30 Ruth Thomson Laws, interview with the author, June 2004.

31 "News of the Church: Three New Nurses for China," n.d., MWPC.

32 Mavis Knight Weatherhead, communication with the author, 11 May 2008.

33 Murray McCheyne Thomson, *A Daring Confidence: The Life and Times of Andrew Thomson in China, 1906–1942* (Ottawa: Murray Thomson, 1992), 188–89.

34 Marion F. Menzies Hummel, *Memoirs of a Mishkid*, comp. and ed. Elizabeth Mittler (Beamsville, ON: Elizabeth Mittler, 2001), 18.

35 Robert McClure, interview by Peter Stursberg, Toronto, 14 July 1976, Library and Archives Canada (hereafter LAC), MG 31, series D78, vol. 44, file 44-29.

36 Munroe Scott, *McClure: The China Years of Dr. Bob McClure* (Toronto: Canec Publishing, 1977), 9.

37 McClure, interview by Stursberg.
38 Mavis Knight Weatherhead, interview with the author, November 2006.
39 Copland, *Moon Cakes*, 51.
40 Scott, *McClure*, 23.
41 Copland, *Moon Cakes*, 5.
42 Scott, *McClure*, 10.
43 Hummel, *Memoirs*, 26.
44 Ibid.
45 Thomson, *Daring Confidence*, 188.
46 Ibid.
47 See Linfu Dong, *Cross Culture and Faith: The Life and Work of James Mellon Menzies* (Toronto: University of Toronto Press, 2005).
48 Hummel, *Memoirs*, 29.
49 Ibid., 94–95.
50 Ibid., 31.
51 McClure, interview by Stursberg.
52 Edward W. Said, *Orientalism* (New York: Pantheon, 1978); Franz Fanon, *The Wretched of the Earth* (New York: Grove Press, 2004).
53 Murray McCheyne Thomson, *Mother, God Bless Her! A Memoir Based on the Letters and Stories of Margaret Mackay Thomson, 1881–1973* (Ottawa: Murray Thomson, 2005), 10.
54 Ibid.
55 Ibid.
56 Copland, *Moon Cakes*, 45.
57 The dates for Dorothy and Mary Boyd are estimated; they have not been verified.
58 Hummel, *Memoirs*, 101.
59 David McCasland, *Eric Liddell: Pure Gold* (Grand Rapids, MI: Discovery House, 2001), 153.
60 Scott, *McClure*, 62.
61 Letter from Margaret Thomson (Daokou) to Betty Thomson (Toronto), 15 June 1934, MWPC.
62 Ibid.
63 Ibid.
64 Letter from Andrew Thomson (Daokou) to Betty Thomson (Toronto), 22 May 1935, MWPC.
65 Ibid.
66 Ibid.
67 Letter from Margaret Thomson (Daokou) to Betty Thomson (Toronto), 22 May 1935, MWPC.
68 Board of Overseas Missions, "Reverend Andrew Thomson, M.A., B.D., D.D.," 1948, UCCA Bio Files; Letter from Margaret Thomson (Daokou) to her children (Toronto), 23 September 1934, MWPC.
69 "Toronto General Hospital School for Nurses Graduation Exercises Programme," 22 May 1935, MWPC.
70 Letter from Andrew Thomson (Daokou) to Betty Thomson (Toronto), 15 June 1935, MWPC.
71 Letter from Margret Thomson (Beidaihe) to Betty Thomson (Toronto), 22 June 1935, MWPC.

72 Letter from Mary Stanley (Beijing) to Mrs. Taylor (Toronto), 16 January 1941, UCCA 83.058C, box 58, file 7, series 3.

Notes to Chapter 2

1 Murray McCheyne Thomson, *A Daring Confidence: The Life and Times of Andrew Thomson in China, 1906–1942* (Ottawa: Murray Thomson, 1992), 182.
2 Ibid., 181.
3 Ibid.
4 Ibid.
5 Margaret Brown, "History of the Honan (North China) Mission of the United Church of Canada, Originally a Mission of the Presbyterian Church in Canada" (unpublished, n.d.), UCCA, 112: 1.
6 Marnie Copland, *Moon Cakes and Maple Sugar* (Burlington, ON: G.R. Welch, 1980), 43.
7 Sonya Grypma, *Healing Henan: Canadian Nurses at the North China Mission, 1888–1947* (Vancouver: University of British Columbia Press, 2008).
8 Murray McCheyne Thomson, *Mother, God Bless Her! A Memoir Based on the Letters and Stories of Margaret Mackay Thomson, 1881–1973* (Ottawa: Murray Thomson, 2005), 13.
9 Ibid.
10 Ibid.
11 Murray Thomson, interview with the author, Ottawa, June 2004.
12 Thomson, *Daring Confidence*, 40. Rev. George Leslie MacKay had gone to Formosa earlier, but remained on the fringes of China missions.
13 Thomson, *Daring Confidence*, 44.
14 The title Murray Thomson gave to his biography about his father, Andrew Thomson.
15 Thomson, *Daring Confidence*, 136.
16 Ibid.
17 Ibid., 137.
18 Ibid., 138.
19 Ibid.
20 Ibid.
21 Ibid., 117.
22 Ibid., 117–18.
23 Ibid., 118.
24 Ibid.
25 Ibid.
26 Ibid.
27 Ibid., 118–19.
28 Ibid., 119.
29 Ibid., 120.
30 Ibid.
31 Ibid.
32 Rhonda Anne Semple, *Missionary Women: Gender, Professionalism and the Victorian Idea of Christian Mission* (Rochester, NY: Boydell, 2003); Ruth Compton Brouwer, *Modern Women, Modernizing Men: The Changing Missions of Three Professional*

Women in Asia and Africa, 1902–69 (Vancouver: University of British Columbia Press, 2002).

33 Thomson, *Mother*, 17.

34 Thomson, *Daring Confidence*, 18.

35 Thomson, *Mother*, 53.

36 See Thomson, *Mother*.

37 Marion F. Menzies Hummel, *Memoirs of a Mishkid*, comp. and ed. Elizabeth Mittler (Beamsville, ON: Elizabeth Mittler, 2001), 104. Dr. Edna Guest was a highly respected physician celebrated in a *Canadian Medical Association Journal* article in 1989 for her accomplishments, particularly her role in women's health care issues, including the treatment of venereal disease. See Shabir Bhimji and Rose Sheinin, "Dr. Edna Mary Guest: She Promoted Women's Issues Before It Was Fashionable," *Canadian Medical Association Journal* 141 (1989): 1093–94. More recently, however, Edna Guest is painted in a less favourable light by one of her former patients, whose memoir of her experiences at the Andrew Mercer Reformatory for Females includes a depiction of Edna Guest as an angry and oppressive physician whose approach to the physical examination of young women borders on pathologic. See Velma Demerson, *Incorrigible* (Waterloo, ON: Wilfrid Laurier University Press, 2004).

38 Undated, unsigned letter, apparently from Margaret Thomson to her daughter Betty (shortly before Betty was to make a speech on her arrival at the North China Mission), c. 1938, MWPC.

39 Ibid.

40 Ibid.

41 Ibid.

42 Ibid.

43 Thomson, *Mother*, 65.

44 Alvyn Austin, *Saving China: Canadian Missionaries in the Middle Kingdom, 1888–1959* (Toronto: University of Toronto Press, 1987), 6.

45 For a fuller discussion of the shift from evangelical to professional aims, see Grypma, *Healing Henan*.

Notes to Chapter 3

1 Munroe Scott, *McClure: The China Years of Dr. Bob McClure* (Toronto: Canec Publishing, 1977), 101.

2 Ibid, 106.

3 Ibid, 108.

4 Ibid, 142.

5 Letter from Betty Thomson (Beijing) to her "Folks" (Toronto), 4 June 1939, MWPC.

6 Letter from Betty Thomson (Beijing) to her "Folks" (Toronto), 14 May 1939, MWPC.

7 Ibid.

8 Letter from Betty Thomson (Beijing) to her "Folks" (Toronto), 28 May 1939, MWPC.

9 Ibid.

10 Letter from Betty Thomson (Beijing) to her "Folks" (Toronto), 4 June 1939, MWPC.

11 Ibid.

12 Letter from Betty Thomson (Beijing) to her "Folks" (Toronto), 14 May 1939, MWPC.

13 Ibid.

14 Ibid.

15 Letter from Betty Thomson (Beidaihe) to her "Folks" (Toronto), 15 August 1939, MWPC.

16 Ibid.

17 Letter from Davina Menzies (Beidaihe) to Mrs. Taylor (Toronto), 15 August 1939, UCCA 83.058C, box 58, file 26, series 3.

18 Letter from Betty Thomson (Beidaihe) to her "Folks" (Toronto), 15 August 1939, MWPC.

19 Ibid.

20 Sonya Grypma, *Healing Henan: Canadian Nurses at the North China Mission, 1888–1947* (Vancouver: University of British Columbia Press, 2008), 148.

21 Ibid., 148–49.

22 Margaret Brown, "History of the Honan (North China) Mission of the United Church of Canada, Originally a Mission of the Presbyterian Church in Canada" (unpublished, n.d.), UCCA, C: 10.

23 Letter by Margaret Gay, "Events in the Autumn of 1939 in Honan," n.d., private collection, courtesy Muriel Gay.

24 According to annals of the Xinxiang Medical School (formerly Weihui hospital), the Canadians handed over the hospital unconditionally to Chinese management after the Anti-British Movement of 1939. A Chinese surgeon, Dr. Duan Mei-Qing, became the hospital director.

25 Grypma, *Healing Henan*, 150.

26 Letter from H.A. Boyd to Forbes, 29 October 1939, UCCA 83.058C, box 56, file 11, series 3.

27 Ibid.

28 Gay, "Autumn of 1939."

29 Letter from G.K. King to Dr. Armstrong, 14 December 1939, UCCA 83.058C, box 56, file 11, series 3. Margaret Gay reported meeting Dr. Chang a few months later, in West China. Gay, "Autumn of 1939."

30 Grypma, *Healing Henan*, 151.

31 G.K. King, "Events which led missionaries of the United Church of Canada to withdraw from Weihui, Henan, October 12, 1939," (report), UCCA 83.045, box 9, file 56.

32 Andrew Thomson, dressed in Chinese clothing, managed to remain at the small mission centre of Taokow for another seven months. He left Henan in May for Qilu, where he officiated at the wedding ceremony of his daughter Elizabeth in September 1940. Andrew Thomson, "Report, July–December 1940," UCCA 83.045C, box 10, file 163.

33 A. Baxter, foreword to *Interned in China*, by Godfrey Gale (London: Livingstone Press [LMS], 1946), p. iii.

34 "Wedding," (newspaper clipping, n.d.), MWPC.

35 Betty Gale, interview with Margaret Wightman, audio-tape, 198(?), MWPC.

36 Betty Gale, diary, 20 August 1939, MWPC.

37 Ibid., 27 August 1939.

38 Letter from Betty Thomson (Beijing) to her "Folks" (Toronto), 12 September 1939, MWPC.

39 Betty Gale, diary, 2 September 1939.

40 Mary Stanley (Staunton, Virginia), (letter written on the occasion of Godfrey and Betty Gale's fortieth anniversary), 16 October 1980, MWPC.

41 Ibid.

42 Letter from Betty Thomson (Beijing) to her "Folks" (Toronto), 12 September 1939, MWPC.

43 Betty Gale, diary, 6 September 1939.

44 Letter from Godfrey Gale (Jinan) to Betty Thomson (Beijing), 11 September 1939, MWPC.

45 Ibid.

46 Betty Gale, diary, 19 September 1939.

47 Letter from G.K. King to Mrs. Taylor, 14 December 1939, UCCA 85.058C, box 56, file 11, series 3.

48 Report from Helen McDougall (Beijing) to Mrs. Hugh D. Taylor (Toronto), 14 December 1939, UCCA 85.058C, box 56, file 11, series 3.

49 Associated Boards for Christian Colleges in China and the United Committee for Christian Universities in China, "Cheeloo" (n.p.: "The University Press," c. 1937), MWPC.

50 Ibid.

51 By June 1939, forty-seven institutions had moved to Free China, and twenty-one to the foreign concessions of Shanghai. This mass emigration involved thousands of students and hundreds of professors travelling by boat, bus, and/or foot over hundreds of miles of dangerous territory—something C.H. Corbett called "one of the most astonishing phenomena in the struggle against Japan." Cited in Brown, "History of the Honan Mission," 99: 2.

52 Letter from Isabelle MacTavish (aboard the *Gripsholm*) to Mrs. Taylor (Toronto), 8 August 1942, UCCA 83.045C, box 11, file 174.

53 Frances McAll and Kenneth McAll, *The Moon Looks Down* (London: Darley Anderson, 1987), 18.

54 Associated Boards, "Cheeloo," MWPC.

55 The Nationalist Army seizure of Nanjing on 24 March 1927 triggered a mass evacuation of missionaries from all over China out of fear of civil conflict. Altogether 8,300 Protestant missionaries evacuated China in 1937 during what was dubbed "the Great Missionary Exodus"; 3,000 never returned. Grypma, *Healing Henan*, 103.

56 Handwritten note from Godfrey Gale to Betty Thomson, n.d., MWPC.

57 Betty Gale, diary, 24 December 1939.

58 Letter from Betty Thomson (Jinan) to Margaret Thomson (Toronto), 25 December 1939, MWPC.

59 Letter from Andrew Thomson (Daokou) to his family (Toronto), 19 December 1939, MWPC.

60 Letter from Betty Thomson (Jinan) to Margaret Thomson (Toronto), 3 February 1940, MWPC.

61 Letter from Betty Thomson to Rev. G.K. King, 18 January 1940, UCCA 83.058C, box 58, file 36, series 3.

62 Letter from Betty Thomson (Jinan) to Margaret Thomson (Toronto), 3 February 1940, MWPC.

63 Murray Thomson, "The Jinan Tchit Tchat" (newsletter, created as a gift to Betty Thomson for her wedding day), 14 September 1940, MWPC.

64 Letter from Betty Thomson (Jinan) to Margaret Thomson (Toronto), 3 February 1940, MWPC.

65 Letter from Betty Thomson (Jinan) to Mrs. Hugh Taylor (Toronto), 11 February 1940, UCCA 83.058C, file 36, box 58, series 3.

66 Ibid.

67 Letter from Betty Thomson (Jinan) to Margaret Thomson (Toronto), 3 February 1940, MWPC.

68 Ibid.

69 Ibid.

70 Ibid.

71 Ibid.

72 Ibid.

73 Ibid.

74 Letter from Betty Thomson (Jinan) to Margaret Thomson (Toronto), 22 February 1940, MWPC.

75 Letter from Betty Thomson (Jinan) to family (Toronto), 28 May 1940, MWPC.

76 Ibid.

77 Letter from Mrs. Ruth Taylor to Rev. G.K. King, 2 April 1940, UCCA 83.058C, box 56, file 12, series 3.

78 Letter from Betty Thomson (Beidaihe) to her "Folks" (Toronto), 12 August 1940, MWPC.

79 Mavis Knight Weatherhead, correspondence with the author, 11 December 2005.

80 Ibid.

81 Letter from Betty Thomson (Beidaihe) to her "Folks" (Toronto), 12 August 1940, MWPC.

82 Letter from Betty Thomson (Beidaihe) to Margaret Thomson (Toronto), 29 August 1940, MWPC.

83 Letter from Margaret Thomson (Toronto) to "Elizabeth Dearie," 13 September 1940, MWPC.

84 Ibid.

85 "Wedding," (newspaper clipping), n.p., n.d., MWPC.

86 Godfrey Gale (Qingdao) to Margaret Thomson (Toronto), 19 September 1940.

87 Thomson, "Tchit Tchat."

88 Ibid.

89 Jeannette Ratcliffe, Janet Brydon, Clara Preston, Margaret Gay, and Susie Kelsey each served in China for between twenty-two and thirty years.

Notes to Chapter 4

1 Murray McCheyne Thomson, *A Daring Confidence: The Life and Times of Andrew Thomson in China, 1906–1942* (Ottawa: Murray Thomson, 1992), 150.

2 Letter Betty Gale (Qing Dao) to Margaret Thomson (Toronto), 19 September 1940, MWPC.

3 Ibid.

4   Letter from Betty Gale (Jinan) to Margaret Thomson (Toronto), 13 October 1940, MWPC.

5   Ibid.

6   Ibid.

7   Letter from Betty Gale (Qilu) to "Peg" (Toronto), 24 October 1940, MWPC.

8   Letter from Betty Gale (Qilu) to Margaret Thomson (Toronto), 25 December 1940, MWPC. In her diary, written in the late 1920s, Mary Austin Endicott—wife of United Church West China missionary James Endicott—referred both to condoms (freely available in the larger cities like Shanghai) and "the Dutch cap," which was a fitted cervical cap available through one's physician. Presumably the medical community at Qilu, including Godfrey and Betty, had access to both. Shirley Jane Endicott, *China Diary: The Life of Mary Austin Endicott* (Waterloo, ON: Wilfrid Laurier University Press, 2003), 81.

9   Letter from Betty Gale (Qilu) to Margaret Thomson (Toronto), 25 December 1940, MWPC.

10 Letter from Betty Gale (Jinan) to "Gwen" (Toronto?), 5 February 1941, MWPC.

11 Ibid.

12 Ibid.

13 Ibid.

14 Gwen's married name was Edmison. Margaret Wightman, personal communication with the author, December 2008.

15 Letter from Betty Gale (Jinan) to "Gwen" (Toronto?), 5 February 1941, MWPC.

16 Ibid.

17 Ibid.

18 Ibid.

19 Ibid.

20 Dorothy Galbraith, "Missionary in Torpedoed Ship," *North China Herald*, 26 March 1941, 510; see also "Prince Line," The Red Duster, The Merchant Navy Association, http://www.red-duster.co.uk/PRINCE13.htm.

21 Letter from G.K. King to Mrs. Taylor, 3 February 1941, UCCA 83.058C, box 56, file 14, series 3.

22 Ibid.

23 Ibid.

24 Letter from G.K. King to Mrs. Taylor, 7 March 1941, UCCA 83.058C, box 56, file 14, series 3.

25 "March 18, 1941 from Tientsin," (anonymous note), UCCA 83.058C, box 58, file 26, series 3.

26 Letter from G.K. King to Mrs. Taylor, 3 December 1941, UCCA 83.058C, box 56, file 14, series 3.

27 Radiogram from Handley Stockley (Xian) in February 1942 (?) picked up by the Official Listening Post at Ventura, California (a copy was sent to the United Church mission headquarters in Toronto), UCCA 83.045C, box 11, file 174.

28 Letter from G.K. King to Mrs. Taylor, 3 October 1941, UCCA 83.058C, box 56, file 14, series 3.

29 David McCasland, *Eric Liddell: Pure Gold* (Grand Rapids, MI: Discovery House, 2001), 225.

30 Ibid.

31 Dr. Ken McAll, audiotaped interview with Margaret Wightman, 1991, MWPC.

32 McCasland, *Pure Gold,* 225

33 Letter from Norman Knight (addressee unknown, n.d.), UCCA 83.045C, box 9, file 151.

34 Heather Ingham (daughter of Florence Liddell), correspondence with the author, November 2007.

35 Ibid.

36 Letter from Adelaide Harrison to Knight, 18 February 1941, UCCA 83.058C, box 62, file 20, series 5.

37 Cited in letter from Adelaide Harrison to Mrs. Taylor, 7 May 1941, UCCA 83.058C, box 61, file 13, series 5.

38 Ibid.

39 Letter from Mrs. Taylor to G.K. King, 30 September 1941, UCCA 83.058C, box 56, file 14, series 3.

40 Letter from G.K. King to Mrs. Taylor, 23 April 1940, UCCA 83.058C, box 56, file 12, series 3.

41 Ibid.

42 Letter from Mary Boyd to Mrs. Taylor, 16 January 1941, UCCA 83.058C, box 58, file 7, series 3.

43 Ibid.

44 Donald Menzies (grandson of George Wilders), personal communication with the author, 27 February 2007.

45 Letter from Mary Boyd to Mrs. Taylor, 16 January 1941, UCCA 83.058C, box 58, file 7, series 3.

46 Letter from G.K. King to Dr. I. MacTavish, 29 October 1940, UCCA 83.058C, box 56, file 13, series 3.

47 Letter from Mary Boyd to Mrs. Taylor, 16 January 1941, UCCA 83.058C, box 58, file 7, series 3.

48 Letter from G.K. King to Mrs. Taylor, 28 November 1940, UCCA 83.058C, box 56, file 12, series 3.

49 Letter from Mary Stanley (Beijing) to Mrs. Ruth Taylor (Toronto), 16 January 1941, UCCA 83.058C, box 58, file 7, series 3.

50 Ibid.

51 Ibid.

52 Ibid.

53 Betty Gale, diary, 29 June 1941.

54 Sonya J. Grypma, "China Nurse Jean Ewen: Embracing and Abandoning Communist Revolutionaries," *Journal of Historical Biography* 9 (2011): 37–68.

55 Letter from Mary Stanley (Beijing) to Mrs. Ruth Taylor (Toronto), 16 January 1941, UCCA 83.058C, box 58, file 7, series 3.

56 "Beginnings," The Wilder-Stanley Saga, http://reced.org/dmenzi/Wilders/wilder -Stanley.htm.

57 His full name is Charles Johnson ("John") Stanley. John Stanley was the son of missionaries Charles Stanley and Louise Hathaway, grandson of missionaries Charles Alfred Stanley and Ursula Johnson. Charles Alfred Stanley was the first American missionary to reach North China, where he lived until his retirement in

1909. Information courtesy Sandra Miller Long (correspondence), 1 August 2008. See also "Beginnings," http://reced.org/dmenzi/wilders/wilder-Stanley.htm.

58 Letter from Gertrude S. Wilder (Beijing) to "Durand and Ursula," 9 August 1941, in "The Wilders, 1941: Forebodings of a World at War," (unpublished compilation of documents, n.d.), 31, http://reced.org/dmenzi/Wilders/Downloads.htm.

59 Hugh Hubbard and Mabel Hubbard, eds., "Postscript," *The Watchman* 14, no. 2 (1 November 1941), in "The Wilders, 1941," 51.

60 Ibid., 51–52.

61 Ibid., 52.

62 Letter from Elizabeth Gale (Qilu) to her "Folks" (Toronto), 11 June 1942, MWPC. According to this letter, Mary Stanley was due with her second child on 15 June 1942.

63 Letter from Gertrude Wilder (Beijing) to "Theodore," 7 December 1941 (with an addition by George Wilder and a postscript written on 9 December 1941), in "The Wilders, 1941," 61–62.

64 Ibid., 64.

65 Ibid., 65.

66 "Movements of Honan Missionaries," April 1941, UCCA 83.058C, box 56, file 14, series 3; G.K. King, "Had to Guard Writing While in Hands of Japs, Missionary Says Here," *The Globe and Mail* (Toronto), 28 August 1942, UCCA83.058C, box 56, file 15, series 3. According to Betty Gale's diary, John Menzies Lewis was born on 23 February 1941.

67 Letter from the Acting Under-Secretary of State for External Affairs to Mrs. Taylor, 13 March 1941, UCCA 83.058C, box 56, file 14, series 3.

68 While the mission board "gave in" to Dr. MacTavish's decision to stay, they continued to urge Davina Menzies to quit China.

69 Letter from G.K. King to Mrs. Taylor, 3 October 1941, UCCA 83.058C, box 56, file 14, series 3.

70 Letter from Margaret Thomson (Toronto) to "Andrew and Godfrey" (Jinan), 30 March 1941, MWPC. The names of the two children are in the Ash Camp list in Greg Leck, *Captives of Empire: The Japanese Internment of Allied Civilians in China, 1941–1945* (Bangor, PA: Shandy Press, 2006).

71 Letter from G.K. King to Mrs. Taylor, 3 December 1941, UCCA 83.058C, box 56, file 14, series 3.

72 Letter from G.K. King to Mrs. Taylor, 7 March 1941, UCCA 83.058C, box 56, file 14, series 3.

73 Letter from Margaret Thomson (Toronto) to "Andrew and Godfrey," 30 March 1941, MWPC.

74 Letter from Margaret Thomson (Toronto) to "Dad, Godfrey—Elizabeth (?)," 5 April 1941, MWPC.

75 "Movements of Honan Missionaries," April 1941, UCCA 83.058C, box 56, file 14, series 3.

76 Betty Gale, diary, 23–28 February 1941.

77 Barb Putnam, personal communication with the author, 6 October 2003.

78 Frances McAll and Kenneth McAll, *The Moon Looks Down* (London: Darley Anderson, 1987), 20.

79 Godfrey Gale, introduction to Betty Gale, "The Journal of Betty Gale: A Personal Account of Four Years of Civilian Internment in Occupied China" (Unpublished journal, July 1941–September 1945), MWPC.

80 McAll and McAll, *Moon Looks Down*, 7.

81 Frances McAll, *Hurdles are for Jumping* (Oxford: New Cherwell Press, 1998), 64–65.

82 Ken McAll, interview with Wightman. McAll recalled in great detail the furniture and belongings they left behind, including an ornate dining table and sideboards, delicately carved furniture, and rare silverware. They never saw their belongings again, nor were they reimbursed for their loss.

83 McAll and McAll, *Moon Looks Down*, 19.

84 Letter from Margaret Thomson (Toronto) to "Dad, Godfrey—Elizabeth (?)," 5 April 1941, MWPC.

85 Letter from Margaret Thomson (Toronto) to "Elizabeth," n.d. (probably 8 April 1941), MWPC.

86 Letter from Margaret Thomson (Toronto) to "Andrew, Elizabeth and Godfrey," 27 April 1941, MWPC.

87 Letter from Betty Gale (Jinan) to Mrs. Gale (England), 11 May 1941, MWPC.

88 Letter from Margaret Thomson (Toronto) to Betty Gale (Jinan), 25 May 1941, MWPC.

89 Letter Betty Gale (Jinan) to Mrs. Gale (England), 3 July 1941, MWPC.

90 Ibid.

91 Ibid.

92 Letter from Margaret Thomson (Toronto) to "Dad, Elizabeth and Godfrey" (Jinan), 9 July 1941, MWPC.

93 Letter from Betty Gale (Jinan) to Mrs. Gale (England), 3 July 1941, MWPC.

94 Ibid.

95 Letter from Margaret Thomson (Toronto) to "Dad, Elizabeth and Godfrey" (Jinan), 4 October 1941, MWPC.

96 Letter from Margaret Thomson (Toronto) to "Dad, Elizabeth and Godfrey" (Jinan), 9 July 1941, MWPC.

97 Ibid.

98 Letter from Margaret Thomson (Toronto) to "Dad, Elizabeth & Godfrey" (Jinan), 3 August 1941, MWPC.

99 Letter from Betty Gale (Jinan) to Mrs. Gale (England), 9 August 1941, MWPC.

100 Letter from Margaret Thomson (Toronto) to "Dad, Elizabeth and Godfrey" (Jinan), 3 August 1941, MWPC.

101 Betty Gale, diary, 17 July 1941.

102 Betty Gale, "Journal," 17 July 1941.

103 Ibid., 30 July 1941.

104 Letter from Betty Gale (Jinan) to Mrs. Gale (England), 9 August 1941, MWPC.

105 Betty Gale, "Journal," 28 July 1941.

106 McAll and McAll, *Moon Looks Down*, 21.

107 Godfrey Gale, preface to Betty Gale, diary.

108 Godfrey Gale, "Pacific War" (unpublished memoir/diary, n.d.), MWPC.

109 McAll and McAll, *Moon Looks Down*, 20.

110 Ibid.
111 Letter from G.K. King (Beijing) to Mrs. Taylor (Toronto), 7 March 1941, UCCA 83.058C, box 56, file 14, series 3.
112 "Map of Military Operations in China on November 1, 1938," *North China Herald*, 9 November 1938, 225.
113 "Special writer," "Japanese North China Failure," *North China Herald*, 5 February 1941, 47.
114 Ibid.
115 Ibid.
116 McAll and McAll, *Moon Looks Down*, 20.
117 "Honan Drive and Southward Move," *North China Herald*, 19 February 1941, 274.
118 Letter from Betty Gale (Jinan) to Mrs. Gale (England), 4 September 1941, MWPC.
119 "New Rules for Travel in North China," *North China Herald*, 11 June 1941, 404.
120 Letter from Betty Gale (Jinan) to Mrs. Gale (England), 4 September 1941, MWPC.
121 Ibid.
122 Letter from Margaret Thomson (Toronto) to "Dad, Elizabeth and Godfrey" (Jinan), 14 September 1941, MWPC.
123 Letter from Margaret Thomson (Toronto) to "Dad, Elizabeth and Godfrey" (Jinan), 27 September 1941, MWPC.
124 Letter from Margaret Thomson (Toronto) to "Dad, Elizabeth and Godfrey" (Jinan), 1 December 1941, MWPC.
125 Letter from Betty Gale (Jinan) to her "Folks," 20 October 1941, MWPC.
126 Betty Gale, diary, 17 October 1941.
127 Letter from Betty Gale (Jinan) to her "Folks," 20 October 1941.
128 "Report of Cheeloo University Hospital, July 1, 1941 to January 15, 1942." UCCA 83.045C, box 11, file 176.
129 Ibid. The other nurses identified were: Marjorie Alderman (Director of Nursing Service), Geneva E. Miller (Director of Nursing Education), Ruth M. Danner (Public Health), Florence Evans (Charge of Surgical Supplies), Chao K'un (Supervisor), and Li Pao Chen (Instructor).
130 Miss Fuller, "Annual Report Qilu University," April 1940, UCCA 83.058C, box 57, file 14, series 3.
131 Godfrey Gale, "Pacific War."
132 Letter from Betty Gale (Jinan) to her "Folks," 20 October 1941, MWPC.
133 Ibid.
134 McAll and McAll, *Moon Looks Down*, 21.
135 "Hospital Employees on Strike," *North China Herald*, 8 January 1941.
136 McAll and McAll, *Moon Looks Down*, 21.
137 Ibid.
138 Ruth M. Danner, "Cheeloo University School of Nursing Report," 1941–42, UCCA83.045C, box 11, file 176.
139 Betty Gale, "Journal," 9 September 1941.
140 Godfrey Gale, "Pacific War."
141 For more on nurses training in China, see Kaiyi Chen, "Missionaries and the Early Development of Nursing in China," *Nursing History Review* 4 (1996): 129–49; and Kaiyi Chen, "Quality Versus Quantity: The Rockefeller Foundation and Nurses Training in China," *Journal of American East Asian Relations* 5, no. 1 (1996): 77–104.

142   "Excellent Work of Wusih Hospital," *North China Herald*, 30 April 1941, 165.
143   Ibid.
144   Miss Fuller, "Annual Report Cheeloo University," April 1940, UCCA 83.058C, box 57, file 14, series 3.
145   Ibid.
146   Ibid.
147   Betty Gale, "Journal," 28 October 1941.
148   Ibid.
149   Ibid.
150   Godfrey Gale, "Pacific War."
151   Ibid.
152   The woman was Miss C.E.M Gale; the attack happened on 6 May 1941. "Shanghai Woman Has Narrow Escape from Death at Sea," *North China Herald*, 23 July 1941, 158.
153   Godfrey Gale, "Pacific War."
154   Letter from Betty Gale (Jinan) to her "Folks" (Toronto), 25 November 1941, MWPC.
155   Ibid.
156   Godfrey Gale, "Pacific War."
157   Letter from Betty Gale (Jinan) to her "Folks" (Toronto), 25 November 1941, MWPC.
158   Cablegrams to and from Korea, Japan, and North China, UCCA 83.058C, box 56, file 14, series 3.
159   Ibid.
160   Godfrey Gale, introduction to Betty Gale, "Journal."
161   Ibid.
162   Ibid.
163   Betty Gale, notebook, 22 January 1945.
164   Godfrey Gale, "Pacific War."
165   Ibid.
166   Betty Gale, "Journal," 7 December 1941.

Notes to Chapter 5

1   The friends were the Nordstroms of the Jinan Post Office. Godfrey Gale, "Pacific War" (unpublished memoir/diary), 7 December 1941, MWPC.
2   Ibid.
3   Betty Gale, diary, 25 December 1941.
4   Betty Gale, "The Journal of Betty Gale: A Personal Account of Four Years of Civilian Internment in Occupied China" (Unpublished journal, July 1941–September 1945), 7 December 1941, MWPC.
5   Ibid.
6   The friends were the Scotts, McAlls, Rowlands, and Amy Watkins. Godfrey Gale, "Pacific War," 7 December 1941.
7   See epigraph to the Introduction.
8   Ibid.
9   Betty Gale, diary, 8 December 1941.
10   Betty Gale, "Journal," 8 December 1941.
11   Letter from Elizabeth Gale (Qilu) to her "Folks" (Toronto), 11 June 1942, MWPC.

12 Godfrey Gale, "Pacific War," 8 December 1941.

13 Ibid., 7 December 1941.

14 See Peggy Abkhazi, *A Curious Cage: Life in a Japanese Internment Camp, 1943–1945* (Victoria, BC: SonoNis Press, 2002), 16.

15 Godfrey Gale, "Pacific War," 7 December 1941.

16 Ibid., 8 December 1941.

17 Ibid.

18 Betty Gale, "Journal," 8 December 1941.

19 Godfrey Gale, "Four Years Under the Japs [*sic*]," (Unpublished manuscript, n.d.), MWPC.

20 Betty Gale, diary, 8 December 1941.

21 Godfrey Gale, "Pacific War," 8 December 1941.

22 Ibid.

23 Ibid.

24 E.V. Lucas, *The Open Road: A Book for Wayfarers*, 1913, Roz Hulze Ltd: Beautiful Books, Maps and Prints, http://www.rozhulse.com/acatalog/books_91190_lucas .htm; Antiquarian Booksellers of North America, http://search.abaa.org/dbp2/ book31741356I.html.

25 Abkhazi, *Curious Cage*, 18.

26 The book, *A Curious Cage* (2002), is a "reproduction" of Pemberton-Carter's wartime journal. After internment, Peggy Pemberton-Carter purchased property in Victoria and, together with her husband, Prince Nicholas Abkhazi, developed a masterpiece garden well known in British Columbia as the Abkhazi Garden.

27 Abkhazi, *Curious Cage*, 52.

28 Ibid.

29 Ibid., 52–53.

30 Ibid., 53.

31 Betty Gale, "Journal," 8 December 1941.

32 Ibid.

33 Ibid.

34 Ibid.

35 "Report of Cheeloo University Work in Tsinan, 1941–1942," UCCA 83.045C, box 11, file 176.

36 Godfrey Gale, "Pacific War", 8 December 1941.

37 Ibid.

38 Betty Gale, diary, 8 December 1941.

39 Betty Gale, interview with Margaret Wightman, audio-tape, 198(?), MWPC.

40 "Report of Cheeloo University Work in Tsinan, 1941–42," 1, MWPC.

41 Godfrey Gale, "Pacific War," 9 December 1941.

42 Ibid.

43 Betty Gale, "Journal," 8 December 1941.

44 Ibid.

45 Godfrey Gale, "Pacific War," 19 December 1941.

46 "Report of Cheeloo University Hospital, July 1, 1941 to January 15, 1942," UCCA 83.045C, box 11, file 176.

47 Godfrey Gale, "Pacific War," 9 December 1941.

48 Ibid.
49 Letter from Isabelle MacTavish (on board the *M.S. Gripsholm* en route to Canada) to Ruth Taylor, 8 August 1942, UCCA 83.045C, box 11, file 177.
50 Ibid.
51 Godfrey Gale, "Pacific War," 10 December 1941.
52 Ibid.
53 Ibid.
54 Ibid.
55 Ibid.
56 Ibid., 11 December 1941.
57 Ibid.
58 Betty Gale, "Journal," 11 December 1941.
59 Ibid.
60 Ibid.
61 Ibid.
62 Ibid.
63 Ruth M. Danner, "Cheeloo University School of Nursing Report, 1941–1942," UCCA 83.045C, box 11, file 176.
64 Ibid.
65 Betty Gale, "Journal," 15 December 1941.
66 Ibid.
67 Godfrey Gale, "Pacific War," 13 December 1941.
68 Ibid.
69 Ibid.
70 Ibid., 15 December 1941.
71 Ibid.
72 Ibid.
73 Ibid.
74 "Church of England Missionary Is Home: Nurse Was Two Years Prisoner of Japanese—Wants to Go Back" (Newspaper article, n.p., n.d., from a page on Susie Kelsey in an alumni scrapbook), WGH/HSCS.
75 Godfrey Gale, "Pacific War," 18 December 1941.
76 Ibid.
77 Ibid., 21 December 1941.
78 Ibid., 23 December 1941.
79 Ibid.
80 Annie V. Scott, "Report of Cheeloo University Hospital, July 1, 1941 to January 15, 1942," UCCA 83.045C, box 11, file 176.
81 "Report of Cheeloo University Work in Tsinan, 1941–1942," UCCA 83.045C, box 11, file 176.
82 Ibid.
83 Scott, "Cheeloo University Hospital."
84 These were Dr. Gualt, Dr. Gell, Dr. MacTavish, and Dr. Scott. Scott, "Cheeloo University Hospital."
85 Letter from A.E. Armstrong (Toronto) to Mrs. Faris (Vancouver), 22 January 1942, UCCA 84.045C, box 11, file 174.

86   Ibid.
87   Letter from Marion Faris (Vancouver) to Rev. A.E. Armstrong (Toronto), 20 March 1942, UCCA 83.045C, box 11, file 174.
88   Ibid.
89   Ibid.
90   Ibid.
91   Ibid.
92   Ibid.
93   "Confidential" letter from Rev. A.E. Armstrong (Toronto) to Mrs. D.K. Faris (Vancouver), 27 March 1942, UCCA 83.045C, box 11, file 174.
94   Letter from Faris to Armstrong, 20 March 1942.
95   "Advice to the Relative of a Man Who Is Missing," LAC, National Defence Fonds (hereafter NDF), microfiche reel C, file 5535–9050.
96   Ibid.
97   Letter from G.K. King to A.E. Armstrong, 21 February 1942, UCCA 83.045C, box 11, file 174.
98   Letter from Isabelle MacTavish (Jinan) to Clara Preston (Chengdu), 2 February 1942, UCCA 83.045C, box 11, file 174.
99   Letter from Clara Preston (Chengdu) to Mrs. Taylor (Toronto), 2 February 1942, UCCA 83.045C, box 11, file 174.
100 An area of two hundred acres in Tianjin leased to the British crown "in perpetuity" since 1860.
101 Letter from Eric Liddell (Tianjin) to Clara Preston (Chongqing), 1 March 1942, UCCA 83.045C, box 11, file 174.
102 Ibid.
103 Ibid.
104 Letter from Winifred Warren (Shanghai) to Mrs. Taylor (Toronto), 4 March 1942, UCCA83.045C, box 11, file 174.
105 Ibid.
106 Letter from Gerald Bell (Chengdu, Sichuan) to Rev. A.E. Armstrong (Toronto), 18 April 1942, UCCA 83.045C, box 11, file 174.
107 A.M. Stephen, *War in China: What It Means to Canada* (Vancouver, BC: China Aid Council and The National Salvation League, 1938), 12. The leftist China Aid Council was started in New York in 1937 with the support of Madame Sun Yat-sen. It sponsored Dr. Norman Bethune's work with Mao Zedong's Eighth Route Army in 1938 and 1939.
108 Stephen, *War in China*, 12.
109 Ibid., 13.
110 A.E. Armstrong and Ruth Taylor, "Thirty Missionaries Now in Enemy Countries," *The United Church Observer*, 15 March 1942, UCCA box 9881.A, 702 PS, microfilm.
111 Ibid.
112 Ibid.
113 Godfrey Gale, "Pacific War," 24 December 1941.
114 Ibid.
115 Ibid.
116 Ibid.
117 Ibid.

118 Ibid.
119 Ibid., 14 December 1941.
120 Ibid.
121 Betty Gale, diary, 14 December 1941.
122 "Report of Cheeloo University Work in Tsinan, 1941–1942."
123 Betty Gale, "Journal," 25 December 1941.
124 Ibid.
125 Godfrey Gale, "Pacific War," 24 December 1941.
126 Ibid., 31 December 1941.
127 Ibid.
128 Ibid., 7 January 1942.
129 Ibid., 13 January 1942.
130 Ibid.
131 Ibid., 14 January 1942.
132 Ibid.
133 Ibid., 26 January 1942.
134 Betty Gale, "Journal," 1 January 1942.
135 Godfrey Gale, "Pacific War," 26 January 1941.
136 Betty Gale, "Journal," 12 March 1942.
137 Ibid.
138 Godfrey Gale, "Pacific War," 5 January 1942.
139 Betty Gale, "Journal," 6 January 1942.
140 Ibid.
141 Betty Gale, diary, 5 January 1942.
142 Godfrey Gale, "Pacific War," 3 May 1942.
143 Ibid.
144 Betty Gale, "Journal," 23 May 1942.
145 Ibid., 24 May 1942.
146 Ibid., 25 May 1942.
147 Ibid.
148 Ibid.
149 Godfrey Gale, "Pacific War," 15 December 1941.
150 Betty Gale, "Journal," 13 April 1942.
151 Betty Gale, "Journal," 10 August 1942; Godfrey Gale, "Four Years," 2.
152 See Leslie Weatherhead, *The Eternal Voice* (London: Student Christian Movement, 1939).
153 Godfrey Gale, "Pacific War," 22 February 1942.
154 Ibid.
155 Ibid.
156 Ibid., 16 April 1942.
157 Ibid.
158 Betty Gale, "Journal," 18 May 1942.
159 Ibid.
160 Ibid.
161 Godfrey Gale, *Interned in China* (London: Livingstone Press, 1946), 10.
162 Ibid.
163 Ibid.
164 Betty Gale, "Journal," 18 May 1942.

165 See especially Greg Leck, *Captives of Empire: The Japanese Internment of Allied Civilians in China, 1941–1945* (Bangor, PA: Shandy Press, 2006); Bernice Archer, *A Patchwork of Internment: The Internment of Western Civilians under the Japanese, 1941–1945* (New York: RoutledgeCurzon, 2004); and Desmond Power, *Little Foreign Devil* (Vancouver: Pangli Imprint, 2006).

166 "Report of Cheeloo University Work in Tsinan, 1941–1942."

167 Godfrey Gale, "Pacific War," 21 January 1942.

168 "Report of Cheeloo University Work in Tsinan, 1941–1942."

169 Ibid.

170 Letter from Alfred Rive (Department of Foreign Affairs, Ottawa) to Colonel Clarke (Department of National Defence, Ottawa), 13 May 1942, LAC, NDF, microfiche reel C, 5070–4498. The *Gripsholm* was used as a US-Japanese exchange ship. She sailed the first leg of the journey from North and South America, and then the *Asama Maru* and *Conte Verde* sailed the second leg onward to Japan. They were to meet at Lourenço Marques, where the evacuees would be exchanged. Bruce Elleman, *Japanese American Civilian Prisoner Exchanges and Detention Camps, 1941–45* (London: Routledge, 2006), 24.

171 Andrew Thomson, "The Voyage Home," October 1942, 1 (Unpublished report), UCCA 83.058C, box 56, file 15, series 3.

172 Betty Gale, "Journal," 6 April 1942.

173 Letter from Elizabeth Gale (Qilu) to her "folks" (Toronto), 11 June 1942, MWPC.

174 Betty Gale, "Journal," 23 May 1942.

175 Letter from Gale to her "folks", 11 June 1942.

176 Ibid.

177 Letter from Godfrey Gale to (unknown), 13 June 1941 (*sic*—should be 1942), MWPC.

178 Betty Gale, "Journal," 13 June 1942.

179 Betty Gale, diary, 13 June 1942.

180 Letter from Elizabeth Gale (Qilu) to her "folks" (Toronto), 11 June 1942, MWPC.

181 Ibid.

182 Letter from Godfrey Gale (Jinan) to "My dear Mother," 13 June 1941 (*sic*—should be 1942), MWPC.

183 "Had to guard writing while in the hands of Japs [*sic*], missionary says here," *Globe and Mail*, 28 August 1942, UCC 83.058C, box 56-15, series 3.

184 Betty Gale, "Journal," 17 July 1942.

185 Ibid., 7 August 1942.

186 Ibid.

187 Frances McAll and Kenneth McAll, *The Moon Looks Down* (London: Darley Anderson, 1987), 28.

188 Betty Gale, "Journal," 7 August 1942.

189 Betty Gale, diary, 8 August 1942.

190 Betty Gale, "Journal," 11 August 1942.

191 Ibid.

192 Ibid.

193 Letter from Elizabeth Gale (Shanghai) to "My dearest folks" (Toronto), 11 February 1943, MWPC. In this letter Betty wrote, "Dad, we heard from the Red Jewel today (he often writes) and he is now a policeman, or at least he is training to be one!"

194 Godfrey Gale, "Four Years," 3.

Notes to Chapter 6

1 The CCC did not become an official internment camp until May 1943. While it would probably be more appropriate to call these people "refugees," since there was no Japanese categorization for this abandoned group, they are referred to here as internees.

2 Betty Gale, diary, 12 August 1942.

3 Godfrey Gale, "Pacific War" (unpublished memoir/diary), 15 August 1942, MWPC.

4 Some, like Sir Arthur Blackburn, who was Councillor of the British Embassy in Chongqing, simply accepted that "a special exchange arrangement was made for me and my wife" by the Swiss Consul General that allowed them an unexpected spot on the *Kamakura Maru* on 17 August 1942. A. Blackburn, "Hong Kong, December 1941–July 1942," http://sunzi1.lib.hku.hk/hkjo/view/44/4401660.pdf.

5 Desmond Power, personal communication with the author, 26 February 2007.

6 Letter from Betty Gale (Shanghai) to her "Folks" (Toronto), 16 August 1942, MWPC.

7 Ibid.

8 Betty Gale, "The Journal of Betty Gale: A Personal Account of Four Years of Civilian Internment in Occupied China" (Unpublished journal, July 1941–September 1945), 14 August 1942, MWPC.

9 Ibid.

10 Ibid.

11 Ibid.

12 Letter from Winifred Warren (Shanghai) to Mrs. Taylor (Toronto), 1 January 1943, UCCA 83.045C, box 11, file 180.

13 Betty Gale, "Journal," 22 January 1943.

14 Ibid., 25 September 1943.

15 Postcard from Dr. and Mrs. G.L. Gale (British) (Columbia Country Club, Shanghai) to Rev. and Mrs. A. Thomson (Toronto), 31 October 1942, MWPC.

16 Letter from AFA (Dr. Armstrong?) (Toronto) to Rev. Bruce Copland (Sichuan), 24 November 1942, UCCA83.045C, box 11, file 177.

17 Ibid.

18 Betty Gale, diary, 7 February 1943.

19 Betty Gale, "Journal," 9 February 1943.

20 Ibid.

21 S.W. Jackson, Introduction in Peggy Abkhazi, *A Curious Cage: Life in a Japanese Internment Camp, 1943–1945* (Victoria, BC: SonoNis Press, 2002), 13.

22 Ibid.

23 Ibid., 14.

24 Ibid., 16.

25 Oliver Lyndsay and John R. Harris, *The Battle for Hong Kong, 1941–1945: Hostage to Fortune* (Hong Kong: Hong Kong University Press, 2005), 40.

26 Ibid.

27 Ibid.

28 Betty Gale, "Journal," 5 November 1942.

29 Ibid.

30 Betty Gale, diary, 5 November 1942.

31 Letter from Elizabeth Gale (Shanghai) to "My dearest Folks" (Toronto), 11 February 1943, MWPC.

32 Ibid.

33 Betty Gale, interview with Margaret Wightman, audio-tape, 198(?), MWPC.

34 Broadcasts from Japan Concerning Treatment of Internees, 21 April 1943, LAC, NDF, microfiche reel C, 5342, file HQS 9050 (33–37), 45.

35 Ibid., 47.

36 Betty Gale, "Journal," 8 March 1943.

37 Ibid.

38 Letter from Elizabeth Gale (Shanghai) to "My dearest Folks" (Toronto), 9 March 1943, MWPC.

39 Greg Leck, "Nominal Rolls—Weihsien Camp (1943–1945)," in *Captives of Empire: The Japanese Internment of Allied Civilians in China, 1941–1945* (Bangor, PA: Shandy Press, 2006), 655–84. Susie Kelsey is not in the nominal rolls, having been repatriated in 1943.

40 Frances McAll and Kenneth McAll, *The Moon Looks Down* (London: Darley Anderson, 1987), 32.

41 Betty Gale, "Journal," 10 March 1943.

42 Ibid., 12 March 1943.

43 Ken and Frances McAll, audio-taped interview with Margaret Wightman, 1991, MWPC.

44 Letter from Godfrey Gale (Jinan) to Betty Thomson (Beijing), 11 September 1939, MWPC.

45 McAll and McAll, *Moon Looks Down*, 36.

46 Ken and Frances McAll, interview with Wightman.

47 Betty Gale, "Journal," 12 March 1943.

48 Leck, *Captives of Empire*, 187.

49 Ibid.

50 Probably meaning for children's sports. Godfrey Gale, in Betty Gale, "Journal," 12 March 1943.

51 The Japanese set up several banks in China during the war. The Central Reserve Bank in central and south China (1941–1945) was one of the most prominent. Its currency experienced high inflation through the war.

52 "Swiss Consul Report: Inspection of the Internment Camps at Yangchow, China," LAC, NDF, reel C534, file HQS 9050 (33–37), 5–7 July 1943.

53 Betty Gale, "Journal," 21 March 1943.

54 McAll and McAll, *Moon Looks Down*, 37.

55 Ibid., 37–38.

56 Ibid.

57 Ibid., 38.

58 Ibid.

59 Ibid.

60 Betty Gale, "Journal," 24 March 1943.

61 Leck, *Captives of Empire*, 503.

62 McAll and McAll, *Moon Looks Down*, 38.

63 Betty Gale, "Journal," 23 March 1943. According to Greg Leck, the camp representative was Edward Read of the Asiatic Petroleum Company. Leck, *Captives of Empire*, 503.

64 Betty Gale, diary, 23 March 1943.

65 It is not clear if this was an internee or a Japanese officer, but most likely it was an internee with police experience.

66 Betty Gale, "Journal," 24 March 1943.

67 Ibid.

68 Betty Gale, interview with Wightman; Ken McAll, interview with Wightman.

69 Betty Gale, "Journal," 20 June 1943.

70 In *The Moon Looks Down*, Frances McAll identifies the woman. Her demographic information is thus traceable from camp records. In deference to Betty Gale's preference to leave the woman unnamed, I have done so here, too.

71 Betty Gale, "Journal," 20 June 1943.

72 Betty Gale, diary, 27 March 1943.

73 Betty Gale, Journal, 27 March 1943.

74 Ken McAll, interview with Wightman.

75 Betty Gale, "Journal," 29 March 1943.

76 McAll and McAll, *Moon Looks Down*, 36.

77 Ibid., 37.

78 Frances McAll, interview with Wightman.

79 Ibid.

80 Abkhazi, *Curious Cage*, 81.

81 Ibid., 66.

82 Ibid., 86.

83 Ibid., 71.

84 Ibid.

85 Ibid., 69.

86 Ibid., 71.

87 Ibid.

88 Ibid., 69.

89 Ibid.

90 Ibid., 70.

91 Ibid.

92 Betty Gale, "Journal," 1 April 1943.

93 Ibid., 24 June 1943.

94 Ibid.

95 Ibid., 14 April 1943.

96 McAll and McAll, *Moon Looks Down*, 40.

97 Ibid.

98 Betty Gale, "Journal," 2 August 1943.

99 Ibid., 30 April 1943.

100 The woman was Marion Brotchie. Betty Gale, "Journal," 17 July 1943.

101 Betty Gale, "Journal," 15 August 1943.

102 Ibid., 7 April 1943.

103 Ibid., 4 August 1943.

104 Sodium amytal contains amobarbital sodium, which is a barbiturate causing drowsiness and used to induce sleep.

105 Betty Gale, interview with Wightman.

106 Ibid.

107 Betty Gale, diary, 4 August 1943.

108 Betty Gale, "Journal," 6 August 1943.

109 Abkhazi, *Curious Cage*, 67–68.

110 See above: Broadcasts from Japan Concerning Treatment of Internees, 21 April 1943.

111 Abkhazi, *Curious Cage*, 67–68.

112 Ibid.

113 From Washington to "Foreign Office" (Japan?), 2 September 1942, received 6 September 1942, LAC, NDF, microfiche reel C, 5070–4498.

114 International Committee of the Red Cross. "What Is International Humanitarian Law?" Advisory Service on International Humanitarian Law, July 2004, http://www.icrc.org/eng/assets/files/other/what_is_ihl.pdf.

115 Charles Roland, *Long Night's Journey into Day: Prisoners of War in Hong Kong and Japan, 1941–1945* (Waterloo, ON: Wilfrid Laurier University Press, 2001).

116 Letter from Ernest L. Maag (Delegate in Canada of the International Committee of the Red Cross) to the Department of External Affairs (Ottawa), 15 October 1942, LAC, NDF, microfiche reel C, 5333, file HQS 9050.

117 Letter from Elizabeth Gale (Shanghai) to Mrs. Andrew Thomson (Toronto) (on a stationery form created by the International Committee of the Red Cross), 21 January 1943, MWPC.

118 Ibid., 7 April 1943.

119 Ibid., 17 April 1943.

120 Also honoured with a D.D. degree were missionaries G.E. Bott of Japan, G.G. Endicott of West China, and United Church Moderator Dr. Sclater. The ceremonies were held in the Eaton Memorial Church in Toronto. Letter from AFA (Dr. Armstrong?) (Toronto) to Bruce Copeland (Sichuan), 24 November 1942.

121 Letter from "Mother, Father, Muriel, Murray, Margaret, Geo and Andy" (Toronto) to "Elizabeth, Godfrey and Margaret" (Yangzhou), 23 August 1943, MWPC.

122 McAll and McAll, *Moon Looks Down*, 42.

123 Betty Gale, diary, 5 July 1943.

124 McAll and McAll, *Moon Looks Down*, 42.

125 "Inspection of the Internment Camps at Yangchow, China, 5th, 6th, and 7th of July, 1943 by the Swiss," (stamped 6 May 1944), LAC, NDF, reel C, 5342, file HQS 9050 (33–37).

126 Ibid.

127 Ibid.

128 Ibid.

129 Ibid.

130 Ibid.

131 Ibid.

132 Betty Gale, "Journal," 17 September 1943.

133 Ibid., 24 September 1943.

134 Ibid., 29 September 1943.

135 Frances McAll did not have the same qualms about identifying Mrs. M: she did so in an interview with Margaret Wightman in 1991. Until then Wightman did not know the name of her mother's internment nemesis.

136 According to Betty Gale, the missionaries were: Godfrey, Betty, and Margaret Gale; Ken, Frances, and Eli McAll; Jean Gillison; Anne MacKeith; Marion (Ginger) Anderson; and George Robinson. Interview with Wightman.

Notes to Chapter 7

1 Swiss Consul (Emile Fontanel), "Confidential Report on the Inspection of the Civilian Assembly Centre at Pootung by the Swiss," 22 June 1943, Department of External Affairs, LAC, NDF, C5342, file HQS 9050 (33–37).
2 Ibid.
3 Godfrey Gale, "Pootung," notes in Betty Gale, "The Journal of Betty Gale: A Personal Account of Four Years of Civilian Internment in Occupied China" (Unpublished journal, July 1941–September 1945), MWPC.
4 Swiss Consul, "Confidential Report," 22 June 1943.
5 Godfrey Gale, "Pootung."
6 Ibid.
7 This was the official count by the Swiss Consul in August 1944. Godfrey and Betty reported 1,150 as the number in Pudong Camp.
8 Betty Gale, "Journal," 1 October 1943.
9 Betty Gale, diary, 1 October 1943.
10 Ibid., 6 October 1943.
11 Betty Gale, interview with Margaret Wightman, audio-tape, 198(?), MWPC.
12 Betty Gale, diary, 2 October 1943.
13 Betty Gale, "Journal," 6 October 1943.
14 Ibid.
15 Ibid.
16 Ibid., 3 July 1944.
17 Ibid., 6 October 1943.
18 Letter from Anne Norman (née Baker) to the Gales, October 1980, MWPC.
19 Godfrey Gale, "Free at Last," *The Missionary Monthly* (November 1945): 485–86, MWPC.
20 Swiss Consul, "Confidential Report," 27–29 September 1944, LAC, NDF, reel C, 5342, file HQS 9050 (33–37).
21 Shanghai was divided into districts or concessions, representing the various foreign interests in the treaty port. The French Concession, for example, was in a different part of Shanghai than the British Concession. Chinese residents were confined to districts designated for them. The area beside the tobacco warehouse had been a Chinese district.
22 Betty Gale, "Journal," 3 August 1943.
23 Jean Gillison, Anne MacKeith, and Marion (Ginger) Anderson (LMS missionaries), interview with Margaret Wightman, Lomas House, Worthing, Sussex, 1991. (Ninety-four-year-old Ethel Taylor was to join them for the interview, but she had a fall and could not attend.)
24 Frances McAll, audio-taped interview with Margaret Wightman, 1991.
25 Gillison, MacKeith, and Anderson, interview with Wightman.
26 Betty Gale, "Journal," 22 October 1943.
27 Ibid., 3 October 1943.
28 Ibid., 25 October 1943.
29 Ibid., 26 February 1944.
30 Ibid.
31 Betty Gale, interview with Wightman.
32 Frances McAll, interview with Wightman.

33 Betty Gale, "Journal," 8 February 1944.

34 Ibid., 31 October 1943.

35 Ibid., 28 May 1944.

36 Although Betty called the man "Morris" his given name would have been Maurice. According to the nominal rolls in Greg Leck, *Captives of Empire: The Japanese Internment of Allied Civilians in China, 1941–1945* (Bangor, PA: Shandy Press, 2006), 611, Maurice Bernard Weill, husband of Esther, died on "Mar 30 1944." It is likely that this is the person Betty is referring to, and that he died on 30 May. Maurice was 37; Esther was 31. Esther was released to Shanghai in October 1944.

37 Ken McAll, audio-taped interview with Margaret Wightman, 1991.

38 Ibid.

39 Betty Gale, interview with Wightman.

40 Ibid.

41 Swiss Consul, "Confidential Report," 27–29 September 1944.

42 Letter from Joan and John Jackson (Warwicks, England) to Margaret, Kendall, and Patricia (Toronto) on the occasion of Godfrey and Betty Gale's fortieth wedding anniversary, MWPC.

43 Betty Gale, "Journal," 12 July 1944.

44 John J. Mulheron, ed., *The Medical Age: A Semi-monthly Journal of Medicine and Surgery* 3 (1885): 428.

45 Swiss Consul, "Confidential Report," 27–29 September 1944.

46 Betty Gale, "Journal," 11 August 1944.

47 Ibid.

48 Ibid., 13 August 1944. Betty Gale identifies the woman by her full name in her notebook. Betty Gale, notebook, 12 August 1944. According to official camp records, this woman had two daughters aged 28 and 19.

49 Betty Gale, notebook, 12 August 1944.

50 Although Betty Gale later recalled that there were five pregnancies among unmarried girls, since one had married after discovering that she was pregnant, it is not clear whether this means that there were five or six of these pregnancies in Pudong Camp.

51 Betty Gale, "Journal," 26 August 1944.

52 Ibid., 12 November 1944.

53 Ibid.

54 Ibid.

55 Ibid., 26 October 1943.

56 Ibid., 29 October 1943.

57 Ibid.

58 Swiss Consul, "Confidential Report," 22 June 1943.

59 Frances McAll, *Hurdles Are for Jumping* (Oxford: New Cherwell Press, 1998), 68.

60 Betty Gale, "Journal," 24 February 1944.

61 Ibid.

62 McAll, *Hurdles*, 70.

63 Ibid.

64 Ibid.

65 Betty Gale, notebook, 21 August 1944.

66 Betty Gale, notes, n.d., 14, from William Sewell, *Strange Harmony* (London: Edinburgh House, 1946).

67 Betty Gale, "Journal," 26 October 1943.

68 Ibid.

69 Gillison, MacKeith, and Anderson, interview with Wightman.

70 Ibid.

71 Frances McAll, interview with Wightman.

72 Ken McAll, interview with Wightman.

73 Betty Gale, "Journal," 23 May 1944. Betty Gale's notebook, written on 16 June 1944, corroborates what she later wrote in her journal.

74 Betty Gale, "Journal," 23 May 1944.

75 Ibid.

76 Ibid.

77 Ibid.

78 Frances McAll, interview with Wightman. McAll heard this story from the ex-internee at a reunion decades later.

79 Betty Gale, "Journal," 1 February 1944.

80 Ibid., 23 May 1944. Mr "Z" may be either Chester Zackiewicz, a 26-year-old American able seaman, Timothy Zucchi, a 32-year-old American bellboy, or Josef Zwerenz, a 41-year-old room steward: all three were crew members of the captured *SS President Harrison.*

81 Betty Gale, "Journal," 23 May 1944.

82 Ibid.

83 Ibid., 24 May 1944.

84 Leck, *Captives of Empire,* 343–45. Although we do not know what happened to these particular prisoners, Leck notes that internees who were caught attempting to escape were beaten (some to death) or sent to prison (e.g., Ward Road Gaol).

85 Ken McAll, interview with Wightman.

86 Betty Gale, diary, 5 November 1943.

87 Betty Gale, "Journal," 6 November 1943.

88 Ibid., 20 October, 1944.

89 Ibid., 14 April 1945.

90 Ibid., 28 March 1944.

91 Ibid., 30 March 1944.

92 Ibid.

93 Swiss Consul, "Confidential Report," 27–29 September 1944.

94 Ibid.

95 Betty Gale, notebook, 12 September 1944.

96 Swiss Consul, "Confidential Report," 27–29 September 1944.

97 Betty Gale, "Journal," 8 January 1944.

98 Ibid., 11 January 1943.

99 Ibid., 13 January 1943.

100 Betty Gale, notebook, 24 August 1945.

101 Betty Gale, "Journal," 18 November 1943.

102 Ibid., 4 January 1944.

103 Gillison, MacKeith, and Anderson, interview with Wightman.

104 Betty Gale, "Journal," 29 July 1944.

105 Swiss Consul, "Confidential Report," 27–29 September 1944.

106 Ibid.

107 Ibid.

108 Betty Gale, "Journal," 19 December 1943.
109 Ibid., 30 January 1944.
110 Ibid.
111 Ibid., 31 December 1943.
112 Ibid., 22 October 1943.
113 Ibid.
114 Ibid., 7 April, 1944.
115 Ibid.
116 Ibid., 11 April 1944.
117 Ibid., 22 July 1944.
118 Ken McAll, "Pootung Incident," (unpublished poem written for the occasion of Betty and Godfrey Gale's fortieth wedding anniversary celebration), October 1980, MWPC.
119 Betty Gale, "Journal," 16 August 1944.
120 Betty Gale, notebook, 16 April 1944.
121 Betty Gale, "Journal," 15 April, 1944.
122 Ibid., 20 December 1944.
123 Ibid., 21 December 1944.
124 Ibid., 26 December 1944.
125 Ibid., 17 February 1945.
126 Ibid., 15 January 1944.
127 Ibid.
128 Ibid., 26 April 1944.
129 Betty Gale, notebook, 16 June 1944.
130 Betty Gale, "Journal," 11 June 1944.
131 Ibid., 23 June 1944.
132 Ibid.
133 Ibid.
134 Frances and Ken McAll, interview with Wightman.
135 Frances McAll, interview with Wightman.
136 Betty Gale, notebook, 23 July 1944.
137 Ibid., 12 August 1944.
138 Betty Gale, "Journal," 12 August 1944.
139 Ibid., 11 November 1944.
140 Ibid.
141 Ibid., 13 January 1945.
142 Ibid.
143 Ibid., 21 January 1945.
144 Ibid., 23 January 1945.
145 Ibid., 5 February 1945.
146 Ibid., 16 April 1945.
147 Ibid., 17 April 1945.
148 Betty Gale, notebook, 16 April 1945.
149 Sonya Grypma, *Healing Henan: Canadian Nurses at the North China Mission, 1888–1947* (Vancouver: University of British Columbia Press, 2008), 187.
150 Betty Gale, "Journal," 29 April 1945.
151 Ibid., 3 May 1945.

152 Ibid., 20 May 1945.
153 Betty Gale, notebook, 3 May 1945.
154 Betty Gale, "Journal," 3 July 1945.
155 Ibid., 5 July 1945.
156 Ibid., 22 July 1945.
157 Ibid.
158 Ibid., 25 July 1945.
159 Ibid.
160 Ibid., 26 July 1945.
161 Ibid.
162 Betty Gale, notes, n.d. (c. 1955).
163 Ibid.
164 Betty Gale, "Journal," 6 August 1945.
165 Betty Gale, notebook, 11 August 1945.
166 Betty Gale, "Journal," 10 August 1945.
167 Ibid.
168 Ibid., 11 August 1945.
169 Ibid., 12 August 1945.
170 Ibid., 13 August 1945.
171 Betty Gale, notebook, 13 August 1945.
172 Betty Gale, "Journal," 13 August 1945.
173 Betty Gale, notebook, 14 August 1945.
174 Ibid., 16 August 1945.
175 Ibid.
176 Betty Gale, "Journal," 15 August 1945.
177 Ibid., 16 August 1945.
178 Betty Gale, notebook, 26 August 1945.
179 Betty Gale, "Journal," 19 August 1945.
180 Ibid., 25 August 1945.
181 Ibid.
182 Ibid., 1 September 1945.
183 Betty Gale, notebook, 12 October 1945.
184 Ibid.
185 Margaret Wightman, personal communication with the author, 14 April 2011.
186 Letter to Margaret (Gale) Wightman from Muriel Box, n.d. (on the occasion of Godfrey and Betty Gale's fortieth wedding anniversary), MWPC.
187 Letter from Florence (Liddell) Hall to Betty and Godfrey, 18 October 1980 (on the occasion of Godfrey and Betty Gale's fortieth wedding anniversary), MWPC.
188 Ibid.

Notes to Conclusion

1 Hamish Ion, "'Much Ado about Too Few': Aspects of the Treatment of Canadian and Commonwealth POWs and Civilian Internees in Metropolitan Japan, 1941–1945," *Defence Studies* 6, no. 3 (2006), 293.
2 Greg Leck, *Captives of Empire: The Japanese Internment of Allied Civilians in China, 1941–1945* (Bangor, PA: Shandy Press, 2006), 26.

3 Betty Gale, Mary Stanley, Georgina Lewis, and Hilda McIllroy were Canadian nurses. North China missionary Winifred Warren was at Lunghua Camp and Bertha Hodge was at Weixian Camp. All but McIllroy had gone to China as WMS missionaries with United Church of Canada's North China Mission. Canadian missionaries repatriated in 1943 were George and Edna King and Susie Kelsey from Weixian Camp, and Harrison Mullett from Stanley Camp.

4 The broader issues identified and discussed by Ion were the influences of humanity on warfare, just penalties for war crimes, and differing perspectives of war across cultural boundaries. Ion, "'Much Ado.'"

5 The totals were: Thomsons, 36 years; Menzies, 46 years; Boyds, 35 years; Mackenzies, 31 years; and McClures, 50 years.

6 Ruth Compton Brouwer, "Shifts in the Salience of Gender in the International Missionary Enterprise during the Interwar Years," in *Canadian Missionaries, Indigenous Peoples: Representing Religion at Home and Abroad*, ed. Alvyn Austin and Jamie S. Scott (Toronto: University of Toronto Press, 2005), 153. Brouwer is citing J.H. Oldham writing to John R. Mott on 18 November 1924. See also Commission of Appraisal, with William Ernest Hocking, Chair, *Re-Thinking Missions: A Laymen's Inquiry after One Hundred Years* (New York: Harper, 1932).

7 "Religion: Re-Thinking Missions," *Time*, 28 November 1932, http://www.time.com/time/magazine/article/0,9171,744802,00.html#ixzz1MxACE48d.

8 See J.G. Ballard, *Empire of the Sun* (London: V. Gollancz, 1984); Desmond Power, *Little Foreign Devil* (Vancouver: Pangli Imprint, 1996); Pierre Boulle, *The Bridge over the River Kwai*, trans. Xan Fielding (New York: Vanguard, 1954).

9 Ion, "'Much Ado.'" 294.

10 Charles Roland, Long Night's Journey into Day: Prisoners of War in Hong Kong and Japan, 1941–1945 (Waterloo, ON: Wilfrid Laurier University Press, 2001), 45.

11 Ion, "'Much Ado,'" 296.

12 See Dominck LaCapra, "Redemptive Narratives," excerpt from interview by Amos Goldberg, Jerusalem, 9 June 1998, Shoah Resource Center, http://www1.yadvashem.org/odot_pdf/Microsoft%20Word%20-%203870.pdf.

13 Letter from Betty Gale (Pudong) to Margaret Thomson (Toronto), 11 February 1945, MWPC.

14 Ibid.

15 Ibid.

16 Ibid.

17 Mona Gail Oikawa, cited in Pamela Sugiman, "'Life is Sweet': Vulnerability and Composure in the Wartime Narratives of Japanese Canadians," *Journal of Canadian Studies* 43, no. 1 (2009): 210.

18 Sugiman, "'Life is Sweet.'"

19 Godfrey Gale, "Four Years Under the Japs [*sic*]," (Unpublished manuscript, n.d.), 7, MWPC.

20 Betty Gale, notes, n.d. (c. 1955), 14.

21 Sugiman, "'Life is Sweet,'" 210.

22 Ibid., 199.

23 Ibid.

24 Viktor E. Frankl, *Man's Search for Meaning* (New York: Washington Square, 1984), 121.

25 Ibid., 126.
26 According to the nominal rolls in Leck's *Captives of Empire*, 543, Charles and Hattie Love Rankin were both missionary doctors with the Fundamentalist Mission, and were not repatriated until August 1945. This differs from the account in Chaff et al. (1977), which listed Hattie's husband as a lawyer-turned-missionary with the Fundamentalist Mission, and had them in an internment camp for thirty months. See Sandra L. Chaff et al., *Women in Medicine: A Bibliography of the Literature on Women Physicians* (Metuchen, NJ: Scarecrow Press, 1977), 594.
27 Hattie Love Rankin, *I Saw It Happen to China, 1913–1949* (Harrisburg, PA: Mount Pleasant Press, 1960).
28 Cited in Chaff et al., *Women in Medicine*, 594.
29 Sugiman, "'Life is Sweet,'" 210.
30 Edward W. Said, *Orientalism* (New York: Pantheon, 1978).
31 Bernice Archer, *A Patchwork of Internment: The Internment of Western Civilians under the Japanese, 1941–1945* (New York: RoutledgeCurzon, 2004).
32 Ibid., 190–91.
33 Ibid., 224.
34 See John Watt, "Breaking into Public Service: The Development of Nursing in Modern China, 1870–1949," *Nursing History Review* 12 (2004), 67–96; Yong Wang, "Mission Unfinished: The United Church of Canada and China, 1925–1970" (PhD dissertation, University of Waterloo, ON, 1999); Yuet-wah Cheung, *Missionary Medicine in China: A Study of Two Protestant Missions in China before 1937* (Lanhan, MD: University Press of America, 1988).
35 In Henan Province, the Canadian impact is best seen through the continuance of former Canadian mission hospitals at Anyang and Weihui, now part of large medical establishments. The hospital at Weihui, now called the First Affiliated Hospital of Xinxiang Medical University, celebrated its 110th anniversary in 2006. Visiting a church at the site of the former mission at Anyang in 2003, I was told that there were, at that time, 80,000 Christians in Anyang.
36 This was the slogan of the Student Volunteer Movement for Foreign Missions, a movement that swelled in 1866 after it held its first international convention in Liverpool. John R. Mott, *The Evangelization of the World in This Generation* (New York: Student Volunteer Movement for Foreign Missions, 1905).
37 From Yves Lequin (1980) and Watchtel (1986), in Pamela Sugiman, "Memories of Internment: Narrating Japanese Canadian Women's Life Stories," *Canadian Journal of Sociology / Cahiers de sociologie* 29, no. 3 (2004): 369–70.
38 See Committee of Appraisal, *Re-Thinking Missions*.
39 Ruth Compton Brouwer, "When Missions Became Development: Ironies of 'NGOization' in Mainstream Canadian Churches in the 1960s," *The Canadian Historical Review* 91, no. 4 (2010): 662–93.
40 Sonya Grypma, "Withdrawal from Weihui: China Missions and the Silencing of Missionary Nursing, 1888–1947," *Nursing Inquiry* 14, no. 4 (2007): 306–19.
41 Alvyn Austin and Jamie S. Scott, *Canadian Missionaries, Indigenous Peoples: Representing Religion at Home and Abroad* (Toronto: University of Toronto Press, 2005), 5.
42 Ibid., 4.
43 Alvyn Austin, *Saving China: Canadian Missionaries in the Middle Kingdom, 1888–1959* (Toronto: University of Toronto Press, 1987), 308.

44 Kendall Gale and Patricia Gale MacDonald, both born in Canada.
45 "Canada Accepts Japan's Apology for Hong Kong PoWs," CBC News, 8 December 2011, http://www.cbc.ca/news/canada/story/2011/12/08/japan-apology-canada.html. Of the 1,975 Canadians sent to Hong Kong, 1,050 died or were wounded during the battle or in prison camps afterward.
46 Sugiman, "Memories of internment," 384.
47 Ion, "'Much Ado,'" 311.
48 Ibid.
49 For example, see Ria Koster, ed., "Kumpulana: Memories of Dutch-Canadian Survivors of Japanese Prison Camps during World War II," 2010, http://www.kumpulana.ca; David Lea, "Bittersweet Reunion for Japanese Internment Camp Survivors," *Oakville Beaver*, 1 April 2010, Inside Halton, http://www.insidehalton.com/insidehalton/article/659612.

Bibliography

Primary sources were obtained from both public (archive) and private (family) collections. Both are detailed in the Notes. Publicly available sources are listed here for the ease of readers wishing to do further research.

Archive Collections

Alumnae Association of the Winnipeg General Hospital
Alumnae Journal, 1914–42.
Alumnae Scrapbook.
WGH Yearbook Blue and White, class of 1923.

Glenbow Museum
Red Cross Files, 1941–45.

Grey Sisters of the Immaculate Conception of Pembroke Archives
Grey Sisters in China 1929–52.

Library and Archives Canada
Department of National Defence: Prisoner of War fonds.
Peter Stursberg Fonds (interview of Dr. Robert McClure) MG 31, series D78, vol. 44, file 44-29.

United Church of Canada Archives
Brown, Margaret. *History of the Honan (North China) Mission of the United Church of Canada, Originally a Mission of the Presbyterian Church in Canada.* Volumes 1–4. N.d. (1500 pages).
Norman MacKenzie Papers. Accession no. 89.155C FA 316.
Presbyterian Church in Canada Woman's Missionary Society 1876–1927. Accession no. 79.205 C; fonds 127, FA 226; boxes 12, 19.
United Church of Canada Biographical Files (Bio Files).
United Church of Canada Board of Overseas Missions. Accession no. 83.045C; fonds 502, FA 186; series 4/3: China (Henan) Mission 1912–1952; boxes 1–3, 5–10, 12, 13, 16–18, 40, 41.
United Church of Canada Board of World Missions. Accession no. 83.041; fonds 503, FA 321; series 5: China 1888–1969; box 3.
United Church of Canada Microfilm Collection. BX 9001; A40 PS microfilm 25.
United Church of Canada Photograph Collection (Graphic Files).

United Church of Canada Woman's Missionary Society. Accession no. 83.058C; fonds 505, FA 90; series 3: China (Henan) 1925–1955; boxes 56–58.
United Church of Canada Woman's Missionary Society. Accession no. 83.058C; fonds 505, FA 90; series 5: China (West) 1935–1952; boxes 61–63.

University of Alberta J.W. Scott Library
Balme, Harold, and Milton T. Shauffer, "An Enquiry into the Scientific Efficiency of Mission Hospitals in China," 1–39. Presented at the *Annual Conference of the China Medical Missionary Association*, 21–27 February 1920, Beijing (microfiche).

Vancouver General Hospital Alumnae Association
Vancouver General Hospital Training School Annual, 1926.

Wellington County Museum and Archives
Brydon (Eramosa township) Family File.
"Going to Mission Field," *Fergus News Record*, 19 July 1917.

Xinxiang Medical College (First Affiliated Hospital), Weihui, Henan, People's Republic of China
"The General Situation in the Newly Established Period (1896–1948) of the First Affiliated Hospital of Xinxiang Medical College." Unpublished history of Huimin Hospital.

Books, Articles, and Dissertations

Abkhazi, Peggy. *A Curious Cage: Life in a Japanese Internment Camp, 1943–1945.* Victoria, BC: Sono Nis Press, 2002.
Archer, Bernice. *A Patchwork of Internment: The Internment of Western Civilians under the Japanese, 1941–1945.* New York: RoutledgeCurzon, 2004.
Armstrong, A.E., and Ruth Taylor. "Thirty Missionaries Now in Enemy Countries." *The United Church Observer*, 15 March 1942.
Associated Boards for Christian Colleges in China and the United Committee for Christian Universities in China. "Cheeloo." N.p.: "The University Press," 1937.
Austin, Alvyn. *Saving China: Canadian Missionaries in the Middle Kingdom, 1888–1959.* Toronto: University of Toronto Press, 1987.
Austin, Alvyn. "Wallace of West China." In *Canadian Missionaries, Indigenous Peoples: Representing Religion at Home and Abroad*, edited by Alyvn Austin and Jamie S. Scott, 111–33. Toronto: University of Toronto Press, 2005.
Austin, Alvyn, and Jamie S. Scott. *Canadian Missionaries, Indigenous Peoples: Representing Religion at Home and Abroad.* Toronto: University of Toronto Press, 2005.
Australian Government Department of Veterans' Affairs. "Australia's War 1939–1945: Nurses Recovered." http://www.ww2australia.gov.au/behindwire/found.html.
Balme, Harold, and Milton T. Shauffer, "An Enquiry into the Scientific Efficiency of Mission Hospitals in China." Presented at the Annual Conference of the China Medical Missionary Association, Beijing, 21–27 February 1920.
Beaton, Janet. "Canadian Missionary Nurses in China: 1894–1951." Paper presented at the 14th Annual Conference of the Canadian Association for the History of Nursing, 9 June 2001.

Beaton, Kenneth. *Serving with the Sons of Shuh: Fifty Fateful Years in West China, 1891–1941.* Toronto: United Church of Canada, 1941.

Bhimji, Shabir, and Rose Sheinin. "Dr. Edna Mary Guest: She Promoted Women's Issues Before It Was Fashionable." *Canadian Medical Association Journal* 141 (1989): 1093–94.

Boschma, Geertje, Sonya Grypma, and Florence Melchior. "Reflections on Researcher Subjectivity and Identity in Nursing History." In *Capturing Nursing History: A Guide to Historical Methods in Research,* edited by Sandra B. Lewenson and Eleanor Krohn Herrmann, 99–122. New York: Springer, 2008.

Boschma, Geertje, Margaret Scaia, Nerrisa Bonifacio, and Erica Roberts. "Oral History Research." In *Capturing Nursing History: A Guide to Historical Methods in Research,* edited by Sandra B. Lewenson and Eleanor Krohn Herrmann, 79–98. New York: Springer, 2008.

Boulle, Pierre. *The Bridge over the River Kwai.* Translated by Xan Fielding. New York: Vanguard, 1954.

Brouwer, Ruth Compton. *Modern Women, Modernizing Men: The Changing Missions of Three Professional Women in Asia and Africa, 1902–69.* Vancouver: University of British Columbia Press, 2002.

Brouwer, Ruth Compton. *New Women for God: Canadian Presbyterian Women and India Missions, 1876–1914.* Toronto: University of Toronto Press, 1990.

Brouwer, Ruth Compton. "When Missions Became Development: Ironies of 'NGOization' in Mainstream Canadian Churches in the 1960s." *The Canadian Historical Review* 91, no. 4 (2010): 662–93.

Brush, Barbara L., Joan E. Lynaugh, Geertje Boschma, Anne Marie Rafferty, Meryn Stuart, and Nancy J. Tomes. *Nurses of All Nations: A History of the International Council of Nurses, 1899–1999.* Philadelphia: Lippincott, 1999.

Cameron, Elspeth. "Truth in Biography." In *Boswell's Children: The Art of the Biographer,* edited by R.B. Fleming, 27–32. Toronto: Dundurn Press, 1992.

Caughey, Ellen. *Eric Liddell: Olympian and Missionary.* Uhrichsville, OH: Barbour, 2000.

Chaff, Sandra L., Ruth Haimbach, Carol Fenichel, and Nina B. Woodside. *Women in Medicine: A Bibliography of the Literature on Women Physicians.* Metuchen, NJ: Scarecrow Press, 1977.

Chen, Kaiyi. "Quality Versus Quantity: The Rockefeller Foundation and Nurses Training in China." *Journal of American East Asian Relations* 5, no. 1 (1996): 77–104.

Chen, Kaiyi. "Missionaries and the Early Development of Nursing in China." *Nursing History Review* 4 (1996): 129–49.

Christensen, Erleen J. *In War and Famine: Missionaries in China's Honan Province in the 1940s.* Montreal: McGill-Queen's University Press, 2005.

Chueng, Yuet-wah. *Missionary Medicine in China: A Study of Two Canadian Protestant Missions in China before 1937.* Lanhan, MD: University Press of America, 1988.

Chung-tung, Liu. "From San Gu Liu Po to 'Caring Scholar': The Chinese Nurse in Perspective." *International Journal of Nursing Studies* 28, no. 4 (1991): 315–24.

Commission of Appraisal, with William Ernest Hocking, Chair. *Re-Thinking Missions: A Laymen's Inquiry after One Hundred Years.* New York: Harper and Brothers, 1932.

Copland, Marnie. *Moon Cakes and Maple Sugar.* Burlington, ON: G.R. Welch, 1980.

Cruikshank, Kathleen. "Education History and the Art of Biography." *American Journal of Education* 107, no. 3 (1999): 231–39.

D'Antonio, Patricia. "Nurses—and Wives and Mothers: Women and the Latter-day Saints Training School's Class of 1919." *Journal of Women's History* 19, no. 3 (2007): 112–36.

D'Antonio, Patricia. "Revisiting and Rethinking the Rewriting of Nursing History." *Bulletin of the History of Medicine* 73 (1999): 268–90.

Demerson, Velma. *Incorrigible.* Waterloo, ON: Wilfrid Laurier University Press, 2004.

Dong, Linfu. *Cross Culture and Faith: The Life and Work of James Mellon Menzies.* Toronto: University of Toronto Press, 2005.

Doona, Mary Ellen. "Linda Richards and Nursing in Japan." *Nursing History Review* 4 (1996): 99–128.

Dowd Hall, Jacquelyn. "Second Thoughts: On Writing Feminist Biography." *Feminist Studies* 13, no. 1 (1987), 19–37.

Elleman, Bruce. *Japanese American Civilian Prisoner Exchanges and Detention Camps, 1941–45.* London: Routledge, 2006.

Endicott, Shirley Jane. *China Diary: The Life of Mary Austin Endicott.* Waterloo, ON: Wilfrid Laurier University Press, 2003.

Endicott, Stephen. *James G. Endicott: Rebel out of China.* Toronto: University of Toronto Press, 1980.

Esselstrom, Erik W. *Crossing Empire's Edge: Foreign Ministry Police and Japanese Expansionsim in Northeast Asia.* Honolulu: University of Hawai'i Press, 2009.

Ewen, Jean. *China Nurse, 1932–1939: A Young Canadian Witnesses History.* Toronto: McClelland and Stewart, 1981.

Fanon, Franz. *The Wretched of the Earth.* New York: Grover Press, 2004. [1963]

Fitzpatrick, M. Louise. "Historical Research: The Method." *Nursing Research: A Qualitative Perspective*, 2nd ed., edited by Patricia Munhall and Carolyn Oiler Boyd, 364–70. New York: National League for Nursing Press, 1993.

Frankl, Viktor E. *Man's Search for Meaning.* New York: Washington Square Press, 1984. [1959]

Frazer Smith, James. *Life's Waking Part: Being the Autobiography of Reverend James Frazer Smith, Pioneer Medical Missionary to Honan, China, and Missionary to Central Asia.* Toronto: T. Nelson, 1937.

Gagan, Rosemary. "The Methodist Background of Canadian WMS Missionaries." *Canadian Methodist Historical Society Papers* 7 (1990): 115–36.

Gagan, Rosemary. *A Sensitive Independence: Canadian Methodist Women Missionaries in Canada and the Orient, 1881–1925.* Montreal: McGill-Queen's University Press, 1992.

Gale, Betty. "The Journal of Betty Gale: A Personal Account of Four Years of Civilian Internment in Occupied China, July 1941 to September 1945." Unpublished manuscript, n.d.

Gale, Godfrey. "Four Years under the Japs [*sic*]." Unpublished manuscript, n.d.

Gale, Godfrey. "Free at Last." *The Missionary Monthly* (November 1945): 485–86.

Gale, Godfrey. *Interned in China.* London: Livingstone Press, 1946.

Gale, Godfrey. "Pacific War." Unpublished manuscript, n.d.

Gerwurtz, Margo S. "'Their Names May Not Shine': Narrating Chinese Christian Converts." In *Canadian Missionaries, Indigenous Peoples: Representing Religion at Home and Abroad*, edited by Alvyn Austin and Jamie S. Scott, 134–51. Toronto: University of Toronto Press, 2005.

Grundmann, Christoffer. *Sent to Heal! Emergence and Development of Medical Missions.* Landham, MD: University Press of America, 2005.

Grypma, Sonya J. "China Nurse Jean Ewen: Embracing and Abandoning Communist Revolutionaries." *Journal of Historical Biography* 9 (2011): 37–69.

Grypma, Sonya. "Critical Issues in the Use of the Biographic Method." *Nursing History Review* 13 (2005): 171–87.

Grypma, Sonya. *Healing Henan: Canadian Nurses at the North China Mission, 1888–1947.* Vancouver: University of British Columbia Press, 2008.

Grypma, Sonya. "James R. Menzies: Healing and Preaching in Early 20th-Century China." *Canadian Medical Association Journal* 170, no. 1 (2004): 84–85.

Grypma, Sonya. "Missionary Nursing: Internationalizing Religious Ideals." In *Religion, Religious Ethics and Nursing,* edited by M. Fowler, B. Pesut., S. Reimer-Kirkham, and R. Sawatzky, 129–50. New York: Springer, 2011.

Grypma, Sonya. "Neither Angels of Mercy nor Foreign Devils: Re-Visioning Canadian Missionary Nurses in China, 1935–1947." *Nursing History Review* 12 (2004): 97–119.

Grypma, Sonya. "Withdrawal from Weihui: China Missions and the Silencing of Missionary Nursing, 1888–1947." *Nursing Inquiry* 14, no. 4 (2007): 306–19.

Hulheron, John J., ed. *The Medical Age: A Semi-monthly Journal of Medicine and Surgery.* Detroit, MI: George S. Davis, 1885.

Hummel, Marion F. Menzies. *Memoirs of a Mishkid.* Compiled and edited by Elizabeth Mittler. Beamsville, ON: Elizabeth Mittler, 2001.

Ion, A. Hamish. "'Much Ado about Too Few': Aspects of the Treatment of Canadian and Commonwealth POWs and Civilian Internees in Metropolitan Japan, 1941–1945." *Defence Studies* 6, no. 3 (2006): 292–317.

Jeffrey, Betty. *White Coolies.* Sydney: Angus and Robertson, 1985. [1954]

Kelsey, Susie. "In a Concentration Camp in China." *Canadian Nurse* 40, no. 7 (1944): 480–82.

Kip, Ka-che. "China and Christianity: Perspectives on Missions, Nationalism, and the State in the Republican Period, 1912–1949." *Missions, Nationalism, and the End of Empire,* edited by Brian Stanley, 132–43. Grand Rapids: Eerdmans, 2003.

LaCapra, Dominck. "Redemptive Narratives." Excerpt from interview by Amos Goldberg. Jerusalem, 9 June 1998. Shoah Resource Center. http://www1.yadvashem.org/odot_pdf/Microsoft%20Word%20-%203870.pdf.

Leck, Greg. *Captives of Empire: The Japanese Internment of Allied Civilians in China, 1941–1945.* Bangor, PA: Shandy Press, 2006.

Lyndsay, Oliver, and John R. Harris. *The Battle for Hong Kong, 1941–1945: Hostage to Fortune.* Hong Kong: Hong Kong University Press, 2005.

MacKay, George Leslie. *From Far Formosa: The Island, Its People and Missions,* 4th ed. New York: Fleming H. Revell, 1895.

Maxwell, Grant. "Partners in Mission: The Grey Sisters." In *Assignment in Chekiang: Seventy-One Canadians in China, 1902–1954,* 126–42. Scarborough, ON: Scarboro Foreign Mission Society, 1984.

McAll, Frances. *Hurdles Are for Jumping.* Oxford: New Cherwell Press, 1998.

McAll, Frances, and Kenneth McAll. *Moon Looks Down.* London: Darley Anderson, 1987.

McCasland, David. *Eric Liddell: Pure Gold.* Grand Rapids, MI: Discovery House, 2001.

Mott, John R. *The Evangelization of the World in This Generation*. New York: Student Volunteer Movement for Foreign Missions, 1905.

Nelson, Sioban. "The Fork in the Road: Nursing History vs. the History of Nursing?" *Nursing History Review* 10 (2002): 175–88.

New, Peter Kong-Ming, and Yuet-wah Cheung. "Early Years of Medical Missionary Work in the Canadian Presbyterian Mission in North Honan, China, 1887–1900." *Asian Profile* 12, no. 5 (1984): 409–23.

Norman, Elizabeth M. *We Band of Angels: The Untold Story of American Nurses Trapped on Bataan by the Japanese*. New York: Random House, 1999.

North China Herald. "Dorothy Galbraith, Missionary in Torpedoed Ship." 26 March 1941.

North China Herald. "Honan Drive and Southward Move." 19 February 1941.

North China Herald. "Hospital Employees on Strike." 8 January 1941.

North China Herald. "New Rules for Travel in North China." 11 June 1941.

North China Herald. "Shanghai Woman Has Narrow Escape from Death at Sea." 23 July 1941.

Power, Desmond. *Little Foreign Devil*. Vancouver: Pangli Imprint, 1996.

Rankin, Hattie Love. *I Saw It Happen to China, 1913–1949*. Harrisburg, PA: Mount Pleasant Press, 1960.

Roland, Charles. *Long Night's Journey into Day: Prisoners of War in Hong Kong and Japan, 1941–1945*. Waterloo, ON: Wilfrid Laurier University Press, 2001.

Ross Kerr, Janet C. "Nursing History at the Graduate Level: State of the Art." *Canadian Bulletin of Medical History* 11, no. 1 (1994): 230–36.

Said, Edward W. *Orientalism*. New York: Pantheon, 1978.

Scott, Munroe. *McClure: The China Years of Dr. Bob McClure*. Toronto: Canec Publishing, 1977.

Semple, Rhonda Anne. *Missionary Women: Gender, Professionalism and the Victorian Idea of Christian Mission*. Rochester, NY: Boydell, 2003.

Sewell, William. *Strange Harmony*. London: Edinburgh House Press, 1946.

Spence, Jonathan D. *Search for Modern China*. New York: W.W. Norton, 1990.

Stephen, A.M. *War in China: What It Means to Canada*. Vancouver: China Aid Council and The National Salvation League, 1938.

Stursberg, Peter. *The Golden Hope: Christians in China*. Toronto: United Church Publishing House, 1987.

Sugiman, Pamela. "'Life is Sweet': Vulnerability and Composure in the Wartime Narratives of Japanese Canadians." *Journal of Canadian Studies* 43, no. 1 (2009): 186–218.

Sugiman, Pamela. "Memories of Internment: Narrating Japanese Canadian Women's Life Stories." *Canadian Journal of Sociology / Cahiers canadiens de sociologie* 29, no. 3 (2004): 359–88.

Thomson, Murray McCheyne. *A Daring Confidence: The Life and Times of Andrew Thomson in China, 1906–1942*. Ottawa: Murray Thomson, 1992.

Thomson, Murray McCheyne. *Mother, God Bless Her! A Memoir Based on the Letters and Stories of Margaret Mackay Thomson, 1881–1973*. Ottawa: Murray Thomson, 2005.

Time. "Religion: Re-Thinking Missions." 28 November 1932. http://www.time.com/time/magazine/article/0,9171,744802,00.html#ixzz1MxACE48d.

Wang, Yong. "Mission Unfinished: The United Church of Canada and China, 1925–1970." PhD diss., University of Waterloo, ON, 1999.

Watt, John. "Breaking into Public Service: The Development of Nursing in Modern China, 1870–1949." *Nursing History Review* 12 (2004): 67–96.

Weatherhead, Leslie. *The Eternal Voice.* London: Student Christian Movement, 1939.

Wexler, Alice. "Emma Goldman and the Anxiety of Biography." In *The Challenge of Feminist Biography: Writing the Lives of Modern American Women,* edited by Sara Alpern, Joyce Antler, Elisabeth Israels Perry, and Ingrid Winther Scobie, 34–50. Urbana, IL: University of Illinois Press, 1992.

Wilder-Stanley Saga. Website. http://reced.org/dmenzi/Wilders/wilder-Stanley.htm.

Index